The Practical / Vocational Nurse and Today's Family

SECOND EDITION

DORIS HASLER, B.S., M.S., Formerly, Instructor
School of Practical Nursing
Indianapolis Public Schools, Indianapolis, Indiana

With the Collaboration of LOU PEVETO SCOTT, R.N., B.S.
Head, Department of Practical Nursing
Pensacola Junior College, Pensacola, Florida

MACMILLAN PUBLISHING CO., INC.
New York

COLLIER MACMILLAN PUBLISHERS
London

Copyright © 1972, Doris Hasler Cartwright

Printed in the United States of America

All rights reserved. No part of this book may be reproduced or transmitted in any form or by any means, electronic or mechanical, including photocopying, recording, or any information storage and retrieval system, without permission in writing from the Publisher.

Earlier edition entitled *The Practical Nurse and Today's Family* copyright © 1964 by Doris Hasler

Macmillan Publishing Co., Inc.
866 Third Avenue, New York, New York 10022

Collier-Macmillan Canada, Ltd.

Library of Congress catalog card number: 73-176057

Printing   7 8 9   Year   7 8 9

Affectionately Dedicated
To My Mother
Zena Harlan Hasler
and
To the Memory of My Father
A Great Teacher
E. A. Hasler

PREFACE

As an important member of the health team, today's practical nurse plays numerous roles. She works in many areas — hospitals, industry, doctor's offices, public health services and agencies, and private duty in the home. A one-year course of study must be greatly concentrated to prepare her adequately for these various duties. To help her achieve the background and knowledge required to appreciate today's family, this book has been written, tracing the growth and development of the family from its beginning to its final years. Insofar as possible, nontechnical language has been used to convey scientific information in order to provide a readily comprehensible text.

The practical nurse needs to see her patient as a member of a family whose life is altered by illness. She should be prepared to work harmoniously and sympathetically with the patient's family, learn its health problems, and find ways in which to assist it.

Nursing comprises total patient care with emphasis upon rehabilitation. As the purpose of hospitalization now is to help the patient get well and then to teach him how to stay well, the nurse's role has added responsibilities. An understanding of the patient's family life will enable her to assist more effectively with rehabilitation and in teaching good health habits.

The family has changed greatly in recent decades. The nurse should know how the changes in family living affect nursing. Because broken homes tend to create problems, a strong and secure family life is both a preventive of and an antidote to many social problems.

Part I, "The Nurse and the Beginning Family," deals with the importance of good family life and the need for the newlywed to adjust to each other and to the arrival of their first baby.

Part II, "Normal Development," contains a description of the normal growth processes. It is written as a supplement and correlates to the student's knowledge of the human body and its functions.

It is assumed that the student received instruction in maternal and child nursing elsewhere in the curriculum; therefore, the discussion of the well baby emphasizes family relationships and the aspects of baby care — such as the laundry — that may not be included in other courses.

Part III, "The Baby, Toddler, and Preschool Child," proceeds from the premise that every child is an individual. The most valuable criterion for appraising a child is to compare him with himself over a period of time. The nurse does not have sufficient time to make such a comparison. He is a stranger to the nurse who is entrusted with his care. If she knows what to expect of well children at certain ages, she will be more reasonable in her expectations of her young patient and will more readily recognize abnormal behavior, arrested development, symptoms of illness, and evidence of recovery.

The Developmental Skill-Age Inventory (see page 315) is a reliable tool for those who want to compare a child's progress with the specific age at which children usually master each skill. The scoring may be done in a short time by evaluators who need not be trained as developmental experts.

The increasing influence of the community on the family, the tremendous changes in today's urban life, and the family's use of community resources are discussed in Part IV, "The Family in the Middle Years," as well as in other parts of the book. The student nurse learns about community health services in the class on personal and community health; hence Chapter 20, "Community Resources: Laws and Agencies Affecting the Family," is not intended to be a complete description of all the health services in a community. The expansion of practical nurses on public health agency staffs focuses the need for nurses to understand the different factors molding city life, as discussed in Chapter 19. The nurse is not expected to solve the gigantic problems facing the country, but her supportive action can be a positive factor.

A good nurse can be a tremendous influence in the lives of schoolchildren and adolescents. A brief description of the health problems and the major personal problems of the schoolchild and the adolescent is given in Chapters 15, "The Six- to Twelve-Year-Old." and 16, "The Adolescent." Because children grow and learn in many ways, diversions and play activities merit special consideration for each age group. Physical growth and development during adolescence are so closely related to social, emotional, and personal growth that all phases of development are considered in Chapter 16.

The care of adult patients consumes a large proportion of practical nursing hours; hence Chapter 18, "The Mature Adult," has been greatly expanded in the second edition of this book.

In Part V, "The Family in the Later Years," the author strives to give the student information that will give her greater insight into the elderly. The number of persons living past the age of 75 years continues to increase. Graduate practical nurses are much needed in nursing homes, geriatric hospital units, and homes for the aged. Knowledge of body structure and function will be an asset to the student reading Chapter 23, "Physical Changes with Age."

When the nurse understands the physical changes involved in the aging process, she can more readily adapt nursing techniques, skills, and interpersonal relationships to the care of the elderly. With the increasing elderly population have come new problems for each community and for the country as a whole. The student is encouraged to think in terms of solving the problems.

In the classes on foods, nutrition, and diets, the student nurse learns about food necessities for a well-balanced diet and how to modify them for therapeutic purposes. Good nutrition, in the fullest sense, means more than consuming essential foodstuffs in the required amounts; it means the appropriate utilization

Preface

of food in the body. This book attempts to guide the student to recognize that food needs differ with age, and to suggest ways to create interest in proper food that will appeal to the baby, toddler, schoolchild, adolescent, adult, and elderly person. The discussion is not a substitute for, but a supplement to, the study of normal and therapeutic nutrition.

At the end of each chapter are questions for discussion; lists of books, magazines, and pamphlets for additional reading; and recommended audiovisual aids. Complete addresses for the companies distributing audiovisual aids are given on p. 330.

The author sincerely hopes that the practical nurse, proudly accepting the responsibilities and obligations of her profession, will contribute toward healthful living, both in her community and in her own family life.

I wish to express my gratitude to the many people who assisted in one way or another with the preparation of this book.

Mrs. Lou Scott, collaborator, Head of the Department of Practical Nursing, Pensacola Junior College, gave many hours of her time to preview the films and filmstrips. She wrote the audiovisual comments, read the manuscript with a critical eye, and offered many valuable suggestions.

Mrs. Louise DuBose, secretary of the Department of Practical Nursing, Pensacola Junior College, gave invaluable assistance with the mechanics of collaboration. The faculty and staff of the Department of Practical Nursing, Pensacola Junior College, are all to be thanked: Mrs. Maria Cotsonis, Mrs. Pauline Taliaferro, Miss Delores Raynor, Mrs. Katherine Goldsmith, Mrs. Joyce Higginbotham, Mrs. Suzanne Ray, and Mrs. Laura McClammay.

Sincere thanks go to Dr. Gerald Alpern, Director of Research, Child Psychiatry Services, Indiana University Medical Center, for his helpful comments regarding adolescent delinquents and child guidance clinics. Dr. Alpern and Dr. Thomas J. Boll made an important contribution to this book by giving permission to include in the Appendix an adapted version of their Developmental Skill-Age Inventory.

To Sister M. Elaine, O.S.F., R.N., Saint Mary's Franciscan Hospital, Philadelphia, I wish to express my thanks for her gracious consent to reproduce her illustration in Chapter 2, and for her inspirational words of encouragement.

For help in the revision, I wish to thank Miss Rosemary Haboush, R.N., Miss Verna J. Coons, R.N., and Mrs. Helen Miller, all of the School of Practical Nursing, Indianapolis Public Schools.

My gratitude to Mr. Alexander Munro, Senior Citizens Center, Indianapolis; Mr. Harry A. Radliffe, Assistant Superintendent, Indianapolis Public Schools; and Mr. Pershing Meyers, Assistant Superintendent, Indianapolis Public Schools.

Special thanks to typists Miss Frances Anderson and Mrs. Lois Greenwalt.

I wish to express my gratitude again to certain people who helped with the writing of the first edition of this book, and whose ideas and pertinent remarks are incorporated in the second edition. My thanks to Mr. Robert G. White, Mrs.

Marguerite Klein Clark, Mrs. Helen Layton Moor, Mrs. Helen Rowan, Mrs. Alice Grubbs, Mrs. Oneida Jackson, Mrs. Leanna Farrell, Mrs. Gladys Buckwalter, and Mr. Henry Van Swearingen.

My sincere appreciation to Mr. T. P. McConahay, editor, College and Professional Division of The Macmillan Company, for his patience and guidance in the revision of this book.

D. H.

CONTENTS

PART I/The Nurse and the Beginning Family

1   The Practical Nurse and Today's Family   3
2   Successful Family Life   10
3   The Newlywed   19
4   Parenthood: Arrival of the Baby   28

PART II/Normal Development

5   Normal Child Development   37

PART III/The Baby, Toddler, and Preschool Child

6   The Well Baby   53
7   The Two-Year-Old   64
8   The Three-Year-Old   73
9   The Four-Year-Old   81
10   The Five-Year-Old   88
11   The Toddler, the Preschool Child, and Food   98
12   Fears, Hospitalization, and the Young Child   107
13   Recreation for the Sick Child   117

PART IV/The Family in the Middle Years

14   The Family with Schoolchildren   129
15   The Six- to Twelve-Year-Old   133
16   The Adolescent   152
17   The Young Adult   174
18   The Mature Adult   184
19   The Nurse, the Family, the Community   197
20   Community Resources: Laws and Agencies Affecting the Family   208

PART V/The Family in the Later Years

21   Nursing and the Aging Population   225
22   Social and Emotional Needs of Older People; Useful Activity   236
23   Physical Changes with Age   251
24   Mental and Personality Changes with Age   264
25   Good Hygiene for Elderly People   273
26   Finances of Older People   287
27   Community Responsibility and Resources for the Aged   297

APPENDIX

    Alpern-Boll Developmental Skill-Age Inventory   315
    Addresses for Audiovisual Aids   330
    General References   332

INDEX   333

PART I / *The Nurse and the Beginning Family*

CHAPTER 1 / THE PRACTICAL NURSE AND

TODAY'S FAMILY

In time of illness today's practical nurse is the person closest to the patient and to the patient's family. The rapid advancement in medical knowledge, equipment, and techniques have not replaced the essential human element — the bedside nurse. The sick person and his family need support and understanding. The practical nurse — in the hospital, home, or clinic — is often the key person of the human element: nursing care. To the patient and his family, she may even be their link to all medical care. This presents great responsibility and challenge.

Is the patient truly benefiting from modern medical knowledge and scientific research? Is the helpless individual treated with genuine thoughtfulness and consideration? And do we understand how the patient's emotional attitude and his relationship to his family can help or hinder his recovery?

The content of this book is concerned with the last question — to help the practical nurse see her patient as an individual with hopes, feelings, ambitions, and problems, and as a person who is part of a family. Remember, when the patient leaves the hospital, he goes back to his family.

Let us eliminate the reasons underlying the remark I have heard: "Nurses have the reputation of giving good care to the patient, but to heck with the family."

With changes in the function of hospitals and the goal of medical care, the role of the nurse has expanded. It is now important both to help the patient to get well and to teach him how to stay well. To accomplish these two goals, the family needs consideration. During serious illness, nursing should mean total and complete care of the patient — and this involves the patient's family. In progressive patient care, home care of the patient is the final step — and this too involves the family. To teach the patient how to stay well, the nurse may have to win the cooperation of the family, and perhaps also to instruct family members.

As we note the changes in family life, we see that a study of family life today includes a study of the larger family circle — the community. An informed nurse can be a stabilizing force in her community as well as in her own home.

Your patient's family may be in the beginning years, in the middle years, or in the later years of the family life cycle.

The Family in the Beginning Years

Your patient may be newly married and part of a very new family. Adjusting to each other during the first few months of marriage is extremely important to the individual and to the success of the marriage. The wise nurse understands this.

You will spend many days as a student nurse taking care of newborn babies and of the new mothers. If you understand the changes that a new baby, especially the first baby, brings into the lives of the parents, you will be more likely to give good complete nursing care. The nurse can also guide a mother with other children at home in planning how she can help them to accept the new baby. Just being brothers and sisters does not ensure love. We *learn* to love, just as we learn to be a good parent and we learn to be a nurse.

Of particular interest to the nurse is the family with toddlers and preschool children. As a student practical nurse, you will spend from three to six weeks of your clinical experience in pediatrics. An understanding of well children is a prerequisite to working with sick children.

A nurse needs to be well informed on how children grow and develop; how they form good habits of eating, sleeping, dressing, cleanliness, and toilet control; and how they develop intellectually, emotionally, and socially. The nurse who knows what to expect of children at certain ages will be less likely to expect too much or too little from her young patient. Hospitalization can be a frightening experience to the child. A true understanding of what makes the small child afraid will enable the nurse to help her patient adjust to the hospital experience with as little real emotional damage as possible. Parents today may justifiably question some ironclad hospital rules that seem to be made for adults only.

The Family in the Middle Years

When children enter school, the family becomes more involved in community affairs. The patient with school-age children, or the schoolchild himself, does not want to "miss out." A nurse who is well versed in good health habits herself can be an effective teacher of good health habits. Particularly the children will look upon you, the nurse, as someone who knows how to maintain good health.

The teenage patient is a very special person. Not a child, not an adult, he is painfully aware of any differences he may have from his peer group. To be left out of school events is a real tragedy. The nurse needs to look through a teenager's eyes to understand what illness can mean to him. The tactful nurse will realize that the home illness of another family member can be of monumental consequence to the teenager. The "generation gap" may be real.

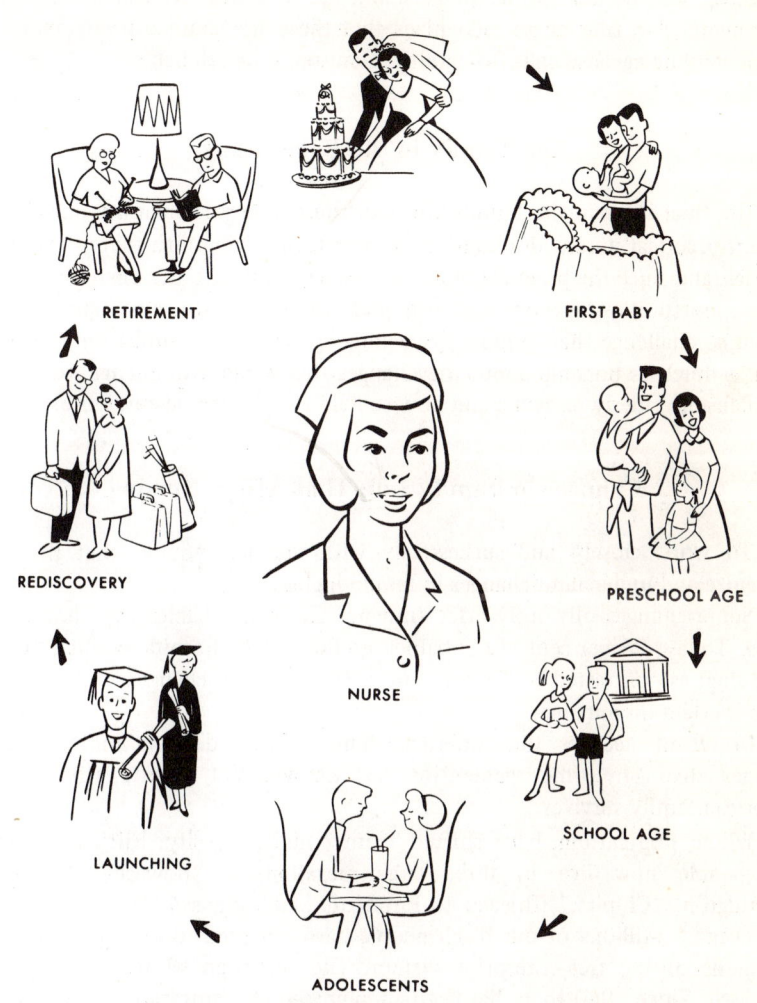

Figure 1. *The life cycle of the patient's family.*

Family finances are strained the most during the teenage and the "launching" stage. Sending a son or daughter to college, getting the son started in business, giving the daughter a big wedding — these are all large expenses for the family. Then along comes illness, and you, the nurse, enter. Financial matters become more difficult.

After the children are independent comes the stage in the family life cycle called the "empty nest" or rediscovery, which probably did not exist 50 years ago. This can be a second honeymoon to the couple; or the wife can feel lonely,

5

depressed, and useless, while the husband has a feeling of failure and lack of attainment. The true nurse recognizes that these are genuine problems for the couple. Middle age also calls for careful attention to health habits.

The Family in the Later Years

The final stage in the family life cycle merits the particular attention of the student practical nurse. More and more people are living into their eighties and nineties, and since the practical nurse is especially suited to their care, this means work opportunities for more and more practical nurses. Nursing elderly people is a genuine challenge that requires great nursing skill. Every student nurse should learn as much as possible about the changes that come with old age, techniques for managing elderly patients, and how to help elderly people enjoy life.

Changes in Family Life That Affect Nursing

To work closely and successfully with families requires that the nurse recognize and understand changes in family living.

Some changes obviously affect nursing. Formerly, babies were born in the home. Today, 96 per cent of the babies are born in the hospital with a physician attending, as contrasted to 56 per cent in 1940.[1] Other changes are less obvious in their effect on nursing.

In recent decades the American family has undergone more sweeping changes than any other generation has known. Yet despite criticism, the American family survives.

Whole populations have shifted from country to city. Fifty per cent of our people now live in three large megalopoles: "Bowash," Boston to Washington; "Chipits," Chicago to Pittsburgh; and "Sansan," San Francisco to San Diego.[2] Millions of our black people have migrated to the North and into the perils of the free-enterprise system. The suburban white population has increased. Since 1960 there has been an increased concentration of black people in the central cities, and white people in the suburbs.[3] Both urban and suburban life are different from rural living, yet many of our institutions are based on rural attitudes. In urban life families often lack the support of relatives, familiar community customs, and common opinions. (More differences will be noted in Chapter 19.) The population shift has coincided with the emergence of adolescents as a conspicuous group. Many nurses contact daily the problems that stem from the shift from rural to urban life.

[1] *Statistical Bulletin*, Metropolitan Life Insurance Company, March 1961, p. 2.
[2] *Family Service Highlights*, April–May 1968, p. 119.
[3] *U.S. News and World Report*, April 24, 1967, p. 115.

The Practical Nurse and Today's Family 7

Many people are living better today, and the expanded middle class includes minority groups. The middle-class families have more money to spend for medical and dental care, education, travel, second homes and recreation, even though costs for housing, food, and taxes have risen. Young families do not recall hard times. Jobs are plentiful. Debt is no longer a disgrace; mortgages are considered assets. Thrift as a virtue has lost its appeal. Yet even the affluent people lack a former necessity: service of a cook, maid, or handyman. If you contact the home as private duty or public health nurse, you will not see service people except for an occasional cleaning woman. Yet the family will be remarkably self-sufficient. The man of the house will be able to devise the rehabilitation device needed; the children can assist with the housework.

The affluence has not reached one-fifth of our nation's people, the poor people. Because children of the poor grow up in a meager environment, lacking basic educational skills, proper health care, and even good nutrition, the poor man's child does not reach his full potential when he becomes an adult. He either earns a minimum living or depends on a welfare check. Thus his children are likely to follow the same path. Attempts to break the cycle of the hard-core poor people have focused attention on their problems. No easy solutions are in sight. Help must be given to young people – the very young. Nor is there a clear, simple solution to the problems of racial integration. The educated nurse who understands basic family and community problems can be a bigger help toward reaching solutions than the uninformed nurse.

Improved communication today has made the world seem smaller. We know what is happening in Sydney, Australia, or Biafra, Nigeria. We also see on television how the affluent live, note the products they buy. Is it small wonder that the less privileged minority groups become impatient? Television has tremendous impact on the family.

Your patient today will be an informed person. Even 25 years ago, nurses did not tell the patient about his condition and his treatment. Today he will ask. He has read about the new drugs, the latest research on leukemia, and the heart transplants. It is the duty of the nurses to be extremely diplomatic when answering the patient's questions and reassuring him.

More people are married and have children, but the actual size of families has decreased. Before World War I, big families were the rule in America. The size of families decreased in the 1920's and 1930's, then rose again after World War II. After the peak in 1957 the birthrate declined but not the number of babies born. The total U.S. population increases every year as it has since the first census of 1790, but the sharp drop in birthrate since 1957 has slowed population growth much below earlier predictions. "Population explosion" may no longer be accurate.[4] Economic pinch felt by large families, new and more efficient methods of birth control, and the changed attitudes of organized

---

[4] *U.S. News and World Report*, March 11, 1968, pp. 57–58; and June 24, 1968, pp. 63–64, from U.S. Census Bureau.

religion toward birth control – all have influenced parents to plan smaller families. The Japanese people managed to limit a dangerous potential of "population explosion" on their islands. Population growth is about zero (births balancing death) in Japan, Sweden, Norway, England, and France.[5]

Nurses should recognize and know the facts regarding one baby boom that still rises in America: illegitimate births. In 1966, 8.4 per cent of all births were illegitimate. Nearly 1 in 20 of all white births was illegitimate; for nonwhites a little more than 1 in 4 births was illegitimate.[6]

America has become a nation on the move. We learn that one family in five moves each year, often going to a different state. This makes for flexibility, but it also encourages disruption of fixed values. Houston is not the same as San Francisco. Montana's customs differ from those in Connecticut. Parents attempt to make the home strong enough to support the family. The family becomes a tightly knit unit, with the members greatly dependent emotionally and socially on one another. The loss of one member of the group breaks the pattern of life. In your nursing career, you may contact many families who are completely alone in the community.

In fact, the typical family today is the small nuclear family: mother, father, and the children. We see fewer grandparents, aunts, cousins, as part of the family circle. The small nuclear family is far more dependent on the community than in grandparents' day. They look to the schools to educate the children, to the church to furnish religion instruction, and often to the community for recreation.

As the family becomes more democratic and companionable, we see less of the authoritative family along the patriarchal and matriarchal lines. The family roles are more flexible, less rigid. Sometimes these changes are not well understood, and confusion results. Mother is not always sure of her role, and father is not always sure of his role.

Yesterday's codes of good conduct do not fit today's way of life, and new codes of conduct are less clearly defined. Exactly what code of good conduct is right and what is wrong is frequently left to the individual. Young people can be overwhelmed and thus act unwisely. Practice in making decisions and learning to use freedom responsibly begins in babyhood. Young people today have greater freedom, more privileges, and fewer chaperones. We have also seen a rise in juvenile delinquency, and a rise in crime throughout the country.

In the overall picture, however, most of the changes in family living are improvements. We are living longer and better. We have a greater understanding of the small child, and no longer regard him as a miniature adult. We try to help young people accept freedom with responsibility. We are probing human relationships and attempting to improve them. We are striving to help all Americans participate fully in the best that our country has to offer.

Yes, the nurse needs to remain alert to changes within the family.

[5] *U.S. News and World Report*, June 12, 1967, pp. 64–65.
[6] *U.S. News and World Report*, June 24, 1968, pp. 63–64.

Questions for Discussion

1. Has your own family's contact with nurses been pleasant or unpleasant?
2. Which stages of the family life cycle are most difficult physically? Most expensive? Why?
3. In what ways do you live differently from your grandparents?
4. Has the population in your community increased or decreased during the past ten years?
5. How can the nurse help to strengthen moral standards in her community?

Additional Readings

Duvall, Evelyn Millis. *Family Development*, 4th ed. Chap. 5, "Trends in Family Orientation and Child Rearing." Philadelphia: J. B. Lippincott Company, 1967.

Esau, Margaret, and others. *Practical Nursing Today*. Chap. 12, "Family Structure and Relationships." New York: G. P. Putnam's Sons, 1957.

Recommended Audiovisual Aids

FILMSTRIP

Is There a Typical Family? (43 frames, Filmstrip of the Month Club, Color, 1959)

This filmstrip shows family patterns in various cultures, including Moslems, Eskimos, and American – past and present. It points out that families are not typical, and illustrates some of the variables.

FILM

Family Circles (30 min., McGraw-Hill, B&W, 1949)

Although not recently produced, this film may be available and the subject content is pertinent. The film points out that the enlarged family circle of today includes the school and the community. The experiences of three children illustrate how parental indifference, lack of imagination, and emotional conflict at home can interfere with a child's success at school. The good home is also shown.

CHAPTER 2 / SUCCESSFUL FAMILY LIFE

Good home life is the heart of success for the individual and for the nation. Our country's future lies with strong, sturdy individuals: the products of good homes. Today's predominantly urban society seems to require a stronger, more resolute, and better equipped individual than yesterday's rural society. Good family life was never more important than it is today.

As far back as history reveals, human beings have lived in families. Efforts to abolish or dissolve the family have always failed. Certainly families differ throughout the world, and are constantly changing. But the family exists.

The Family as a Social Group

From the illustration "The Family as the Unit of Society" you can trace the family and its relationships as a social group. Each spoke of the wheel represents contacts of the family members with society. For example, adequate, convenient transportation is crucial to the functioning of the family. Contacts made with bus drivers, train employees, air travel personnel, and others are all contacts of the family with other members of society. At the hub of the wheel is the family, with each member influencing, and being influenced by, every other family member.

Effect of the Family on Your Patient

The nurse can hardly escape noticing the relationship of the patient to his family. Of course, she does not interfere, but she needs to realize that the patient is affected.

The incentive to get well is one of the intangible factors. The patient determined to return to his home and to his loved ones seems to have an advantage, other things being equal, over the patient who simply does not care.

A patient worried about his family or finances is likely to become tense and anxious. He may be an uncooperative patient. Tension, anxiety, and a lack of cooperation will impede recovery.

Family conflict or inner tension may actually cause illness. It may cause a person in a weakened physical condition to get worse. More and more, doctors relate certain illnesses to emotional stress. If the stress cannot be expressed

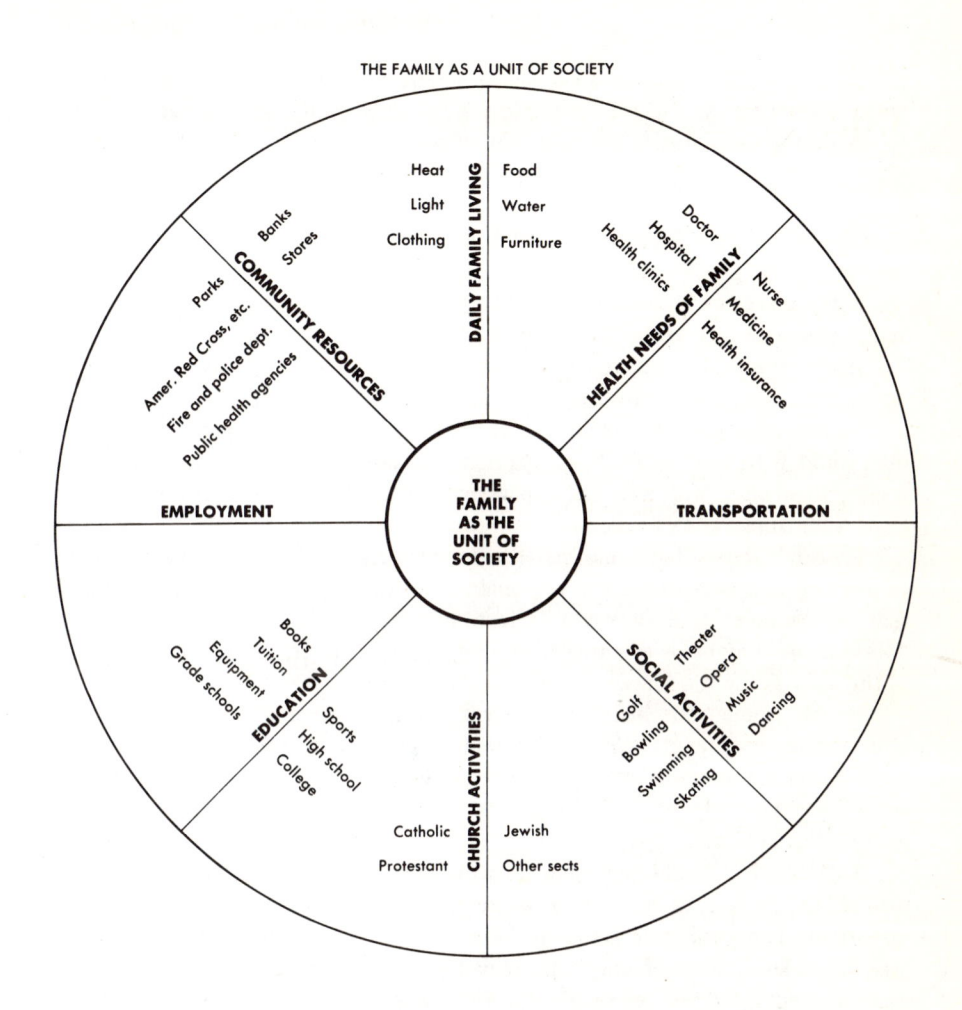

Figure 2. *Courtesy of Sister M. Elaine, St. Mary's Hospital, Philadelphia, Pa.*

through words, some organ of the body may suffer. The organs of respiration are often affected. Asthma attacks have been linked to personal problems that seem impossible to solve.

Astounding advances have been made in treating diseases, deformities, and physical illnesses. Not as much progress has been made in dealing with problems of human relationships, human attitudes, and human behavior. The technology of medicine is being solved better than its sociology.

The bedside nurse assumes a critical role in helping the patient to benefit from scientific achievements. Health is related to the way the patient views his

11

life situation and to the way he reacts to it. This is interwoven with his relations with his own family. In order to effectively reassure and guide the patient back to health, the nurse must understand the importance of good home life.

Importance of Family Influence

Many places of business today are very impersonal. You are given a number, and you are rated in terms of work produced or results obtained.

In the home, the individual gains his identity. The family says, "You are important." You are loved for *who* you are, not *what* you are.

Family life shapes the child into the adult he will become. Surrounding the little child with love, warmth, companionship, and understanding helps him to grow into an adult with a feeling of personal worth. If he has respect for himself, respect for others comes easier.

Research shows that babies raised in an institution with attention given only to physical needs are lacking in personality and development.[1] Children need a rich environment with a warm, affectionate mother and lots of attention. "Mothering" may be as essential to the intellectual and emotional development of the baby as the food he eats and the air he breathes.

In the home, the little child learns what people are like — good, bad, affectionate, indifferent. He acquires values and sets standards that hold for many years. Undesirable attitudes, such as "Get as much as you can" or "The world owes you a living," are difficult to alter. The goal to give, not receive, is learned best at home.

The family should set, and expect adherence to, standards, but not manipulate. In fact, as children grow into adolescence, the "cutting process" is important. The youngster gradually becomes more responsbile for himself and less dependent on his family. His added privileges and greater freedom are accompanied by more responsibility. He needs to practice self-discipline and self-control. If the routines of healthful living are now habits, he continues to observe them.

Both the child and the adult derive feelings of security — or insecurity — from their home life. Basic security gives the individual the courage to face the outside world with all its challenges and problems.

Not All Homes Are Good Homes

As a student nurse you learn the *ideals* of good patient care, healthful living, and good care of children. You may be shocked to see a little child admitted to

---

[1] Boyd R. McCandless, *Children: Behavior and Development*, 2nd ed. (New York: Holt, Rinehart and Winston, 1967) p. 45.

the pediatric ward who has been neglected – malnourished, unclean, not toilet-trained, and sometimes even bearing evidences of physical abuse. Then you realize that some homes are poor places to rear children.

Everywhere one hears statements that refer to poor home training. An elementary school teacher described her discipline difficulties with 36 lively eight- and nine-year-olds. "The ones from broken homes, those with poor home training, are impossible. They keep the entire classroom in an uproar and prevent the other children from learning effectively."

Many families give marvelous care to the baby and preschool child, but fail to offer adequate guidance and supervision to the older child. When this occurs, often the father is absent from the home. The mother alone cannot discipline the older children.

A religious social worker explained that to some people the word "Father" evokes unpleasant memories. Instead of praying, "My Father in Heaven," he substituted words such as "My Savior."

Another social worker made pointed, definite statements about dating practices. She scored heavily the parents of 12- and 13-year-old girls who encourage the girl to date a 16-year-old boy because the boy can drive a car and thus relieve the parents of chauffeuring responsibilities. The social worker also emphasized the importance of an adult's being in the house during a teenager's party. "The one adult keeps the party respectable."

Everywhere one sees evidences of family breakdowns.

Unhappy Family Life Is Costly

One state department of public welfare announced that a survey showed the greatest cause of dependency on public support was *family breakdown:* divorce, separation, and desertion. Of persons receiving state assistance to dependent children, 45.2 per cent came from broken families.[2]

Family breakdown has been described as "America's number one problem" and as being "as destructive as any disease."[3] These figures may be cited: The illegitimacy rate has tripled since 1938; one of four marriages ends in divorce; the delinquency rate has nearly tripled since 1940; and more than 200,000 people are admitted annually to mental hospitals.

All these problems in human relationships can be traced to breakdowns in family relationships.

---

[2] Indiana State Department of Public Welfare, as stated in *Kaleidoscope*, publication of Family Service Association of Indianapolis, June, 1962.
[3] From the fiftieth anniversary publication of *Highlights*, national publication of Family Service Association of America.

Evaluating Success of the Family

If a family stays together, this is not necessarily an indication of success. Divorce was not socially acceptable 100 years ago, but this did not mean that all families were happy or that all family life was good.

Happiness is one indication of successful family life. The family members get along well together. They do things together, not because they have to, but because they want to. Mutual respect, love, and affection are present. They enjoy the same friends. They are probably a healthy family. The wage earners are able to do their work, and they contribute to community life. They have a substantial place in the community.

A truly scientific evaluation of family success is difficult. How does the man rate as a father, a provider, a homemaker, and a husband? How does the woman rate as a wife, a mother, a homemaker, and a person? One aspect may conflict with another. For instance, a man has to decide how much of his time to devote to business and how much to reserve for his family. Perhaps taking a second job, "moonlighting," may permit him to provide better financially for his family. But will the extra money compensate when the five-year-old says, "Daddy, we never get to see you"? This decision must often be made.

Many families rate success in terms of material possessions and social status. They compare their way of life with a previous period, and if they have "bettered themselves," or moved up the social ladder, they feel successful.

Another way of appraising family life is by the social contribution of the family and its members. In a published study of 60,000 American families,[4] the authors based success on number of children, infrequency of divorce and desertion, lack of interference by police, and keeping children in school.

In families rated as poor, the children quit school without jobs or without serious intent to get work. The boys drifted until summoned for military service. The girls waited for "something to happen." These groups were claimed to be the chief source of juvenile delinquency.

The good families allowed into their homes and circles of intimate friends only those other families remarkably like themselves. Family friends with similar values and ideals helped the children accept parental ideals. Also, children were encouraged to proceed further in their education. The actual number of high school graduates, college students, and technically trained people increased. The study pointed to many broken families, and many more very good families. The bad families seemed to be getting worse. The good families were increasing and getting better.

This has been termed as rating family life by minimum criteria, by how well

---

[4] Carle C. Zimmerman and Lucius F. Cervantes, *Successful American Families* (New York: Pageant Press, 1960).

Successful Family Life

the family attained the goals set by society. Duvall[5] defines family success by how well the family encourages and assists its members to achieve developmental tasks. A family is successful if all members get support, acceptance, and opportunities to progress, mature, and move smoothly into the next stage of life. Admittedly, some stages of the family life cycle present more difficulty than others. Families are like individuals in that success leads to more success, while failures tend to lead to more failures. Certainly if a family is meeting the basic needs of its members at each stage in life, that family's home life might be considered successful.

Toward Good Family Life

Good family life means different things to different people. Since our outlook on life tends to reflect our own personal experiences, it is easy to evaluate all family living in terms of our own family life. The student nurse needs to remember that there are great variations among good homes. There are many good ways of bringing up children. But we do find some of the basic characteristics over and over again.

In the good home, there is love — love that is felt and expressed. It is easy to express love to the helpless baby and to the dependent toddler. Sometimes it is not so easy, but ways can be found, to express affection and love for the ten-year-old boy or the adolescent girl.

Large groups of college students were asked to rate the factors that made their early home life happy or unhappy.[6] Most important to the students was their parents' having had a happy marriage. Second, the students mentioned their parents' expression of love for them. Other items mentioned had to do with family unity and family approval of each other. Most of the factors mentioned are within the power of all parents to provide. They do not depend on income.

A good home means sharing of work, sharing of responsibilities, and sharing of recreation. If the father is a golf enthusiast, perhaps he needs to find some recreation that he can truly share with his school-age sons. If the work of the home is done in the spirit of cooperation, children acquire a pleasant attitude toward work.

When each person is recognized as an individual in the home, his projects, activities, and interests are important to the others. The child's school is actually his working world and his occupation. When his parents show him that they think his schoolwork is important, they help him to respect the dignity of work.

---

[5] Evelyn Millis Duvall, *Family Development*, 4th ed. (Philadelphia: Lippincott, 1967) p. 47.

[6] Judson T. Landis and Mary G. Landis, *Personal Adjustment: Marriage and Family Living*. 4th ed. (Englewood Cliffs, N.J.: Prentice-Hall, 1966) p. 355.

The mature student practical nurse, with a family, has said that when she sits down to study her homework, the children are more willing to study theirs. When they see that their mother is working hard to attain her goal, they can understand that they may have to work too.

Even though each person in the home is recognized as an individual, he needs to learn that rules and regulations help him to respect the rights of others. We all have to follow rules. The little child learns this early if his home has discipline, discipline with affection.

Everyone needs new experiences. Family-approved new experiences help children to learn right from wrong and help them to grow into responsible adults.

In the good home, parents are aware of the problems of their children. The children learn to respect the rights of their parents. They do not expect their parents to do all the sacrificing.

Family members need to be able to talk to each other. Sometimes it is an effort to keep open the channels of communication, but it is worthwhile.

Family Guidance

For centuries and centuries, man has looked to a higher power, a higher being, for guidance in the problems of daily living. The guideposts may be found, but do we really follow them? Do we really want to accept what we know is right?

Study your own Bible, your own source of religious beliefs, and notice how many statements apply directly to family living. It is all there — love, faithfulness, loyalty, tolerance, foregiveness, sympathy, patience, accepting imperfections, recognizing the rights of each person — the list is endless.

A family that actually strives to live by these principles is following the right road to a rich family life. Research has shown a close association between family religiousness and success in family living.[7]

If we would only *do* what we know is right, many great personal tragedies would be averted. We all make mistakes. Perhaps it is a matter of relativity.

The wife who has been deserted, the husband who has deserted, the mother with the illegitimate child, the juvenile delinquent — these people need to be accepted as they are and encouraged to strive to live better lives. All of us can do better.

The child who grows up in a warm, loving home with parents who are kind, giving, and secure in their own feelings — this child has a truly good start toward being a useful, responsible citizen.

---

[7] Judson T. Landis: "Religiousness, Family Relationships, and Family Values in Protestant, Catholic, and Jewish Families," *Marriage and Family Living,* 22: 341–47 (Nov., 1960).

Questions for Discussion

1. Bring to class newspaper clippings (1) that describe evidences of family breakdown and (2) that show evidences of family solidarity or successful family living.
2. Describe physical illnesses that are believed to be related to emotional problems.
3. Do emotions affect digestion of food? If so, how?
4. Set up a code or method for evaluating the success of a family.

Additional Readings

Duvall, Evelyn Millis. *Family Development*. 4th ed., pp. 47–50. Philadelphia: J. B. Lippincott Company, 1967.

Janet, Sister Mary. "How are We Forming Ideals and Attitudes in Youth," in *Survey Papers*. Golden Anniversary White House Conference on Children and Youth, p. 67.

Landis, Judson T., and Mary G. Landis. *Personal Adjustment: Marriage and Family Living*, 4th ed. Chap. 27, "The Successful Family." Engelwood Cliffs, N.J.: Prentice-Hall, Inc., 1966.

Mead, Margaret, and Ken Heyman. *Family*. New York: The Macmillan Company, 1965.

Zimmerman, Carle C. and Lucius F. Cervantes. *Successful American Families*. New York: Pageant Press, Inc., 1960.

Recommended Audiovisual Aids

FILMS

A Family Affair (31 min. International Film Bureau, B&W)
A family can work together, for the good of all. In this film, the parents are worried because the son wants to become an actor, not a lawyer, and the 16-year-old daughter is dating a 20-year-old boy. The family service counselor helps the father to understand that his son's choice need not repeat his own decision, that is, a routine job with security in place of creativity. The father realizes that his life could now include some creativity. The mother can become less tense and less strict, for the benefit of all the family.

Families First (20 min., New York State Department of Commerce, B&W, 1948)
This film contrasts the results of good and bad family life. The children who grow up in a family atmosphere of love and serenity become responsible citizens, as contrasted with the children who grow up amidst friction and emotional instability.

FILMSTRIP

Awareness: Insight into People (54 frames, record 20 min., J. C. Penny Co., 1969)
  This three-part filmstrip with accompanying record defines and explains uses of observation, stereotyping, and empathy. The questions presented requiring audience participation would help the student nurse to understand herself and her patient.

CHAPTER 3 / **THE NEWLYWED**

A stable marriage and a stable home are the concern of everyone. The practical nurse, like every responsible citizen, should recognize the importance of sound preparation for marriage, of selecting suitable marriage partners, and of the newlywed's making good adjustments. As a student practical nurse, and later as a graduate practical nurse, you will work directly with families broken by divorce and separation. When you see the tragedies some people experience, you will realize that efforts to prevent divorce and separation are worthwhile. Averting tragedy is wiser than trying to help people to pick up the threads of a broken family life and proceed from there. The young couple are in love when they marry. What goes wrong? Let us concentrate on what can be done in the right way.

Preparation for Marriage

Many young people are inadequately prepared for the responsibilities of marriage. The movies, the popular magazines, the television advertisements have overglamorized marriage. It is depicted as a perpetual whirlwind of courtship and flowers. All wives continue to be beautiful models of femininity; all husbands continue to be gallant lovers.

These shallow views need to be replaced by a more realistic approach to the depths and the capacities of marriage. A young couple can look forward to a richer life and deeper love as they share work, responsibility, disappointments, and triumphs. They will begin to realize that in giving, you truly receive.

Evelyn Millis Duvall writes:

Married love grows as the marriage progresses. It is built on companionship. It gradually takes the place of romantic love, which arises from dreams and idealisms. Romantic love is sweet and blinding. No marriage is soundly built until married love takes the place of romantic illusions. Many marriages break up quickly because couples are not prepared for a shift in feelings toward each other. They think because they feel differently, their love is gone. Actually, married love can be more satisfying than romantic love. It is sturdier. It emerges as the two people face realities and accept each other for what they are, lovable but still human personalities.

Many factors in the life of a young person prepare him for marriage. The ability to make friends and to get along with people helps toward making a good

[1] Evelyn Millis Duvall, *Building Your Marriage*, Public Affairs Pamphlet No. 113, adapted, pp. 5 and 6.

marriage. If you have a good friend, you try to accept him as he is; you do not try to remake him; you compromise; you build up his feelings of self-worth when possible; you consider how he feels about certain things. These are all good characteristics to extend toward a marriage partner. This also means not being a "doormat." We are uncomfortable around people we take advantage of.

The young man or woman who supports himself, pays his own bills, and manages his own life acquires assets helpful toward building a good marriage. The young woman who economizes on beauty parlor visits in order to save money for a vacation trip is learning to sacrifice toward a larger goal. She will know how to watch for food bargains and to stretch the food dollar when she is a wife.

Adjustments for Every Couple

Generally, a person tends to marry someone similar to himself in temperament, age, background, intelligence, stature, and even appearance. Yet regardless of similarities, every couple has to adjust frequently in many ways. The first year of marriage is a critical time for its success. Divorces and annulments are more frequent during the early years of marriage than at any other time in the family life cycle. Half of divorces come during the first six years of marriage, and recent research shows that actual marriage failures occurred in the first or second year of marriage.[2] If the couple can compromise and adjust while romantic love prevails, they will probably continue doing so.

Establishing household routines merits consideration, time, and thought. Meal planning, grocery shopping, cooking, washing dishes, cleaning, laundry — these things are usually planned around the employment of both husband and wife. The young student nurse who decides to marry while still a student may find herself with two masters. Creating a real home is the highest privilege for a woman, a task not to be slighted. Yet if the new bride has an important test the following day in her class on anatomy, should she neglect her studying or her homemaking or her husband?

Religious views serve as a guide for daily living and a basis for making decisions. Differences in religious faiths merit careful and frank discussion before marriage. It may be easy for a person to think: "I can give up my religion." But after children are born, he may realize that his views are more firmly and deeply rooted than he had thought. He may want the children raised in his faith. The difference may involve choosing between public and parochial schools. Also, what do the grandparents think?

Actually, two people professing the same denomination will have decisions to make. "How often shall we go to church? How much money shall we give?

---

[2] Judson T. Landis and Mary G. Landis, *Personal Adjustment, Marriage, and Family Living,* 4th ed. (Englewood Cliffs, N.J.: Prentice-Hall, 1966), p. 287.

How much time shall we give to the church and church activities?" In the case of dissimilar religions, these differences are even greater.

A functioning religion provides a couple with inner strength, a philosophy of life, and a basis to work out many problems. Religion emphasizes self-discipline, and marriage requires stability in a person. Couples who attend church together and have other outside interests are more likely to succeed at marriage than those who have no purposes outside themselves. As religious beliefs deepen and love for fellow men grows, the couple's love for each other becomes stronger.

In-law relationships can be trying, but with tolerance, patience, and willingness to try to understand, the in-laws can become both family and friends. During the first year of marriage, the couple learns the meaning of the adage: "You marry his (her) family too." Perhaps the wife cannot see that her family is being overcritical of her husband or, with too frequent visits, is infringing on the couple's privacy. The husband may not understand that his mother causes his wife to feel inferior and inadequate, and perhaps he is beginning to compare her cooking unfavorably with his mother's.

Sexual adjustments are important to a successful marriage, but since a happy marriage depends on successful relations in general, this is more than sex in its narrow sense. The young couple who have had good premarital counseling will not expect to attain complete sexual adjustment in the first year of marriage. But as their life together becomes more relaxed, and they begin to have greater confidence in each other, their personal relationship will probably become more satisfactory. If it does not, they should not hesitate to seek counsel.

Money matters will require constant adjustments and continual decisions from the couple. If long-term goals are agreed upon, perhaps less friction will arise. If both the husband and wife believe that saving for a new house or for the education of their children is vitally important, each may be more willing to sacrifice in personal ways.

Disagreement over money is often given as the cause for divorce when perhaps the real problem was something else. When the wife purchases a new coat or a new piece of furniture that she knows her husband will have difficulty paying for, she may be "getting even" for something else. If the husband does not tell his wife about a salary bonus, this also indicates something may be wrong.

Finances during the first year of marriage may be handled more smoothly if the couple have made a tentative budget before marriage and if they have frankly discussed resources and liabilities.

A lack of money for comfortable living may be a factor in the high divorce rate for very youthful marriages. The highest rate of divorce is for childless couples under 20 years of age.

When the wife continues to work after marriage, which is the prevailing custom today, further understanding is needed on the handling of her income. Too many working wives have the attitude: "The husband's money is *our* money; what I earn is *my* money." If the couple establish a standard of living that requires two incomes to maintain, they may be in trouble when one has to stop working — for example, the expectant mother. The ideal is to set aside the wife's income for savings. A new range and a new refrigerator are a form of savings. However, many families need the two salaries for necessities. The ideal cannot always be attained.

Social activities and recreation mutually enjoyed, will help the couple. If they expect that having only each other will be enough, they may be expecting too much of their marriage. During dating and courtship, they doubtlessly shared numerous social and recreational activities. To continue enjoying themselves with other people will further their delight in each other.

Many people believe that "togetherness" can be overemphasized. A woman may still enjoy spending one evening a week with her club. The fisherman may still like to go fishing with his fishing buddies or alone. He will come home a happier husband because he has been fishing.

Friends of the couple should be enjoyed by both. This does not mean that each must dearly love all of the other's friends. But the wife is asking for trouble if she consistently and frequently invites to dinner the couple her husband dislikes. She might see them occasionally, but not at all times. If the husband has a buddy that his wife dislikes, he might enjoy his company on a bowling night or at some all-male function.

In reality, the couple may be making new friends. They will mature as a couple, and their interests will change and expand. They will want friends with similar interests.

Jealousy is difficult to analyze. Supposedly, if one feels secure about the love of the mate, and is self-confident, jealousy has no basis. Certainly men in the working world and women who go to work each day have friends of the opposite sex. This need not be a basis for jealousy. Of the successful people you know, do not most of them get along well with all people — both men and women? The nurse who has risen to the position of director of nurses gets along well with nurses under her supervision and with the hospital administrators, doctors, salespeople, and men in many professions. If her husband has faith in her, he will not object or be jealous.

The training and disciplining of children can be a constant source of friction to the couple, or they can support each other. They need to present a united front before the children, regardless of private disagreements. If this lack of complete harmony bothers parents, they might be consoled to know that when only one parent raises the child — as in the case of the divorced mother — the absence of the second parent's criticism and opinion is not necessarily good.

Fortunately, today fewer people believe the theory that warring spouses should have a child to cement their marriage and to bring them closer together.

The Newlywed

A couple who already disagree will only find more cause to disagree. How unfair it is to expect the baby to bring the parents together again.

The little things in a marriage are the constant sources of irritation and may eventually lead to serious trouble. Each person needs to strive to be adaptable, to change himself, and to overlook the faults of the other. Personal consideration may help to keep love alive. A happy marriage is never a gift. Two people who love each other, and are willing to work at their marriage, will usually find that the marriage works for them.

Causes for Marriage Failures

Official causes for divorce as reported in court records do not give the reasons for marriage failures. For example, cruelty is the cause given most often, but why were they cruel to each other?

People do not have to stay together today if they are unhappy. A man can eat his meals in a restaurant and send his shirts to the laundry. A woman can earn her own living. She is not as completely dependent upon a husband as women were many years ago.

Young people who are not prepared for marriage can become quickly disillusioned, and not really work at their marriage. Loneliness is more common today because people move about, change jobs, and have fewer close friends. They expect more of marriage, and are more impatient and less tolerant of mistakes.

Also, they are much more likely to meet and marry someone with a totally different background. Some differences are so great that building a good marriage would be extremely difficult, if not impossible.

Personality may be the most important single factor in marital adjustment. Some personality differences are good. The effervescent, "life of the party" type of woman may be favorably complemented by a somewhat more steady, quiet husband. A too serious husband could be helped to see life in better perspective with a wife whose sense of humor helped him laugh now and then.

Yet extreme differences are difficult to overcome. The tidy, meticulously neat man would be unhappy with a wife who was a careless housekeeper. The conservative woman probably could not adjust permanently to a completely happy-go-lucky husband.

A teenager said to her mother: "I want to marry someone who is *different*."

The mother replied: "Just being a man and a woman is *enough different*."

Age difference between husband and wife does not necessarily mean success or failure in marriage, but a great difference in age would present extra hurdles to surmount. Studies show an increased divorce rate with age differences of 13 years or more. Either husband or wife a few years older does not seem significant.

Educational differences may seem less important than a difference in *intelligence* or general *culture*. A formal education may be had today by most people who have the determination and ability. Perhaps if the couple agrees on the value of education, that is as important as having the same amount of education.

International marriages usually involve other differences, such as climate, a new way of living, different customs, different culture, different religion — all factors important to everyday living. The status of women is quite different in many foreign countries compared with that in the United States. And the community's attitude toward the newcomer is also very important. Some communities graciously and sincerely accept a person quite different from themselves. Other communities may reject or ignore him. It requires extremely mature, self-sufficient, and adaptable people for a sucessful Jewish-Gentile, Chinese-English, or Negro-white marriage.

Dissimilar social and economic backgrounds are extra hazards. An individual's personal habits tend to be formed by the way he has lived. It is not impossible, but it is very difficult, to change one's habits. Studies seem to indicate that a wife may be able to raise her standards more easily than a husband. She may have to see less of her former friends, because all concerned may be uncomfortable or embarrassed if they cannot participate in the social activities.

Immaturity is undoubtedly a contributing factor to many divorces. This is further complicated because clear-cut definitions of the feminine and masculine roles do not exist today. Even mature couples can be confused because the traditional husband-wife roles seem no longer adequate.

All studies agree that responsible individuals with *religious roots* are less divorce-prone and more likely to be happily married. Married couples with no religious affiliations divorce more frequently than do religious pairs.[3]

Broken Families

Divorce may be the only step left when all efforts to keep the family together have failed. Two people have to work at marriage for success. One partner may try earnestly and not wish to admit defeat. The other partner may force the issue or simply quit.

Divorce represents failure, and its effect on individuals involved is immeasurable. Some people are able to profit from their own mistakes, to benefit from unhappy experience, and to proceed to a better life and a more successful second marriage. Other people simply repeat their same mistakes in a

---

[3] Evelyn Millis Duvall, *Family Development*, 4th ed. (Philadelphia: Lippincott, 1967), p. 501.

The Newlywed 25

second marriage that is unhappy, and they continue to meet with frustration and failure.

Divorced people will say that, although it may seem to be the only course of action at the time, divorce itself is not a solution. It only presents a new set of problems.

A child may feel that his world has collapsed. When a child loves both parents, he finds it difficult to understand why he is to live with one parent, not both. His loyalty is divided. Sometimes the child blames himself. Even if the mother tries to speak respectfully of the father, her own hurt or angry feelings make it difficult for her to keep a good image of the father before the children.

Yet some leading psychiatrists and social scientists are beginning to suggest that well-meaning martyrdom of parents does not always help the children. Youngsters from physically intact but emotionally broken homes have shown more emotional problems and delinquency than children of broken homes.[4] There is no simple solution.

Divorce is no longer a social disgrace, and the divorced person is not ostracized from society as he might have been 100 years ago. It is estimated that 10 per cent of the voting population in America has been divorced.[5]

The increase in the divorce rate does not mean that a great increase in marriage unhappiness exists. But the frequency and the legal ease do mean that many couples who might find happiness if they would stay together and work at it now get divorced and remain unhappy apart.

Desertion is fairly common today and, perhaps unfairly, has been described as "the poor man's divorce." The problems are just as great as in divorce, if not more so.

Death is often unexpected, creating difficult adjustments. As a nurse you will see death, and you will see families torn by grief. You must be calm, but try not to become calloused or "hardened" to death.

The widow or widower must learn to live a different life. A mother is concerned about her children and will have to assume the role of the father. She usually has to work and to be away from her children more. The financial responsibility is great. A father left with small children may not be able to afford the salary of a full-time housekeeper. Placing the children in a foster home may be a temporary solution. The social life of either widow or widower is drastically changed. He or she may feel uncomfortable with couples that used to comprise their social circle.

Some people who have lost a husband or wife have said that it called for strength and courage that they did not realize they possessed. Somehow, they got through the time and were able to adjust. One might visualize that these people had support and help from friends and family.

[4] Helen S. Arnstein, *What to Tell Your Child* (Indianapolis: Bobbs-Merrill, 1962), p. 123.
[5] *U.S. News and World Report*, Jan. 3, 1963, p. 44.

Questions for Discussion

1. What are workable methods of handling money in the family? If the wife works, how should the second paycheck be handled?
2. In your community, where are reliable family counseling services available?
3. Differences between husband and wife will arise. What are constructive ways of handling quarrels?
4. What helps one to get along with in-laws?
5. What are the laws regarding marriage and divorce in your state?

Additional Readings

Arnstein, Helen S. *What to Tell Your Child about Birth, Illness, Death, Divorce, and other Family Crises.* Indianapolis: The Bobbs-Merrill Company, Inc., in cooperation with Child Study Association of America, 1962.

Duvall, Evelyn Millis. *Building Your Marriage.* New York: Public Affairs Pamphlet No. 113.

Duvall, Evelyn Millis, and Reuben Hill. *When You Marry.* Rev. ed. Chap. 8, "Newly-Wed." Boston: D. C. Heath and Company, Inc., 1962.

Duvall, Sylvanus M. *Before You Marry.* Chap. 9, "What About Mixed Marriages?" New York: Associated Press, 1959.

Fitzsimmons, Cleo, and Nell White. *Management for You.* Rev. ed., Chap. 13, "Managing Family Income"; Chap. 14, "Spending Family Income." Philadelphia: J. B. Lippincott Company, 1964.

Landis, Judson T., and Mary G. Landis. *Personal Adjustment: Marriage and Family Living.* 4th ed. Chap. 10, "Likes or Opposites in Marriage"; Chap. 16, "What it Means to be Married." Englewood Cliffs, N.J.: Prentice-Hall, Inc., 1966.

Recommended Audiovisual Aids

FILMS

Marriage Is a Partnership (14 min. Coronet, B&W)
   A young couple trying to solve the problems facing them in their first year of marriage — money, sex, in-laws, friends, and social activities — find their most serious problem is learning to understand the in-laws. The in-law situations are well presented.

Marriage Today (22 min., McGraw-Hill, B&W)
   A mature and positive concept of marriage and marriage adjustment is presented. It may be necessary to point out that the couples shown did not arrive at their present adjustment without effort. The film tends to show the ideal marriage, not realities.

The Newlywed

This Charming Couple (20 min., McGraw-Hill, B&W)
   The film opens with the divorce scene, then traces back the courtship, which had danger signals that the couple ignored. Designed to show the unreality of romantic love, the film can also be used to discuss mixed marriages and the importance of fulfilling personality needs in marriage.

Who's Boss (16 min., McGraw-Hill, B&W)
   Not a new film, yet the theme of competition in marriage is still appropriate. It dramatizes the adjustments necessary and the time required to achieve a good balance of partnership and individuality.

FILMSTRIP

Understanding Your Love Feelings. Part IV of Series: Love and the Facts of Life (56 frames, record 22 min., QED Productions, Division of Cathedral Films, Color, 1967)
   This filmstrip would give basis for discussion of such topics as: How do I know it is love? What are the different kinds of love? What are myths surrounding love and marriage? It would particularly help the youthful student nurse to understand her own feelings.

CHAPTER 4 / **PARENTHOOD: ARRIVAL OF**

THE BABY

As a student practical nurse, you will probably spend several weeks caring for new babies and their mothers. You may notice that the mother, especially if this is her first baby, is eager to know how to care for him. She wants to be a good mother. She looks to the nurses for information and instruction, and you should be able to help her when you are a graduate practical nurse.

Later in your practical nursing training, you will study maternal-child nursing, including good prenatal care. Right now, let us consider how this tiny, new baby affects his family.

Preparing Prospective Parents

If the couple have prepared themselves to become parents, they will not expect to be good parents automatically. They will realize that parenthood is a profession requiring training and experience. Most parents learn by raising a child. However, knowing what to expect will give them confidence and help them to succeed.

With the first indication of pregnancy, the wife should see the family physician. He will advise her concerning good care of herself and attempt to detect symptoms of possible trouble. He may recommend an obstetrician, or the wife may ask for his services.

The physician doubtlessly will suggest that the wife attend a formal class on prenatal and baby care (see Fig. 3). Husbands are also urged to attend. If the class is sponsored by the hospital, the prospective parents may tour the maternity section of the hospital and see the labor and delivery rooms. The physician may recommend that the wife attend the class on normal childbirth.

If the family cannot afford regular visits to the physician, he may send the expectant mother to a prenatal clinic.

In some localities, public health nurses may be asked to visit the home, to answer special needs, and to advise the prospective mother on such matters as selecting baby clothes and accessories.

Being informed helps the prospective mother to know what to expect, to have less fear, and to be more relaxed.

Sometimes it is a rude awakening when young parents finally realize what

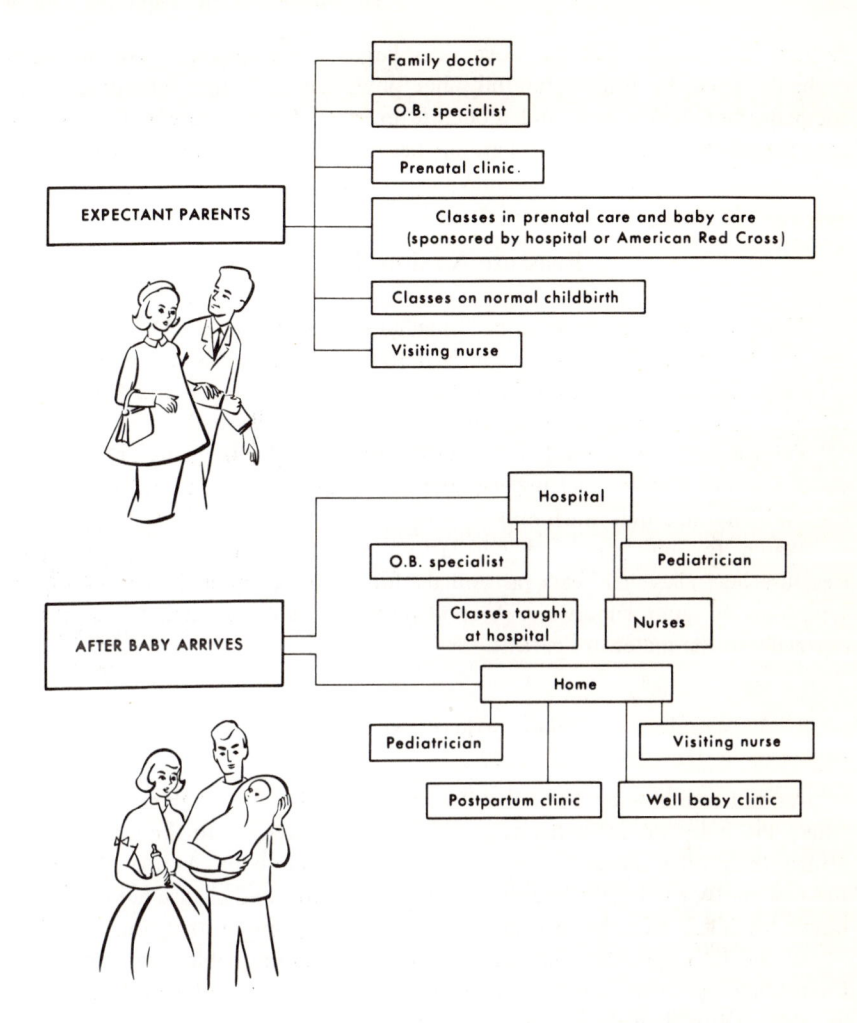

Figure 3. *Community resources. Sources of information for prospective parents.*

parenthood means. The role of parenthood may be assumed more easily and less painfully if the couple anticipate that the tiny newcomer will completely change their lives, that he may be a source of trouble as well as joy, and that he genuinely needs both his father and his mother.

Adjustments During Pregnancy

The wife's pregnancy has already brought many changes into the couple's lives. Visits to the doctor and the baby's layette and equipment cost money.

Perhaps the couple had to move into larger living quarters. The wife has probably tried to follow carefully her physician's recommendations for an adequate diet, added rest, and moderate exercise. Some household tasks may have proved too exhausting for her. She has needed her husband's understanding and support during the times she may have felt depressed.

Reassure Anxious Parents

Your maternity patient taking home her first baby may doubt her ability to care for her child. Overanxiety can be detrimental, or at least a nuisance. One couple grudgingly agreed with the pediatrician who answered their 2 A.M. phone call by saying, "Nothing is wrong with anyone but the parents."

Occasionally a new mother has to stop breast-feeding her baby only because she is not sure that he is getting enough milk. "When I see the bottle half empty, I know he has had that much milk."

Watch for indications of postpartum anxiety in the maternity patient. Reassure her, allay her fears (as you do for all patients), and then report the symptoms to your supervisor. A good nurse consistently teaches health, and especially to the maternity patient.

Help with the New Baby

Your hospital may have the "rooming-in" plan for mothers and babies, where the baby sleeps in the same room with or adjacent to the mother. This affords the mother an early opportunity to care for her baby. At many hospitals, the new mother is taught how to handle, feed, bathe, and change her baby. The nurses teach her, by either private demonstration or group instruction.

If the hospital maintains the central nursery where babies are kept except for feeding, or "visits" to the mother, the new mother can still learn much about her baby that will give her confidence at home.

Services of the visiting nurse may be prearranged, so that the new mother will have help and reassurance when first responsible for bathing, feeding, and dressing her baby. The visiting nurse will answer the mother's questions about caring for herself and will help to interpret individual needs of the baby and the mother. Every baby is different.

Baby Alters Home Life

Despite the changes she has already experienced, your maternity patient can expect more adjustments when she takes her baby home from the hospital.

The baby will interfere with the parents' social life and limit their freedom.

Parenthood: Arrival of the Baby

The entire household will revolve around his feeding time, bath time, and nap time. There will be diapers to wash, formula to prepare, and other demanding tasks. The baby will continue to cost money.

A very young couple may expect these responsibilities, yet not anticipate that their baby will cause arguments. The parents may disagree on how to handle him. The mother is more likely than the father to be informed on the latest methods of child care. Also, grandparents (two sets) may express very definite opinions on how their grandchild should be raised.

Sometimes a new father is unconsciously jealous of the time and attention the baby requires from his wife. He may criticize or call her the "doting mother." The new mother may feel resentful if her husband's first words when returning home from work are "How is the baby?" She may feel that she is "tied down."

Is this immaturity? Possibly overcoming these feelings is a natural step toward maturity.

They are a family now. The baby is more important than themselves. He is an incentive to work, to plan, and to sacrifice. The young couple will find that raising a child can mean continued emotional and spiritual growth. As they give unselfishly, they gain a sense of fulfillment and achievement.

Role of the Father

This sense of fulfillment may be greater if the young couple are aware of each other's needs. The husband should expect his wife to be weak and to need help with the housework. If the mother comes home from the hospital three days after the baby is born, she still needs rest. The new mother should not concentrate so eagerly on acquiring good techniques for handling the baby that she completely neglects her husband.

The ideal situation is for both parents to share in the work and the pleasure of caring for the baby. The baby's sense of security and love comes from being held, fed, bathed, and diapered. His relationship with the world around him begins at birth, and his father should be part of his world. True, the father may seem awkward when first giving the baby a bottle, but perhaps the mother was awkward too. He may be assisting by washing the baby's clothes, but holding his child is more fun. Regardless of how this is accomplished, for the father to feel truly involved with the care of the baby will benefit all concerned.

Not the First Baby

If this is not the first baby for your maternity patient, she will be wondering how the children at home will accept the tiny infant. The baby will change their lives, too. A conscientious mother and father will try to help the little children to accept and love the new arrival and will try to prevent hostile feelings from developing.

The two-year old may find it more difficult to share his mother's attention, time, and affection than does the three-year-old. The two-year-old has decided that he really prefers mother to other people, and a new baby in the family can seem to be stealing his mother's love away from him.

Jealousy shows itself when the child reverts to babyish habits, such as insisting that he have milk from a bottle after he has learned to drink from a cup; wetting when he has learned toilet control; or stuttering when he has been talking well. He may be irritable and completely unmanageable. Sometimes he wants to hurt the baby physically.

Occasionally a child shows no outward signs of jealousy, but wise parents will realize that he has to learn to accept the baby, and they will try to help him do so.

He should have been told earlier (possibly two months in advance) that a new baby was coming. Any change in sleeping arrangements should be made enough in advance for him to welcome a change, not to feel that he was forced to give up *his* bed.

Mothers in the maternity ward often exchange ideas that have proved successful. One mother planned to take a present to the child at home. She also cautioned well-meaning relatives and friends to divide their attention, and even gifts, when they come to see the new baby. Another mother planned for someone else to hold the new baby when she first greeted her two-year-old.

The older children may not realize what a tiny baby is like and should be allowed to look at, touch, or hold him under supervision.

The goal is for the older children to feel that the new baby belongs to them, too, and that they are still important to their mother and father. The older children may bring the diapers to mother or, better yet, pat the baby dry gently with the towel. The father may help sometimes in the care of the baby in order that the mother can spend time with the older children.

A three-year-old might be comforted to hear his father say, "We have to look out for the little baby, *you* and I."

Greatest harm comes when the parents, happy with the new baby, expect that the other children will be happy automatically, and neglect to show consideration for their feelings.

Questions for Discussion

1. Where, in your community, are formal classes given for expectant mothers? Are fathers encouraged to attend?
2. What are the advantages and disadvantages of the hospital "rooming-in" plan for mothers and babies?

Parenthood: Arrival of the Baby

3. How is instruction to new mothers handled in the hospital where you will train as a student?

Additional Readings

Bleier, Inge J. *Maternity Nursing, A Textbook for Practical Nurses.* 2nd ed. Philadelphia: W. B. Saunders Company, 1965.
Duvall, Evelyn Millis. *Family Development.* 4th ed. Chap. 7, "Beginning Families: Expectant Phase." Philadelphia: J. B. Lippincott Company, 1967.
Infant Care. Washington, D.C.: U.S. Department of Health, Education, and Welfare, Children's Bureau Publication No. 8. Rev. 1963.
Landis, Judson T., and Mary G. Landis. *Personal Adjustment: Marriage and Family Living.* 4th ed. Chap. 22, "Approaching Parenthood." Englewood Cliffs, N.J.: Prentice-Hall, Inc., 1966.
Prenatal Care. Washington, D.C.: U.S. Department of Health, Education, and Welfare, Children's Bureau Publication No. 4, rev. 1962.
When Your Baby Is On the Way. Washington D.C.: U.S. Department of Health, Education, and Welfare, Children's Bureau Publication No. 391, 1963.

Recommended Audiovisual Aids

FILMSTRIP

David's Bad Day (36 frames, Stanley-Bowmar Company, B&W)
    A filmstrip that illustrates how the behavior of a child in school is dependent upon his relationships at home. Suggestions are given on how to help a child adjust to a younger child in the home.

FILM

Family Circus (10 min., International Film Bureau, Color)
    A father learns that he cannot give all his attention to the baby without neglecting the older child. A short but excellent film cartoon illustrating sibling jealousy.

PART II / *Normal Development*

CHAPTER 5 / NORMAL CHILD DEVELOPMENT

The nurse is frequently viewed as a "specialist" in child care. To meet these expectations, the practical nurse needs to understand how the infant grows and develops into an adult and how environment influences this development.

An understanding of normal development and normal behavior for the well child is necessary for wise handling of the sick child. Unless the nurse knows what is typical behavior and development at a certain age, she cannot recognize arrested development, abnormal behavior, symptoms of illness, or evidences of recovery.

Many phases of child care are highly controversial, but there is general agreement and knowledge about the growth processes and the developmental sequences during child development.

Your clinical experience in pediatrics will be more meaningful and less difficult if you understand development of the well child.

Maturation and Learning

Development results from maturation and learning.

Maturation is the unfolding of human potentialities, "the neuro-physiological-biochemical changes from conception to death.... Maturity is the physical readiness to learn."[1]

Learning is change resulting from practice, observation, or training.

Some skills the baby learns for himself, and for acquisition of other skills, teaching is necessary. We do not teach the baby to walk, although it helps to permit him freedom of movement, to give him opportunity to practice, and to encourage him. The baby walks when he has had sufficient practice, when he is ready to walk, and when the need exists.

In certain specific skills, teaching is necessary. Just growing up does not mean a child will be able to swim. Practice, training, and motivation are necessary. But if training and practice are to be effective, the child must be sufficiently mature to learn. Too early attempts to teach him to swim may cause him to have fears of the water and later to have difficulty learning to swim when he is sufficiently mature. Almost equally serious is ignoring the child when he is ready to learn. If the bottle-fed baby of six months shows little interest in his bottle, offer him milk in a cup. Later, he may refuse to give up his bottle.

---

[1] Boyd McCandless, *Children: Behavior and Development*, 2nd ed. New York: Holt, Rinehart and Winston, 1967, pp. 118–119.

Many people falsely believe that the earlier a child learns a skill, the better. There is an ideal time to learn everything. The nurse who remembers this principle can reassure anxious parents and will not be likely to expect too much from her young patient.

What is Development?

We glibly say, "The child is developing." A nurse should know that this means more than just growing bigger.

Development may be defined as growth and change, both of structure and of function. Structure refers to the size of the person. Function refers to the ability to act, to move, to think, or to pick up something.

Hence development means increase in the size of a muscle (structure) and increase in strength of hand grip (function).

Not only does the infant get larger, but his body proportions change also. At birth, the baby's head makes up about one-fourth of his body length. At the age of six years, the head is about 90 per cent of the adult size and equals about one-sixth of the child's length. As an adult, the head is approximately one-eighth of the body's length (see Fig. 4).

Sometimes when studying the development of children, we distinguish physical growth, motor development, and social learnings. Physical growth has

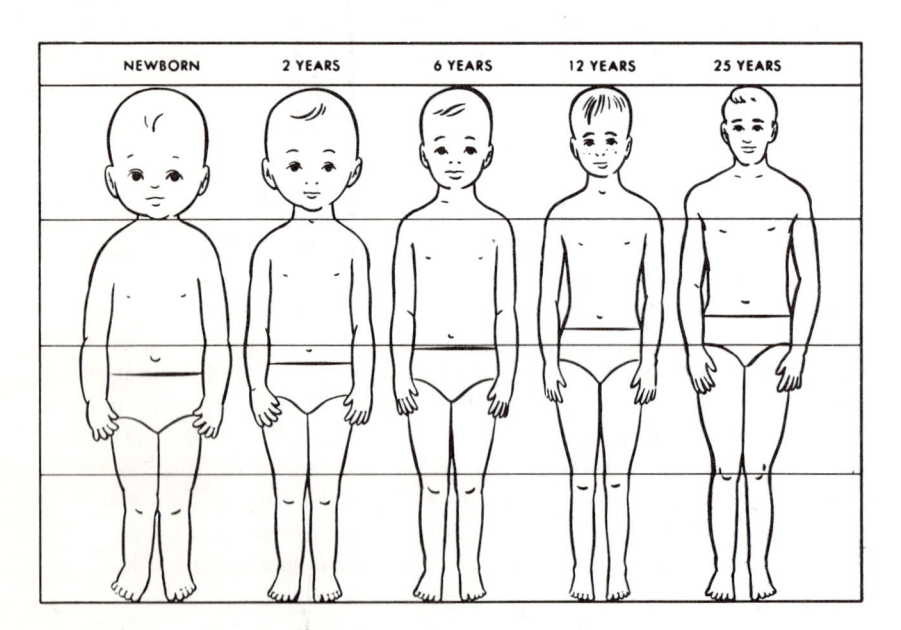

Figure 4. *The body changes form and proportions.*

Normal Child Development

to do with the size, height, and weight of the child. Motor development is the functioning of the child, such as moving about and walking. Social learnings have to do with skills such as getting along with people, controlling the temper, and talking. All of these kinds of development will be considered.

Development is Orderly

Within limits, development is organized and follows a general pattern or sequence. A child will usually sit before he stands, walk before he talks, and gain control of bowel movements before he has the ability to regulate bladder function.

Table 1 shows the average age for certain developments and the variations possible within the normal range. The newborn infant's eyes do not focus

TABLE 1./AVERAGE AGE FOR DEVELOPMENT OF PHYSICAL AND PHYSIOLOGICAL ACTIVITIES*

Developmental Stage	Average Age	Normal Range
Focuses on light	2 weeks	1 to 4 weeks
Lies on stomach, lifts chin	3 weeks	1 to 10 weeks
Birth weight doubled	6 months	5 to 7 months
Rolls from back to stomach	7 months	5½ to 11 months
First tooth erupts	7½ months	4 months to 1 year
Sits alone	7 months (plus)	6 to 11 months
Stands with support	10 months	7½ to 14 months
Creeps (or crawls)	10½ months	7½ to 14 months
Pulls to stand	11 months	7½ to 14 months
Stands alone	13½ months	9 months to 18 months
Walks alone	14 months	10 months to 20 months
Bowel control attained	18 months	12 months to 2½ years
Toilet training (verbalizes needs consistently)	27 to 30 months	18 months to 3½ years
First permanent tooth	6 years	5 to 8 years
First menstruation	12 years, 9 months	10 to 17 years
Menopause in women	48 years (white women)	40 to 50 years (white women)
		35 to 45 years (Negro women)
Climacteric in men		55 to 65 years

*Based on studies by Mary Shirley, Nancy Bailey, and Howard Meredith.

together, and he appears "cross-eyed." Within two weeks, most babies focus their eyes on a light. Some may do this at the age of one week, others at three weeks. We have reason for concern if the baby does not focus his eyes at the age of five weeks. The child who does not talk at the age of three is outside the normal range.

As the child gets older, the normal range of variation increases. The average age of first menstruation is 12 years 9 months, but the normal range is from 10 to 17 years.

An important trend of development you need to know is that *girls mature earlier than boys* but are usually smaller. The girl's skeleton and nervous systems develop somewhat earlier. At birth, the girl is about one month ahead of the boy. At the age of six, the girl's bony structure is about one year advanced over that of the boy of that age. We can expect little girls to learn earlier than little boys such things as walking, talking, toilet control, and self-dressing. Usually, little girls get along better than little boys during their first year of school. Earlier maturing of girls continues through adolescence.

The physical growth records (Chapter 15, Figs. 18 and 19) may be used to compare a child's progress in weight and height with that of other children of his own age and to gain valuable clues to his health. Because development is orderly and continuous, we have a basis for understanding a particular child's growth.

One Kind of Development Influences Another

We may observe a variety of changes that appear to be unrelated, but this is unlikely. One kind of development influences another. "The whole child reacts to his total environment."[2] In other words, the observer may not see the relationship, but it does exist. The little child has to learn many social skills before he plays well with other children his age. He has to learn to share and to take his turn. This may seem unrelated to learning social graces, but it is part of it.

A child may concentrate on one type of learning and remain at a plateau stage with another. The child learning to walk may not progress as rapidly with learning to talk. A large child of 15 months may not be walking while a tiny child the same age is walking. Motor developments of the large child can be retarded by rapid physical growth.

Each Stage of Development Has Characteristic Traits

The growing child normally exhibits traits characteristic of each stage.
Learning to eat has many phases. The baby messing with his food is learning

[2] Robert Watson, *Psychology of the Child*, 2nd ed. New York: Wiley, 1965, p. 78.

Normal Child Development

the texture and the feel of food. He eats large amounts during his first two years, then eats less as he grows more slowly. He actually needs less food, and the mother or the nurse who insists that he eat may actually create a genuine feeding problem. Later, the preadolescent eats everything in sight in the absolute minimum of time. So many things are so very important to him. He cannot waste time at the dinner table. He does not want to wash because he will only get dirty again. Often what parents call "problem behavior" is simply characteristic behavior for the child's age.

Understanding the stages of play will help the nurse who walks into a pediatric ward of strange children. The baby enjoys solitary play with the things around him. Mere motion is play to the toddler. Then he enjoys playing beside another child; this is called "parallel play." Finally, he enters into cooperative play with other children. Each stage of development has characteristic traits; each of these leads to the next performance.

The following chapters will describe more fully the characteristics of each stage of development. If the nurse knows these characteristics, she can distinguish abnormal behavior from what is normal for the child's age. She will not be guilty of expecting too much or too little from a child.

For example, the typical four-year-old has a big imagination. The nurse need not be unduly disturbed if four-year-old Ginny tells a big tale. But she might have reason to be concerned if Ginny is not toilet trained.

Heredity Influences Development

At birth, heredity has decided things about the child, such as the color of his hair, eyes, skin, and his facial characteristics.

Body-build — lean and lanky, short and stocky — is primarily determined by heredity. Today's normal, healthy youngsters will probably grow taller than their parents, but adult height is mostly determined by inherited characteristics. The boy with a father 5 feet 11 inches tall and a mother 5 feet 6 inches tall may grow to be 6 feet or 6 feet 1 inch. The boy whose father is 5 feet 6 inches may reach an adult height of 5 feet 7 inches, but seldom 6 feet. Usually, taller children come from families of taller adults; shorter children have shorter parents and grandparents.

The mental capacity of a child is determined at birth, although environment influences how much of the mental ability is used. We now know that the IQ is not stable throughout a lifetime; that it is affected by education, nutrition, experiences, and other factors.

Intelligence is one of the more important factors correlated to the rate of development. High-grade intelligence is associated with early development; low-grade intelligence with slow development. Positive traits are positively correlated.

The bright child is generally above average in health, size, sociability, and special abilities. His motor and physical development is probably slightly superior to that of the dull child. In fact, IQ tests given to infants are based on motor development.

There is little basis for these popular beliefs: "beautiful but dumb," "all brawn and no brain," "bright people are puny or scrawny." The lower the intelligence, the greater the expectation for retarded physical and motor development. The seriously defective child, the one who cannot go to regular school with other children, will probably be physically handicapped. He may be small in stature and unable to compete in sports.

Similarly, high-grade intelligence has been found to correlate highly with early sexual maturing and low-grade intelligence with late sexual maturing, though there are climatic, racial, and other factors involved.[3]

Although the dull child *is* slow to learn to walk and talk, the term "retarded" must be used with great caution. Sometimes a child with average intelligence is slow learning to walk or talk because other problems are interfering. A nurse may notice some indications of mental retardation, but the physician and the psychologist should diagnose it. If parents overhear the nurse say, "Little Timmy is retarded in walking," they may immediately think: "*That nurse said our Timmy is mentally defective.*"

Interaction of Heredity and Environment

Most developmental factors are influenced by both heredity and environment. Glandular functions play an important role in a child's growth and may be an interaction of heredity and environment. For instance, an overactive thyroid may be inherited, but control may be possible through drugs and nutrition.

The potential for some mental illness may be inherited, but the individual's life may prevent its appearance, or it may precipitate the illness. The causes of one of the most serious mental illnesses, schizophrenia, have been studied frequently. Homes that produced schizophrenic sons or daughters were found to lack warmth, affection, and happiness when compared with homes producing more normal persons.[4] The family of the schizophrenic had failed to offer the boy a satisfactory father-model, or the girl a satisfactory mother-model. This is one example, greatly simplified, of how mental illness can be caused by both heredity and environment.

---

[3] Elizabeth Hurlock, *Child Development*, 4th ed. (New York: McGraw-Hill, 1964).

[4] Boyd McCandless, *Children: Behavior and Development*, 2nd ed. (New York: Holt, Rinehart and Winston, 1967), pp. 474–475.

Normal Child Development

Environmental Influences on Development

Because environment can be either good or bad, we are greatly interested in its influence on the child. A healthy, good environment offers the child greater opportunity to reach his full growth potential and to use his inherited abilities than does a poor environment.

Not only are children growing slightly taller today, but they are also growing up faster and maturing earlier. More thorough knowledge of prenatal care and childbirth, higher standards of baby care, better diets, better medical care — all of these help babies to get a better start in life. Certainly good nutrition helps a child to reach his optimum heredity potential.

Health affects mental, physical, and personality growth. In the pediatric ward, you may notice many evidences of slow development. You will learn both the chronological age and the developmental age of the child. "Johnny is seven years old (chronological age), but he is more like a five-year-old (developmental age)." If chronic or severe illnesses occur during the first three years of life, growth of the long bones may even be stunted.

Later in our study, we will consider in greater detail how to help the child's growth and development by such factors as outdoor play, fresh air and sunlight, sufficient sleep and rest, good eating habits, personal cleanliness, and the like. These seem to be things that we can do something about, but other parts of his environment play an important role in shaping the child's life.

The position in the family — oldest, middle, or youngest child — influences personality development. The oldest and the youngest children usually receive the most attention, with the middle children left to "fend for themselves." Sometimes the youngest child is overprotected and "kept a baby." The oldest child may develop leadership traits, or he may shy away from leadership if too much responsibility is put on him too soon.

Sometimes a second or third child within a family develops more rapidly because he learns from imitating older brothers and sisters. The incentive to learn can be powerful and shows in many ways. The three-year-old will compete with his brother, almost five, and if he cannot get his way physically, he learns another way to win his point.

Generalities are dangerous because so many different factors are involved. Parents learn how to be parents with the first child, and they may feel better equipped to deal with second and third children. Family finances may improve, or they may get worse. In many ways, the presence or absence of brothers and sisters will influence the child.

Parental attitude is extremely important to a child's development. Parents can help a child to accept himself and to think well of himself. If parents reject a child, he may think it is because he is unattractive, weak, or sickly. He forms an image of himself that he dislikes, which in turn has a terrific impact on his personality and his reactions to other people. This is only one example of how parental attitude can influence the child. Other examples could be given.

Skeletal Growth

From conception to maturity, the bones of the body change in length, shape, size, density, hardness, and number. Some of the large bones are mostly cartilage at birth, and some of the small bones appear only after birth. If the baby's bones were hard and rigid, he could never pass down the mother's birth canal to be born. The soft bones gradually become more firm as the cartilage slowly changes to bone, or "ossifies." These softer, more pliable bones of the young child are less resistant to pressure and muscle pull and more liable to deformity than the rigid bones of the adult. For these reasons, we should stress properly fitting shoes, good beds, and good posture. The vertical column, or spine, becomes less flexible as maturity approaches.

The skeleton indicates the body's progress in maturing. Bone development can be evaluated by studying X rays of a child's hand. Since the hand has some 50 points of bone growth, it is a fairly accurate gauge. The term "skeletal age" or "biological age" refers to the level of skeletal development as compared with the normal standards established.

There is a marked relationship between the skeletal age and the age of puberty. A girl who menstruates early, say at 11, will also have reached a greater skeletal age than the majority of girls of her chronological age.

Body Shape and Proportions

The chest is rounded at birth, the neck is short, and the shoulders are high. The first 9 to 12 months, the baby keeps the same general physique, but he gets bigger, as indicated in Figure 4. He begins to lose his chubbiness and become more slender at the toddler stage, ages one to three years. The preschool boy and girl, ages three to five years, are "potbellied." During the years between three and ten, the chest flattens and broadens, and the ribs change from horizontal to an oblique position. The adolescent boy has a concave abdomen, which begins to fill out in the twenties and to expand further in the thirties.

The long bones of the arms and legs are extremely short at birth, remain comparatively short during childhood, and then increase before or during adolescence. At puberty, the legs are four times as long as they were at birth, and at maturity, five times as long. Adult legs make up half the total height of the body, whereas at birth the legs are one-third of the body's length.

Normal Child Development

The Teeth

The first set of teeth (baby or deciduous teeth) begins to form in the jaw about the fifth prenatal month. The lower teeth generally erupt before the upper teeth. The first tooth may appear any time from 3 to 16 months. The eruption of the temporary teeth may be accompanied by discomfort or actual pain, and the baby may lose his appetite and become nervous and irritable. At 20 to 30 months, the first set of 20 teeth is usually in place.

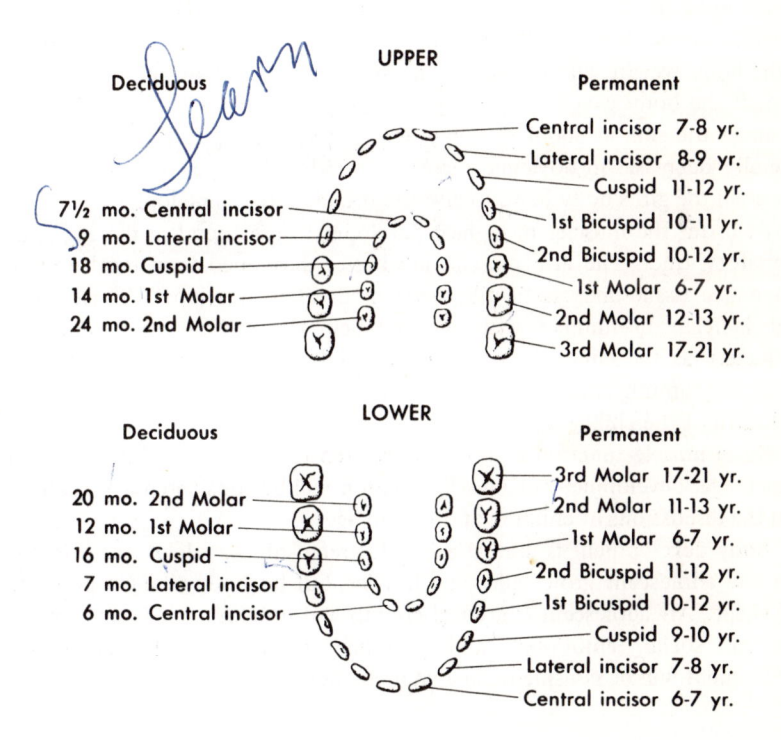

UPPER

Deciduous
- 7½ mo. Central incisor
- 9 mo. Lateral incisor
- 18 mo. Cuspid
- 14 mo. 1st Molar
- 24 mo. 2nd Molar

Permanent
- Central incisor 7-8 yr.
- Lateral incisor 8-9 yr.
- Cuspid 11-12 yr.
- 1st Bicuspid 10-11 yr.
- 2nd Bicuspid 10-12 yr.
- 1st Molar 6-7 yr.
- 2nd Molar 12-13 yr.
- 3rd Molar 17-21 yr.

LOWER

Deciduous
- 20 mo. 2nd Molar
- 12 mo. 1st Molar
- 16 mo. Cuspid
- 7 mo. Lateral incisor
- 6 mo. Central incisor

Permanent
- 3rd Molar 17-21 yr.
- 2nd Molar 11-13 yr.
- 1st Molar 6-7 yr.
- 2nd Bicuspid 11-12 yr.
- 1st Bicuspid 10-12 yr.
- Cuspid 9-10 yr.
- Lateral incisor 7-8 yr.
- Central incisor 6-7 yr.

Figure 5. *Schedule for eruption of teeth.*

There are 32 permanent teeth. They are larger, of better quality, and more durable than the temporary teeth. Generally, permanent teeth cut through the gums without causing discomfort. At every age, girls are usually ahead of boys in the appearance of temporary teeth, shedding of temporary teeth, and eruption of permanent teeth.

Muscle Development

The muscles grow and mature throughout the developmental period. The muscles represent 27 per cent of the body weight at birth. Their growth is proportionate to the whole body growth during the first four years. In the fifth year, the muscles begin to grow more rapidly and account for 75 per cent of the weight increase during that period. After the tremendous spurt of muscular growth during the fifth year, this growth is more gradual until adolescence, when muscular growth increases. Part of the weight gain during adolescence is due to muscle growth. Boys almost double their strength between the twelfth and sixteenth years. Cole[5] reports that at age 15, the muscles represent 32 per cent of the body weight, and at age 16, this has increased to 44 per cent, or almost one-half the body weight. Both boys and girls tend to put on large quantities of fat under the skin at about the time of puberty. After puberty, the fatty tissue generally decreases in boys and increases in girls. The layer of fatty tissue over almost all the girl's body helps to give the rounded, feminine look.

At birth, the muscles of highest development are found in the eye and the respiratory tract. The arm muscles are better developed than the leg muscles. Connective tissue and elastic fibers are moderately developed. These types of fiber increase in number with age and help the muscles to function more adequately as the child matures. Muscle condition is closely related to health, particularly among children. The degree of muscle tone is one measure indicating the health of the child.

Since muscle function is so closely related to the skills a child may acquire at each age, development of muscle function will be considered in greater detail with the discussions of children at different ages.

Body development is dramatically illustrated during adolescence. Not only does the adolescent grow taller and heavier, but his body changes proportions and shape. An adolescent's physical growth and development is so interrelated with his social, emotional, and personal growth that all phases of his development will be considered in a later chapter.

The Developmental Skill-Age Inventory

As a nurse, you need to understand sufficiently the growth and developmental patterns of children so that you can determine if an individual child is average or significantly above or below average in various aspects of his development. The Alpern-Boll "Developmental Skill-Age Inventory" (see the Appendix) will help you to evaluate a child's physical, self-help, social,

[5] Luella Cole, *The Psychology of Adolescence*, 6th ed. (New York, Holt, Rinehart and Winston, 1964), pp. 31, 32.

Normal Child Development

academic, and language skills. Using the inventory will also increase your practical knowledge of the general processes and specific milestones of children's early development. Later in our study, we will consider in detail the baby, the two-year-old, the three-year-old, and so on. The inventory may interest you now, and again during our study of the various ages.

The inventory and its scoring techniques (see page 315) consist of a series of behavioral items that you score simply through a short interview with the child's mother, teacher, or any person familiar with the child. The respondent tells you if the child does or does not perform a certain skill. After the interview, you total the child's score, and then assess his ability in the five developmental areas. Any area in which a child is more than 18 months behind his or her chronological age could be considered indicative of a significant degree of retardation.

The inventory can serve as a useful tool if you are a student nurse working with well children in a day-care center. You will learn more about children if you have specific questions to answer, and if you note carefully a child's ability to perform certain skills. It will help you to avoid expecting too much or too little from a child.

Also, when using the Alpern-Boll technique, you may obtain valuable information concerning the attitudes of your informant. You may notice that the child's mother is overprotective: "Oh, I never let my nine-year-old Johnny adjust the bathwater for fear he will hurt himself." This would indicate rejection: "I'm trying to train Susie not to want cuddling. After all, she's almost four years old." Or infantilization: "No, I've never let him cut his own meat. Are twelve-year-olds usually able to do that?"

The more you work with the inventory, the more confident you will feel in advising parents about their child's development. As a nurse, you try to help parents to know what they can and cannot expect from their children at various ages. You should also be able to advise them what they can do to encourage their child's development in any of the areas – physical, social, academic, self-help, or communication.

Questions for Discussion

1. Compare the development of a child you know quite well (son, brother, nephew or neighbor) with the chart shown.
2. You might find it interesting to compare your body build and physical characteristics with those of your parents and grandparents, or brothers and sisters.
3. Describe a family in which the children exhibit some similar personality traits or a family in which the children are extremely different from one another. Can you explain the similarities or differences? Are the reasons due to environment, heredity, or a combination of both?

4. Using the Alpern-Boll Inventory given in the Appendix, answer the questions about a child that you know well. It would be interesting to rate the same child several months later, during your pediatrics experience or at the finish of your practical nurse training.

Additional Readings

Breckenridge, Marian E., and E. Lee Vincent. *Child Development.* 5th ed. Philadelphia: W. B. Saunders Company, 1965.

Cole, Luella, and Irma Hall. *Psychology of Adolescence.* 6th ed. Part I, "Physical Development." New York: Holt, Rinehart and Winston, Inc., 1964.

Gesell, Arnold. *The Child from Five to Ten.* New York: Harper and Brothers, 1946.

Gesell, Arnold, and others. *The First Five Years of Life.* New York: Harper and Brothers, 1946

Hurlock, Elizabeth. *Child Development.* 4th ed. Chap. 2, "Principles of Development." New York: McGraw-Hill Book Company, Inc., 1946.

Ingalls, A. Joy. *Maternal and Child Health Nursing.* Chap. 19, "Physiological Growth"; Chap. 21, "Ages and Stages." St. Louis: The C. V. Mosby Company, 1967.

McCandless, Boyd R. *Children: Behavior and Development.* 2nd ed. Chap. 9, "Physical Growth and Motor Development." New York: Holt, Rinehart and Winston, Inc. 1967.

Smart, Mollie S. and Russel C. Smart. *Children: Development and Relationships.* 2nd ed. New York: The Macmillan Company, 1972.

Recommended Audiovisual Aids

FILMS

Embryology of Human Behavior (28 min., International Film Bureau, Color, 1951)
   Narrated by Dr. Arnold Gesell, the film explains indications that laws of growth are related to the physical and psychological make-up of the child, and that the child's action system is manifested in patterns of behavior before and after birth. It shows techniques of developmental diagnosis by clinical examinations that contrast children of comparable ages. It illustrates how the needs of children can be interpreted through growth.

Preface to a Life (30 min., U.S. Public Health Service, National Institutes of Health, B&W, 1950)
   An older film with a good message. It shows how a child can develop with different methods of child care: if his father expects too much of him; if his mother fosters overdependency; or if both parents together can give him a warm, gentle home where he can develop his own personality and character. Very good for pointing out the basic principles of child development.

Normal Child Development

Principles of Development (17 min., McGraw-Hill, B&W)
    This film outlines the fundamentals of growth and change from early infancy. After defining the principles of development, it considers the variables that make each child different, such as intelligence, sex, glandular activity, race, nutrition, health, heredity, and parental attitude.

FILMLOOPS

Super-Eight mm. Filmloops (silent) with manual
Growth and Development Series. 14 titles (Prentice-Hall, 1970)
    Titles: Neonate, Part I and Part II; One Month, Part I and Part II; Three Months; Six Months, Part I and Part II; Nine Months, Part I and Part II; One year. Description of other four titles follows:

Growth and Development: Fifteen Months, Part I and Part II
    This filmloop depicts a typical fifteen-month-old toddler's physical growth, interaction with her mother, play abilities, toys, eating abilities, step climbing and descending, and reaction to strangers.

Growth and Development: Eighteen Months, Part I and Part II
    This filmloop depicts an eighteen-month-old boy's physical growth, abilities and interests in toys, right-handedness preference, recognition of animal pictures, climbing, drinking from a glass, and reaction to his security blanket.
Accompanying manual:
    Lange, Crystal, M., and Caroline M. Mertz, *Nursing Skills and Techniques, Instructor's Guide.* Prentice-Hall, Inc., Englewood Cliffs, New Jersey, 1970.

TRANSPARENCIES

Omagine Smith, Home Economics No. 11, Growth and Developmental Patterns. Set of 23 transparencies, 3M Visual Products, 1967
    Titles: Relative body proportions of infant and adult; Average annual growth in early childhood; Motor development – two, three, four, and five years; Intellectual development – two, three, four, and five years; Social development – two, three, four, and five years; Fear; Anxiety; Guilt and anger; Anger and frustration; Disappointment; Envy; Delight and enjoyment; Anticipation; and Affection.

PART III / *The Baby, Toddler, and Preschool Child*

CHAPTER 6 / THE WELL BABY

From babyhood to adulthood the individual follows his own growth pattern, as influenced by heredity and environment. No two children are alike. Yet if the baby is to receive the best of care, his parents and the nurse should understand what a newborn baby is like and what each new development means to the baby.

The Newborn Baby

Parents are often disappointed because the newborn baby is usually not very pretty. His skin is soft, wrinkled, mottled, and red. He has almost no neck. The nose is often misshaped and flattened, but it will soon regain a more normal shape. Sometimes his head and ears are covered with long black hair. A fine downy growth may cover his body, a remaining trace of fetal life. His wobbly head may be lopsided, becoming more symmetrical within 24 to 48 hours after birth. The head has a soft spot on the top (fontanel), where the skull bones are not solidly knit together. He has a very receding chin, which will develop later. His ears are well formed.

At birth, the circumference of the head is greater than the circumference of the chest. The baby's head is proportionately large. His chest is narrow and barrel-shaped. His long, spindly arms and short legs are curled close to the body. His fists are clenched and the fingers are short and stubby. His fingernails and toenails are well developed.

His eyes are grayish blue and do not focus. Sometimes he looks cross-eyed. Within a few days he reacts to light by blinking, frowning, or closing his eyes. He cries without shedding tears. He may have some edema around the eyes, which will subside.

Hearing is probably established within the first few days. When he is startled by a loud, sudden noise, his whole body reacts. Since his nervous system is immature in function, he cannot control his body movements. He twitches and jerks. His sense of touch is the most highly developed sense. He reacts to touch, change of position, temperature, taste (he prefers sweets, dislikes bitters), and to a lesser degree, odors. The baby's sense of pain is less acute than that of older children.

The average birth weight is 7 to 7½ pounds, and the average birth length from 19 to 21 inches. Boy babies average larger in weight and in all measurements than girl babies. The initial loss of weight during the first three or four days can be 6 to 9 per cent of the body weight. The baby usually regains his weight within eight to nine days.

The Baby as an Individual

The baby is a demanding little fellow who does not communicate his wishes very well. The first few days at home may be frustrating to the mother. Baby's movements and reactions are unpredictable. He may scream without apparent reason. He falls asleep at any time. It may not be easy to tell whether he is asleep or awake. Respirations are chiefly abdominal and rapid; the heart rate varies with phases of respiration and activity.

It takes the baby's system about one month to become stabilized. Gesell says: "In a sense, he is not fully born until he is about four weeks of age. It takes that long to attain a working physiological adjustment to his postnatal environment."[1]

The tiny, new baby has a tendency to be most active in the dark and least active in the light. Perhaps the noise and light stimuli lull the baby to sleep, and in the quiet dark, he kicks, stirs, or moves to furnish stimuli. Parents are often relieved when the baby outgrows this tendency, which may not be until he is six months old.

Also during the first three months of life, he is developing a sense of trust in others. As the baby is fed, comforted, and loved, his sense of trust grows. He needs unrestricted love and acceptance. "Mothering" is essential to his growth and development.

From three to four months on, the baby is learning many things. He is beginning to understand that he is separate and apart from mother. He is learning that he can wait. He is beginning to communicate with others. Sometimes at age six to seven months, he reacts differently to strangers, but he is learning that relationship with people can be pleasurable. The one-year-old loves attention.

The baby develops many motor skills during the first year of life. Parents have often needlessly worried because their children did not follow an exact timetable of development. Table 1 (Chapter 5) shows there is an average age for certain characteristics or skills to appear and a range within which a child may vary normally.

Sitting up is a serious physical undertaking for the tiny baby. When he is first propped up into a sitting position, he will tire easily and quickly, that is, within a few minutes. The baby's neck, abdominal, trunk, back, and leg muscles must become sufficiently strong to allow his body to function in the sitting position. When this landmark is reached, at some time around eight months, the child's whole world is changed. He can voluntarily see what is going on without depending on someone to hold him erect.

---

[1] Arnold Gesell and others, *The First Five Years of Life* (New York: Harper and Brothers, 1940), p. 18.

The Well Baby

[handwritten note at top: Motor Control - head sags / May lift head off shoulder / Lift head from bed - 1 mth.]

Standing alone is an incredibly complex and delicate mechanical achievement for the baby. His whole body functions differently. With constant practice, he finally pulls himself up by the side of his playpen or a chair — and then he screams for help because he cannot get down. Sometimes parents are irritated when they do not realize that this is part of the learning process. When he finally starts off alone, he walks for the pleasure of walking. The walk of the baby at 18 months is more like a waddle. He keeps his feet apart for balance, takes short steps, and comes down on the full sole surface. His abdomen protrudes. His arms extend bilaterally from his body. By the time he is two years old, he walks because he wants to get somewhere.

The age from 12 to 20 months brings many problems. He is neither an infant nor a child. He wants to be independent, but he is extremely dependent. He treats other children as objects because he has not yet established his own identity. He is learning many things, such as control of bowel and bladder habits. All learning takes time, and the baby needs someone to love and encourage him.

Learning to Be a Mother

Meeting today's high standards of baby care is not easy.

The new mother would like to know many of the procedures you are learning in practical nurse training. While you are a student practical nurse, you learn how to handle the new infant, how to bathe him, and how to hold him for breast feeding or bottle feeding. You will change diapers for many babies. You may spend several hours in the formula room learning how the baby's formula is prepared.

These are skills and techniques that the infant's mother uses every day. If this is her first baby, she may be awkward. Learning these skills at a time when she is physically weak is not easy. Yet she is pleased with her new baby and eager to show her love. She will learn.

The Feeding Schedule

The pediatrician helps the mother to decide between breast feeding and bottle feeding, or a suitable combination, such as breast feeding and one bottle each day. He prescribes the formula, if needed, and recommends feeding intervals that appear to be best for the particular baby and mother.

At the hospital, the baby was on a schedule based on his weight and condition. Many mothers find it helpful to continue this four-hour or three-hour feeding schedule. If the baby shows that he needs a different feeding schedule, the mother should seek the physician's advice.

Few people today follow yesterday's rigid schedules, which meant that the baby had to be fed at a certain time. If he cried with hunger at 5:45, the mother let him cry until the 6:00 o'clock feeding time.

Many doctors feel that, to a limited extent, the feeding intervals may be left up to the baby during the first few weeks of life. The feeding time will probably be irregularly spaced at first, but gradually the baby settles into a regular pattern of eating and sleeping. This is a version of "self-demand" feeding, which implies that when the baby is hungry he should be fed. The mother should not try to feed him if he is not hungry. Each baby is an individual, and individuals do not always fit identical patterns.

This "self-demand" in feeding seems to be satisfactory when carried out reasonably and adaptably. Today, babies seem to present fewer feeding problems than they did when on rigid schedules. Parents seem more relaxed about their children's eating.

A flexible plan helps the mother to feel that she does not have to rush to feed the baby at the exact appointed time. It helps the baby to learn that he can wait.

The Daily Schedule

When the baby and mother settle into a more or less regular pattern for feeding, a daily routine, adjusted to mother and baby, is established. The mother feels that she can get other tasks done, knowing at what time the baby will need her. The bath time can be in the morning or evening, depending on when the mother feels she can best allot the time. One young mother changed her baby's schedule because she noticed that the baby was always sleeping when the father was at home. She wanted the father to be able to enjoy the baby's waking hours.

At first, the baby will sleep most of the time. Gradually, he will be awake more hours of the day.

Sleeping

The number of hours that the healthy baby sleeps will be about as follows:

The first few weeks	Most of the time except when being fed and bathed
From 2 to 3 months	18 to 20 hours daily
From 4 to 5 months	16 to 18 hours daily
From 6 to 12 months	12 hours at night; morning and afternoon nap
At 2 years	12 hours at night; one long daytime nap

Some babies require more sleep than others. Some will sleep lightly, and some will sleep through many noises. The baby should learn to sleep through

The Well Baby

ordinary household noises, but he should be protected from sudden, loud noises, from drafts and from strong light shining in his eyes. Many new babies sleep much better when swaddled, or wrapped snugly in a light-weight blanket. Hospitals do this for newborn babies, and he may like it at home too. He should be warm and dry.

The crib should be moved out of the parents' room before the baby is six months old. Later, he may resent the change.

Sometime between seven and nine months, many babies have trouble sleeping. This may coincide with respiratory infections, or there may seem to be no physical reason. Perhaps the sleeping difficulties relate to other problems. The baby seems to be in a turmoil because he is more and more aware of the outside world, and he realizes that not every adult is mother. Usually, however, the waking and restlessness taper off by the end of the first year.

Parents can help in several ways. The child should have a fairly consistent sleeping routine. He should see the person who is going to be in the house with him before he goes to sleep. He should not fall asleep in one room and wake up in another room. He needs plenty of time to get ready for bed, and the tempo should slow down before bedtime. He should not be "rushed off" to bed.

The child needs help to accept going to sleep. We cannot leave it to "self-demand," as with eating. The trend today seems to be that eating problems are fewer and sleeping problems are increasing in many families.

Between the ages of 15 and 20 months, a second wave of sleeping problems may appear, but for a different reason. The 18-month-old child is fascinated by the world around him. He rebels at leaving the things he enjoys and the people he loves. He cannot understand that he *needs* sleep. This is why we have to help him to establish a sleep routine.

Baby Clothes

Because the tiny baby will soon outgrow the first garments, the number of garments for the newborn may be limited. The size of the baby's wardrobe depends on the season of the year, the climate, laundering facilities, and the amount of money that can be spent.

A basic minimum layette would include:

- 4 dozen diapers
- 5 or 6 cotton shirts
- 2 carrying or crib blankets
- 1 wool blanket
- 3 to 6 cotton knit nightgowns (or flannel)
- 3 bands (if these will not be supplied at the hospital)

Most mothers will want also:

1 or 2 simple dresses with slips, or rompers
Knitted bootees
1 or 2 wool sweaters
A silk or cotton bonnet

The winter baby should have heavier cotton shirts and suitable clothing for outdoor outings. The wardrobe will be added to as the baby needs more clothes and of a larger size.

Laundering Baby Clothes

The baby's clothes must be washed separately and rinsed thoroughly — these are the two key points to safe laundering of the tiny baby's garments.

A baby's skin is sensitive to many foreign substances that can easily be left in the baby clothes, especially the diapers. Too many people today still believe that diaper rash is a normal hazard of babyhood and is not serious. It is both unnecessary and perilous. In some children, diaper rashes lead to more complicated skin ailments that are difficult to eliminate.

The three most common causes of diaper rashes are (1) Ammonia is formed by the action of bacteria on the urine in the wet diaper. Ammonia is irritating to the skin. (2) Improper washing or rinsing of diapers leaves soap or detergent, which is irritating to the skin. (3) Certain bacteria survive washing and remain in the diaper; these can cause irritation and infection. Washing is not necessarily sterilization.

These causes of diaper rash could be prevented if baby's wet diaper were changed immediately. The wet diaper has ammonia forming on it. Urine increases the irritation from soap or detergent left in the diaper. The wet diaper provides a suitable environment for the growth of any bacteria present. But babies have no respect for the parents' sleep needs when it comes to wetting diapers. So the diapers must be thoroughly cleansed to avoid the conditions that cause diaper rash.

A hospital dermatologist recommends the following to prevent diaper rash:

1. Use mild soap or detergent in soft water, then rinse thoroughly. In an automatic washer, put the diapers through three extra rinses.
2. Soak diapers after each washing in a special antiseptic solution available at drugstores. This solution helps to delay the decomposition of the urine into ammonia.
3. Boil diapers to sterilize them. This kills the skin-irritating bacteria. This should be done after each washing and rinsing, but before soaking in antiseptic solution.[2]

[2] Dr. Louis B. Wexler, dermatologist at Beekman Downtown Hospital and Fordham Hospital, New York City.

The Well Baby

For mothers who find that these procedures take too much time and do not wish to bother with them, the sensible answer is professional diaper service. Professionally processed diapers provide all these health protections for the baby, and the service is convenient for the mother. Many families cannot afford professional diaper service. If the nurse understands the importance of proper diaper care, she can explain and recommend the procedures given here. Following even a part of these recommendations might lessen the likelihood of diaper rash.

Other garments for the baby should also be washed separately and rinsed thoroughly. The baby's garments should never be tossed in with the family washing. The kind of fabric and make of garment will determine its handling. Rinsing should be repeated until the last rinse water is clear.

Safety

During the first year of a baby's life, his safety rests entirely with the people caring for him. As he learns to walk, to express himself, and to remember, we can gradually teach him to safeguard his own person. Preventing accidents from occurring to babies and small children is one of the greatest problems in raising children. In a later chapter, we will consider how to help the preschooler learn to be safety conscious.

Safety for the baby means eternal vigilance from everyone. The baby's family should heed the same safety rules that are drilled into you during your student nurse days. You hear again and again: close all safety pins that you handle; keep one hand on the baby as you change, feed, or bathe him; never, never walk away from the crib with the baby in the crib and the crib side down. The baby can squirm off the bed before he can turn over. (One student nurse was dismissed from training after she let a tiny baby fall out of bed.)

Sleeping bags keep the baby warm and are safe if carefully chosen. Loose blankets or pillows should not be left in the small baby's crib because he may pull them over his face. Clothing that has a drawstring around the neck should be avoided.

Keep all bags or sheets of plastic materials away from the baby. They are extremely dangerous if the baby pulls them over his face. An amazing number of items are carried into the home wrapped in plastic, and it is easy for the baby to get hold of the plastic. Balloons may seem to be a harmless and inexpensive diversion, but may cause a fatality in the hands of an infant. The nurse can help the family to realize that balloons are not for babies.

The habit must be formed of putting away items potentially dangerous to the toddler, such as needles, pins, knives, scissors, household supplies, medicines, and sugar-coated pills. Appliances and cords must be kept out of the range of the creeper or toddler. Unused electrical outlets must be covered. The use of cellophane tape or adhesive tape should be avoided. These the baby can pull off, and remember, at certain times everything goes into baby's mouth.

His toys must be carefully examined for sharp edges or corners and for easily removed parts such as small wheels, bells, pins, or buttons used as eyes on stuffed animals. Paint on articles that can go in the mouth should never contain lead.

The Play Space

Correctly used, the playpen can give the baby both freedom and protection. If he has a variety of toys and can see his mother frequently, the baby may be contented there for an hour or longer. In the summertime, an older baby may enjoy the corner of a porch fenced off as a playpen.

When the child outgrows the playpen, he needs a special area in which to play, such as a room with a gate at the door. If all breakable and potentially dangerous objects are placed out of reach, the child can play with anything and everything as he wishes. This has many advantages. It helps to reduce accidents. It gives the mother a chance to work in peace. It helps to avoid mother-child conflict. Of course, the child should be permitted to go into the rest of the house, or out of doors, with supervision.

Play and Playthings

The tiny baby is stimulated enough when he is fed, changed, and bathed. It is "play" when he is held, talked to, patted, and carried about. His first toys will provide sensory stimulation of color, sound, and texture. The baby's favorite colors are yellow and red. (He likes blue when he is a little older.)

The baby's first playthings may be "*look toys*," a balloon or mobile attached to his crib (see Fig. 6). If it is placed where he can see it, the baby "plays" with his eyes. He will enjoy hitting at the gym set that fastens across the crib before he can reach or grasp a rattle.

Hand toys of different shapes, sizes, textures, and sound effects will teach as well as amuse the baby. As soon as he can hold a plaything, he will put it in his mouth.

Mouth toys should be too large to swallow and safe to suck, bite, lick, and chew. Actually, the baby "eats everything"; so all toys should be watched for sharp points or edges, parts that can come loose, and harmful paint. The child should be able to grasp the toy at any angle.

Cuddle toys of soft texture will satisfy the urge to feel and squeeze. Later he will hug and cuddle them, giving them names.

Educational toys will interest the baby when he sits up, as will blocks. He

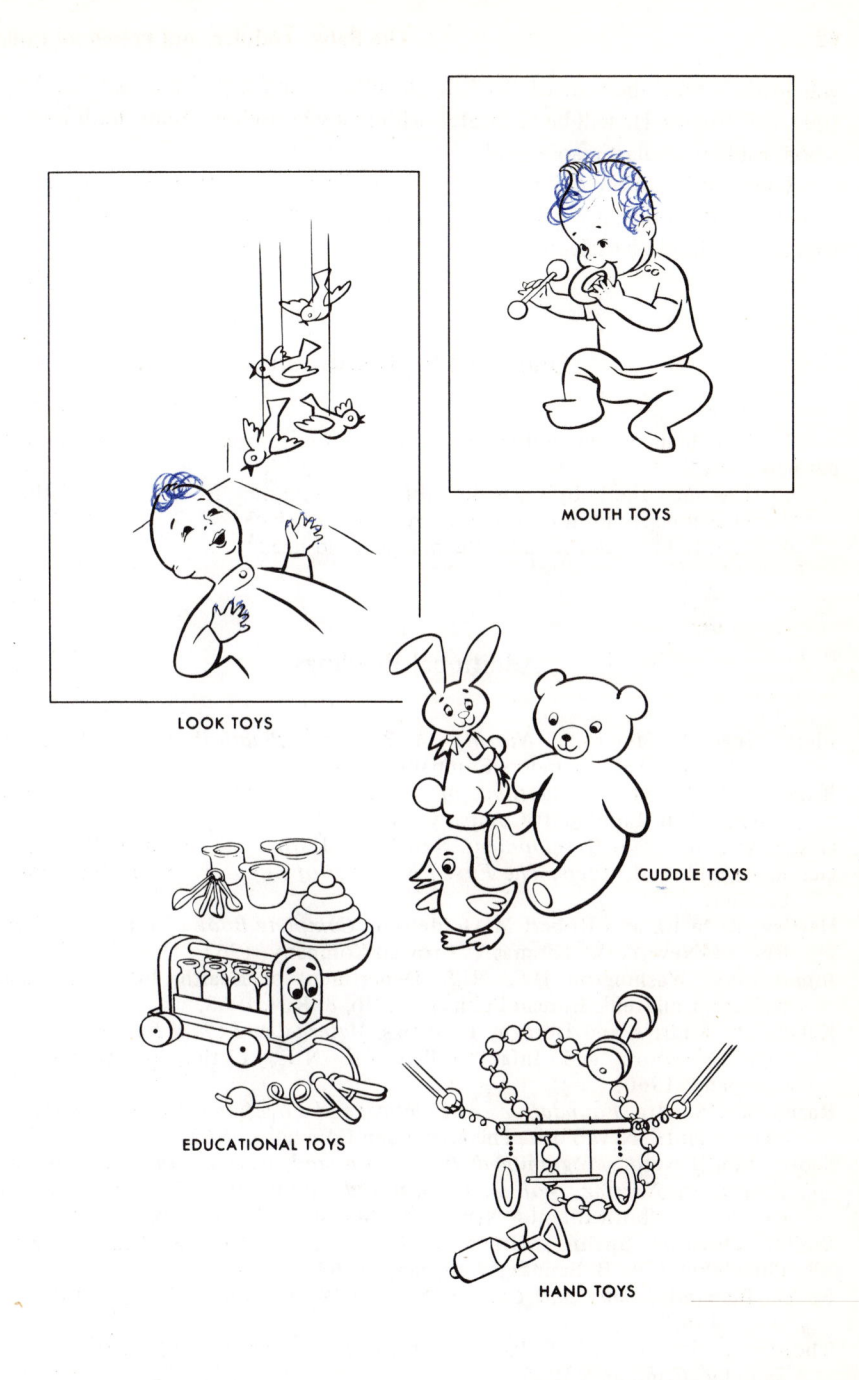

Figure 6. *Baby needs a variety of toys.*

will love to take them apart, fit them together, bang them, and match colors, sizes, and shapes. He will be fascinated with many household items. Bath toys of wood, rubber, or plastic are popular.

When the baby creeps and walks, he is ready for push-and-pull toys and activity toys. Too many toys at one time will confuse the baby. A variety of simple toys should be selected.

Questions for Discussion

1. What helps a new mother to decide whether to breast-feed or bottle-feed her new baby?
2. How may the baby's schedule differ in one home from that in another?
3. What household items are safe toys for the baby?
4. What kind of clothes does the one-year-old need?

Additional Readings

Bleier, Inge J. *Maternity Nursing, A Text for Practical Nurses.* Rev. ed. Philadelphia: J. B. Saunders Company, 1966.

Broadstreet, Violet. *Foundations of Pediatric Nursing,* pp. 117–154. Philadelphia: J. B. Lippincott Company, 1967.

Gesell, Arnold. *Infant Development.* New York: Harper and Brothers, 1952.

Gesell, Arnold, and others. *The First Five Years of Life.* New York: Harper and Brothers, 1940.

Hartley, Ruth E., and Robert M. Goldenson. *Complete Book of Children's Play.* Rev. ed. New York: Thomas Y. Crowell Company, 1963.

Infant Care. Washington D.C.: U.S. Department of Health, Education, and Welfare, Children's Bureau Publication No. 8. Rev. 1963.

Kalafatich, Audrey, and Dorothy R. Meeks. *Maternal and Child Health.* Chap. 7, "The Newborn and Infant." Paterson, N.J.: Littlefield, Adams and Company, 1960.

Rasmussen, Sandra. *Foundations of Practical and Vocational Nursing.* Chap. 43, "The Infant." New York: The Macmillan Company, 1967.

Scott, Lou Peveto. *Programmed Instruction and Review for Practical and Vocational Nursing. Vol. 2: Clinical and Community Nursing.* Chap. 10, Unit 5, "Newborn Infant." New York: The Macmillan Company, 1968.

Smith, Christine Spahn. *Maternal-Child Nursing.* Chap. 6, "The Infant." Philadelphia: W. B. Saunders Company, 1963.

Spock, Benjamin. *Baby and Child Care.* New York: Duell, Sloan, and Pearce, Inc., 1946.

Thompson, Eleanor D. *Pediatrics for Practical Nurses.* Philadelphia: W. B. Saunders Company, 1965.

Your Baby's First Year. Washington, D.C.: Children's Bureau Publication No. 400, 1962.

The Well Baby

Recommended Audiovisual Aids

FILMSTRIPS

Bathing the Baby (36 frames, McGraw-Hill, B&W)
    The filmstrip shows the purpose of the bath, assembling equipment and supplies, preparing the water, safety measures, and proper cleaning of the body.

Feeding the Baby (42 frames, McGraw-Hill, B&W)
    It stresses that the very young infant needs emotional security, and this is attained during feeding when the baby is held by a relaxed person. It gives helpful information on weaning the baby, introducing additional foods and what foods to include at the end of the first year. Illustrations are shown of mealtime behavior at various stages of development.

Keeping Children Safe (35 frames, McGraw-Hill, B&W, 1951)
    Practical illustrations are given of safety measures in the daily care of children, especially the baby. It shows such important safety measures as keeping hand on baby and safety in pinning diapers. Many good illustrations.

Preparing the Formula (46 frames, McGraw-Hill, B&W)
    This filmstrip emphasizes proper sterilization and use of ingredients prescribed by the physician. It shows proper preparation of the formula, including sterilization of bottles and formula separately.

Selecting Children's Clothing (36 frames, McGraw-Hill, B&W)
    Points to consider when selecting proper clothing for the baby and young child are well developed. It discusses selecting clothing for the season of the year, size of layette needed, safety features, and the type and number of garments needed.

TRANSPARENCIES (for overhead projector)

Campbell, Lucille, Home Economics No. 12, *Safety for Children*, Set of 23 transparencies (3M Visual Products, 1967)
    Good illustrations showing danger spots for children, such as climbing on high stool, in bathtub and crib, sunburn, pot handles, outdoor grills, locked in car, baby playing with marbles, people sneezing around baby, leaving poisons within baby's reach, touching electric outlets, climbing down stairs, and immunization.

CHAPTER 7 / THE TWO-YEAR-OLD

The age of two can be a difficult time to be in the hospital — to be away from the mother and father and the set routine that the two-year-old demands. Also, at about two most children prefer their mother and may be shy of strangers. You, the white-frocked nurse, can be a source of terror!

Of course, the two-year-old has made gains in motor and physical development. He is a runabout. He walks, runs, climbs, jumps, balances, and falls. Often he is not sure-footed, and he still does not walk erect. He may lean forward as he runs. He can go up and down stairs now with alternating feet. He can throw a ball, but not direct it. He can turn a doorknob, flush a toilet, and push aside chairs that are in his way.

The two-year-old's lack of really good coordination often leads to trouble. He is curious and gets into everything. He drops things when he does not mean to. He is destructive, and he treats fragile things roughly because he has not learned fine muscular control.

The two-year-old may feed himself clumsily and spill a lot. We expect his appetite to decrease because he is not growing as rapidly as he once did. He does not gain much in weight or height. The average child gains 4 pounds in the third year. He usually has 16 teeth.[1] He may try to use a toothbrush, and this may be a good time for his first dental examination.

He sleeps from 12 to 14 hours each night and still naps in the afternoon. Wise parents make certain that too much excitement and stimulation do not overfatigue the little child and interfere with sound sleep.

He likes to help undress himself and may begin dressing himself. Again, girls are likely to be able to dress themselves at an earlier age than boys. At this age, playing in water is fun.

Toilet Control

Sometimes your two-year-old patient will be toilet trained, sometimes not. Many two-year-olds have fairly good bladder control with frequent lapses occurring. Sometimes bowel control is established at 18 months; sometimes it is only partly attained by two.

At what age can we expect the child to have control of his elimination? On this controversial subject, the public expects the nurse to be well informed and to have an anwer. So think carefully.

Parents usually understand that one child may normally walk at 10 months

[1] The normal range is from 8 to 20 teeth for two-year-olds.

and another at 13 months, that the first tooth may appear at any time from 2 to 12 months. Then why can we not expect that one child may be ready to learn bladder control at 18 months, whereas another child is not yet ready at two years?

Variable factors include the child's physical maturity, his mental development, his health, the attitude of his family, and what is happening around him. The sudden appearance of a new baby brother or sister may turn the youngster's world upside down, and he may not be ready for a new learning.

Of course, wet diapers mean extra work and embarrassment. But embarrassment according to whose standards? This is the one phase of child care that is probably most often subjected to adult standards and to the inaccurate idea that the sooner a child learns something, the better for him.

> Too early training, too much training, or too strict and severe training may be one of the major causes of wetting that persists or that begins after the training period has ended. To shame, punish, threaten, bribe or reward a child for behavior on the toilet is to exert high pressure methods which may cause wetting at a future date.[2]

Fewer mistakes will be made if we consider elimination from the child's point of view, and if we watch for indications that he has sufficiently matured to attempt bladder control. These are indications: if he retains urine for several hours at a time; if he sleeps through the night without wetting; if he notices the difference between wet and dry and wants to be dry; if he is eager to imitate parents and older brothers and sisters; if he can communicate to you; when he gives some signals that he is ready to begin, such as grunting, making noises, wriggling, acting restless, clutching his genitals, or otherwise making his wishes known. The child may begin giving signals between 8 and 15 months for bowel movements and a few months later for urination.

Teaching the child adult words is better than teaching him baby words that he will need to discard later. Avoid words that have other meanings in ordinary conversation and that he might not use when grown because he associates them with the toilet meaning.

Even when children have control fairly well established, occasional lapses will occur. These are normal; hence the word "incident" might be more correct than "accident." However, letting the child think it was an accident is better than shaming him.

A matter-of-fact approach to helping the child learn control is better than an emotional approach. Indeed, our terminology is wrong. We say "training," which implies something one does to another person. This is something the child has to learn for himself. Maturity and environment determine the right time for each child.

---

[2] Nina Ridenour and Isabel Johnson, *Some Special Problems of Children* (New York: Association for Mental Health, 1947), p. 45.

Temper Tantrums

Sometimes we say "the troublesome twos" because often during this year the child has frequent temper tantrums and is in the stage of saying "no" to everything. The reasons are not hard to understand.

The child is learning to think, he can get about more, and he wants to make his own decisions and to explore his expanding world. Yet his muscular coordination has not advanced enough for us to trust him. Also, his ability to think may be superior to his ability to express himself. He may wish to say, "Nurse, I will be glad to eat my lunch after I play here just long enough to try out this little car." But he does not have the ability to say all these words, and he can say "no." So he says "no." Maybe, too, "no" is what he hears most frequently.

How do we handle the child in the "no" stage? First, remember that this is a normal stage. It will pass. In the meantime, try to avoid situations that give the child a chance to say "no." Say, "We are going to do it this way." Let him decide, "Do you want your milk in a glass or a cup?" not, "Do you want milk to drink?"

A continuing negative stage may be a warning that the child needs more independence and more freedom. Limit the controls over him to the most necessary ones. Restricting him excessively, perhaps to suit older members of the family, will result in more outbursts of temper. Let him make choices and give him as much freedom as is reasonable and practical.

Although the temper tantrum may be characteristic of this age, the child must eventually learn that this is not acceptable behavior. Temper outbursts that continue into the school-age years can become genuine behavior problems that require psychiatric help.

The two-year-old with a temper tantrum should be removed from the scene, and not allowed to get what he wants with a tantrum. He should be shown he will be more successful by not getting angry. Yet to deny him love at this time may be denying love when it is needed most.

Providing a new object of interest with an understanding adult close by may be better than complete isolation. When the child loses self-control, he lacks security. Punishment only increases his insecurity.

Preventing temper tantrums in the small child is better for all concerned than attempting to cure them. Hunger, fatigue, lack of play materials and playmates — all provide an opportunity for these outbursts to occur.

Sometimes his resistance to dressing and eating is his way of insisting that "I can do it myself." A firm but still friendly manner will help the child to learn to respect authority and cooperate with you, not become antagonistic. This takes time and patience. He is an individual now!

Retarial—eye blood vessels are broken from shaking up a child.

The Battered Child

The large number of infants and small children under the age of three who are physically abused has, in recent years, become recognized as a national problem. It is realistic to nurses who see the small children that are seriously beaten, burned, and injured.

The nurse wonders what kind of parent will injure his child, and many studies have been made seeking answers. Although more cases have been reported with parents of low income than high income, child beaters have been found in every income level: with IQ's ranging from 70 to 130; from ages 18 to 40 (most in their 20's); unemployed, semiskilled, or professional people; and church members and nonchurch members. It is not true that child abuse occurs only among "bad" people of low socioeconomic status.[3]

Two basic traits seem to characterize the abusive parent.[4] He (she) is unreasonable in his demands and expects performance beyond the ability of the child, such as in toilet training, control of crying, or behavior. Second, the abusive parent appears incapable of "mothering" the helpless child with love, tenderness, and awareness of need. Instead, he feels that the child primarily exists to satisfy his own needs. If the child cannot "mother" him, or does not behave as he thinks that the child should, he strikes out to punish and vents unrestrained anger on him. Later, the child beater may feel regret but seldom guilt. He thinks that the child deserved punishment because the youngster did not meet his own needs and/or did not behave properly.

The creator of the phrase "The battered child syndrome" states that child abuse may be an extreme form of a pattern of child-rearing that is quite prevalent in our culture today.[5] The amount of yelling, scolding, slapping, punching, hitting, and yanking acted out by parents on very small children is shocking.[6] Kempe is optimistic that increased understanding of why child abuse occurs may result in fewer children being "taught to the tune of the hickory stick" and being dealt instead with knowledge of what is reasonable to expect of children at certain ages.

All 50 states now have child abuse laws providing for mandatory reporting of suspected cases. Those reporting are granted "absolute immunity" from prosecution.

However, doctors and social workers directly involved with child abuse are convinced that a merely punitive attitude toward the individual will not prevent

---

[3] Ray E. Helfer and C. Henry Kempe, eds., *The Battered Child* (Chicago: University of Chicago Press, 1968), p. 108.
[4] Ibid., p. 109.
[5] C. Henry Kempe, "The Battered-Child Syndrome," *Journal of American Medical Association*, 181: 17–24, 1962.
[6] Ray E. Helfer and C. Henry Kempe, op. cit., p. 104.

recurrence of abuse. The emotionally disturbed adult who behaves this way needs treatment, treatment from the most experienced personnel available — nurse, social worker, lawyer, law enforcement officer, judge, or physician. The ultimate goal is to improve the home situation so that the child can be safely returned to his parents.

The practical nurse is not expected to be able to manage this complicated problem, but her role can be crucial. The pediatrician or family doctor and the social worker assume the key roles in working with the troubled parent. The physician's first responsibility is to protect the child, and usually begins with admitting him to the hospital. It is important that this be a straightforward admission, for an accusing attitude from staff members will antagonize the parent and make future communication almost impossible.

As the ward nurse, you may find it difficult to maintain an objective, impartial manner toward the parent. You may be less accusing if you realize that the majority of parents who injure their children actually want help.

The nurse should also realize that almost without exception, the abusive parents were themselves abused when small, deprived of mothering in the deep sense of being cared for, although not necessarily deprived of material things. Parental attention was demanding and critical, not loving.

Helfner and Kempe gathered scant but suggestive data of the parents of the abusing parent, that is, the grandparents of the battered child.[7] It appears that the grandparents were themselves subjected to abuse. Unwittingly and unfortunately, this type of child-rearing may have been transmitted from parent to child, through three successive generations. To interrupt this cycle may be a most important accomplishment.

With better understanding of the causative factors of child abuse come methods of prevention. Physicians, social workers, and public health nurses are learning early recognition of cases at a time when families are most receptive to help. Also, questionnaires designed to uncover families with potential for child abuse have been developed.

You need to become familiar with the responsibility of the practical nurse regarding the child abuse law in your state. Your supportive action can be a big contribution.

Learning to Talk

The age of two is often the year of great language development. When the child discovers the power of words, he begins to understand how he can control his world and how he can manage himself in ways that are acceptable to others.

Vocabularies at this age range from 5 words to 1000. The average is 250

---

[7] Ibid., p. 112.

The Two-Year-Old

words. The two-year-old likes to talk to himself and to name things. He uses more nouns than other parts of speech. He may speak in short sentences, and some children learn to recite nursery rhymes.

Encourage a child to talk by talking to him simply, in short sentences that he understands, and make certain that he *needs* to talk. Sometimes a child does not talk because he has no need to talk. He merely grunts, and either Mother or Big Brother knows what he wants. Hearing good English spoken gives him satisfactory models to copy. Some baby talk is merely the child's inability to pronounce words right. Do not laugh at his errors, yet do not encourage baby talk. Often little children will coin new words that can be fun for all the family. Word games, reading aloud to him, singing songs, and playing records — all will help him to understand what talking is. Television programs often replace conversation, but at least the youngster hears words.

If adults pay too much attention to a child's early attempts at speech, or demand perfection of him, he may refuse to talk. Stuttering may begin when he realizes that he does not pronounce the words right and his parents show disapproval. Also, stuttering can be an indication that something is wrong in the child's world, particularly if it appears when he has been talking fairly well. Again, overexcitement, extreme fatigue, emotional upsets — these can be factors in stuttering.

The nurse should try to learn what words the child uses for sleep, milk, toilet, and so forth. Accepting him as he is will help him greatly in a new, strange environment.

Learning to Share

The two-year-old is selfish, not aware of other children's feelings, and does not enjoy group play. He likes to play beside other children (this is called parallel play), but he does not understand cooperative play. He has a very limited sense of time and numbers. To him, "not now" means "never." The conception of taking turns and sharing has to be learned.

The child first learns what "mine" means. To do this, he must own things. We should let him decide himself to give up his toy. If we take it away, the toy is ours, not his. He then has to learn what "not mine" means. Next he finds that some things that are "not mine" are "his" or "hers." After he learns the meaning of time and can take turns, he will see that a possession can be "mine" and "yours" at the same time. Now he can really enjoy playing with other children.

Play Activities and Toys

Play is the child's whole world, so we must consider what it means to him. It is his work, recreation, hobby, way of learning, outlet for emotions, and much more. We say the two-year-old is exploring his world and learning to manage himself physically. His play reflects this.

He wants to investigate everything and to try out all he sees. He wants to sweep, to iron, to hammer, to throw a ball, to see how things fit together. He is likely to use leg muscles a great deal and arm muscles not enough. To encourage development of arm muscles, a pounding set, a small seesaw, a slide, a trapeze and swing set may help. In a sandbox, the child crawls and climbs about, and both arms and legs develop evenly. A sandbox will provide many hours of happy play, either alone or with companions. At first the child digs with a spoon and pours sand into a cup. Later he builds roads and villages, racetracks, or farms, depending on the places he knows about.

Most small children need few purchased toys if allowed to investigate the things around them. Ordinary household items furnish exciting experiences for the two-year-old. Pot lids clang together, he likes to drop clothes-pins in a bottle, tin cans are fun in the sandpile, and pouring water from one container to another is a challenge.

The two-year-old likes push-and-pull toys, a wagon, and a "bicycle" even

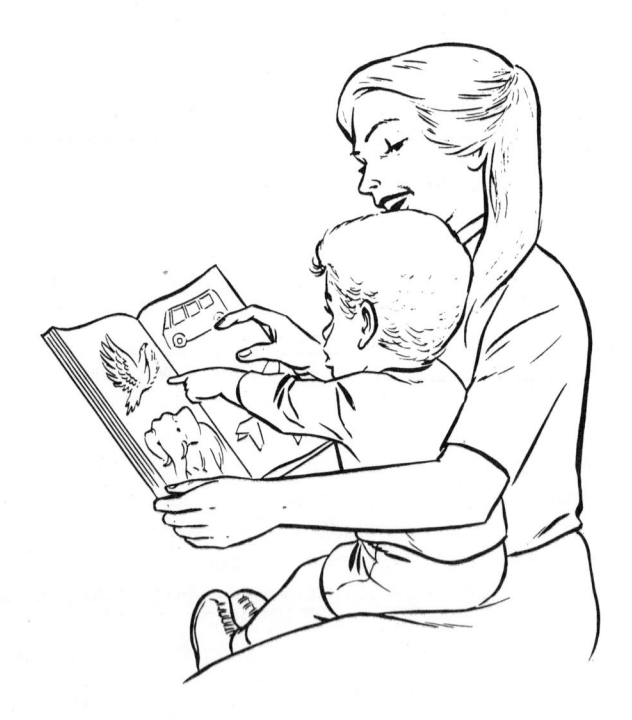

Figure 7. *Encourage the two-year-old to point to and name the objects when reading to him.*

though he cannot push the pedals of the tricycle until nearly three. He likes balls and large, square blocks, Dolls preferred are those representing a baby and the rag doll. The doll is not considered a person yet, and it may be dragged about by the hair. The child loves a toy telephone. Noise toys and simple musical toys are great favorites.

At this age, do not try to distinguish between boys' and girls' toys. When imitative and imaginative play begins, a tea set will thrill a little boy as much as a little girl. The two-year-old needs fewer props for his imaginative play than does the older child.

A satisfactory place to play, both in the house and outdoors, merits attention from the parents. Both the toys and his play space should be carefully checked for safety. Giving him a few well-chosen toys is better than overwhelming him with many toys.

Remember, the two-year-old needs simple toys that do not require fine muscle coordination.

He likes pictures and books of animals, children, and familiar objects.

The simplest of stories will appeal to him; for example, situation stories about children like himself, doing familiar activities.

Questions for Discussion

1. What techniques have you observed that appear successful with a child in the "no" stage?
2. In what ways can the mother or the nurse safely give the two-year-old more independence?
3. Who is likely to learn toilet control earlier — a boy or a girl? Why?
4. Describe a suitable play area for a two-year-old.
5. What are the child abuse laws in your state? What is the responsibility of the nurse?
6. If possible, consult a pediatrician or responsible person with the children's hospital in your area to learn if preventive measures are being taken regarding child abuse. Is help available for the troubled parents?

Additional Readings

Helfer, Ray E., and C. Henry Kempe, eds. *The Battered Child.* Chicago: The University of Chicago Press, 1968.

Langdon, Grace. *Toys for All Children.* New York: American Toy Institute, 1959.

Latham, Helen C., and Robert V. Heckel. *Pediatric Nursing.* Chap. 4, "Toddler and Preschool Child." St. Louis: The C. V. Mosby Company, 1967.

Smith, Christine Spahn. *Maternal-Child Nursing.* Chap. 7, "Preschool Child." Philadelphia: W. B. Saunders Company, 1963.

Spock, Benjamin. *Baby and Child Care.* Rev. ed. New York: Pocket Books, Inc., 1968.

Your Child from One to Six. "From One to Three," pp. 3–27. Washington, D.C.: U.S. Department of Health, Education, and Welfare, Children's Bureau Publication No. 30. Rev. 1967.

Recommended Audiovisual Aids

FILMS

Terrible Two's and Trusting Three's (20 min., McGraw-Hill, B&W, 1950)
    This film pictures normal behavior for children who are two and three years of age. Illustrates positive parent-child relationships.

FILMSTRIP

Teaching Desirable Habits (42 frames, McGraw-Hill, B&W)
    The value of pleasant learning is explained. A child balks when pushed into learning beyond his ability. Suggestions are given on helping a child to learn bowel training (in the second year), to dress himself, to pick up his toys, and to form good sleep habits. It emphasizes techniques such as praising a child for successes, avoiding shaming him, and giving him a choice without asking, "Do you want to?"

FILMLOOP

Growth and Development: Two Years, Part I and Part II (Prentice-Hall, 1970)
    This filmloop focuses on the two-year-old boy's physical growth, abilities, and interests in play — such as climbing a ladder, finger dexterity, coordination in bead stringing and block building, jumping, tricycle riding, drinking from a cup — negativism, and dependence upon the presence of his mother.
    Silent filmloop with manual: Lange, Crystal M., and Caroline M. Mertz, *Nursing Skills and Techniques, Instructor's Guide.* Prentice-Hall, Inc., Englewood Cliffs, New Jersey, 1970.

TRANSPARENCIES

Owens, Gloria. Home Economics No. 20, *Importance and Selection of Toys.* 23 transparencies (3M Visual Products, 1967)
    Very good illustrations with captions explaining how a toy does or does not help the child. Various types of toys are shown, such as imitative toys, large muscle toys, small muscle toys, educational toys, and others. Also explains pride in toy ownership and readiness for a toy, as well as gives tips on care of toys and how to best manage the toy supply.

CHAPTER 8 / THE THREE-YEAR-OLD

The three-year-old is more independent, more stable, and has learned more skills and more words than the two-year-old, but hospitalization can still be difficult for him. Separation from his mother and father can be worse than the illness.

An occasional normal separation from his parents will help him to become a more independent person. A happy, two-hour visit with loved grandparents or a trusted friend will give him extra confidence in himself. Some three-year-olds whine a lot in order to gain attention.

Muscular Development

This is usually a period of slow physical growth. The three-year-old's motor skills are unevenly developed. He is more sure and nimble on his feet than the two-year-old. He runs, skips, marches, and stands on one foot. He catches a ball as well as throws it. He needs a lot of exercise.

The three-year-old shows marked development in large-muscle coordination. He can capably ride a tricycle. However, his small-muscle coordination and his eye-and-hand coordination are not yet well developed. He may have fun with a hand puppet, but not with the marionette operated by strings.

Personal Habits

The three-year-old has a full set of temporary teeth. He eats fairly well alone and can feed himself with little spilling. He drinks from a cup. However, sometimes he does not eat well at the family table. He dawdles. He has a fair appetite, which alters from very good to very poor.

The three-year-old has made progress in toilet control. Bowel control is attained by now, and most children have control for both day and night dryness. Boys may have more problems than girls. Occasional relapses in control are more "normal" than "accidental." The child can usually go to the toilet by himself during the day if his clothes are simple, but he may need help when finished.

The three-year-old can probably wash his hands acceptably and dry them without soiling the towel. He loves to see his success in a low-hung mirror and will try to comb his hair and brush his teeth.

Forming Good Sleep Habits

The lively three-year-old needs an abundance of sleep and rest for his physical well-being. If he has lived by a fairly regular schedule, going to bed and to sleep are routine. The three-year-old usually sleeps the clock around. His daytime nap is probably shortened to an hour.

Because the hospitalized child may find sleep difficult, the nurse should understand the conditions that help children to sleep and how children form good sleep habits.

A quiet time before the afternoon nap or night bedtime will help the child to relax and be more ready for sleep.

If the father's only time to spend with his young child is at bedtime, they should replace active, romping play with a quiet story hour.

Physical conditions influence the benefits a child receives from his sleep. He needs a well-ventilated room, with temperature slightly lowered, his own bed, sufficient bed covers, comfortable night clothes, a drink of water if necessary, and possibly a favorite stuffed toy. If, from babyhood, the child has slept amid the ordinary household noises, his closed bedroom door should be enough protection from noise. A darkened room is also better.

Give the child a few minutes' notice before bedtime so that his play will not be suddenly interrupted. Parents should avoid giving him the feeling that they want him in bed so he will be out of their way. Attend to reasonable requests and give him reassurance that all is well. Children need constant reassurance of their parents' love and affection, and bedtime affords a good opportunity for this. If the bedtime routine has pleasant associations — conversation, a story hour, or music — children will accept it as a matter of course.

Causes for Poor Sleep

Too much excitement, too strenuous a playtime, teasing by adults and older children, exciting parties, too much television — all may prove exhausting to the little child and make sleep difficult. Lack of sleep can result in a cross, irritated child. Repeated sleep loss causes lack of appetite, poor color, and eventually malnutrition.

Disturbed and restless sleep may be caused by too much excitement, or it may indicate that the child has feelings of insecurity and fear that his parents have not recognized.

Bedtime routine is too strict, however, if the child must always have the same toy, sleep in the very same bed, and have his one particular blanket. The child who is accustomed to minor variations in the routine is less likely to be completely upset when his entire routine changes — which happens if he is hospitalized.

Nighttime at the Hospital

Like the child at home, the hospitalized child needs reassurance that all is well and that someone who cares is nearby. Nighttime at the hospital can be awesome with its strange, unaccountable noises, unusual lights, dark shadows on the walls, people walking around, and the bed with side rails.

Sometimes the nurse is actually too busy to get a particular blanket for a child, tuck him in with his own toy, place his shoes on the bedside table, and put a chair by his bed for his mother, who is coming tomorrow. But the night nurse should recognize that these simple nursing chores are important in providing comfort to the child in a strange environment.[1]

If one child needs medicine or treatment in the middle of the night, other children in the room are probably awake and wondering about it. A simple

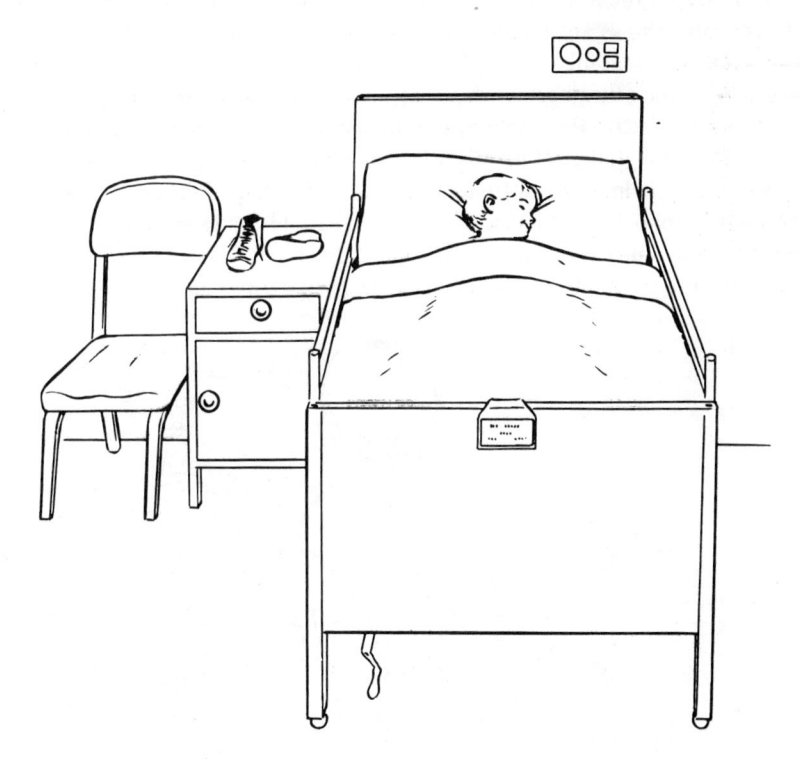

Figure 8. *Sleep at the hospital comes more easily with shoes on the bedside table and a chair placed for the mother's visit next day.*

[1] Beulah B. Muston, "Nighttime Needs of Children," *Am. J. Nursing* (May 1962), p. 82.

explanation will ease the doubt: "Harry was so sick we had to give him extra medicine. Let me get you a drink of water so you can go back to sleep."

The little child needs to know that, night after night, nurses are close by and that morning will come soon.

Learning to Dress

The three-year-old helps with his dressing, as well as undressing. He may manage buttons and zippers, but he cannot always tell the front from the back of his clothes. He may dress himself fairly well one day and poorly the next.

He may hang up his hat and coat if low hooks are provided, Since girls develop more rapidly than boys, the three-year-old girl can often dress herself with little help.

Learning to dress is one way in which a child acquires independence. When the youngster shows an interest, he should be encouraged and permitted to do what he can for himself.

Interest in clothes begins when the one-year-old holds out an arm or leg for his mother to put on the garment. At 15 months he may pull off a shoe, and at 18 months he may take off his stockings or slip out of overalls. The two-year-old is interested in helping to put on clothes as well as take them off. If we make it easy for the child to help himself, the three-year-old can learn to do much of his dressing. The four-year-old can usually dress himself fairly well except for buttons in the back and for shoelaces. The five-year-old learns to tie laces in a

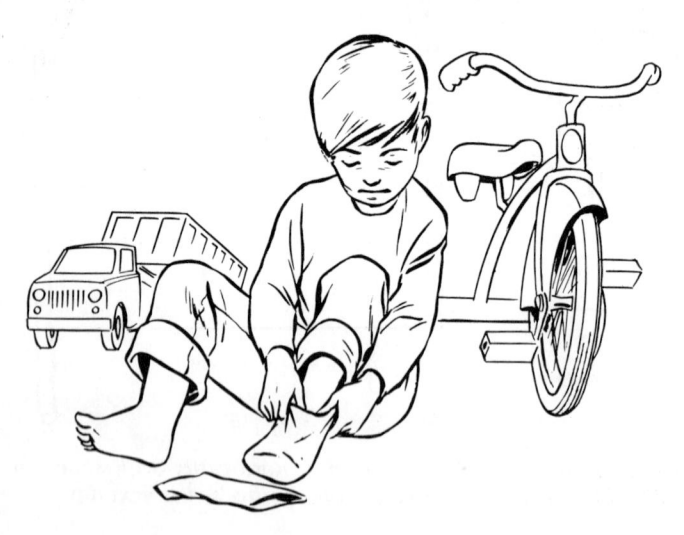

Figure 9. *The three-year-old is learning to dress himself. The right toys aid in his development.*

bow. By school age, children should be able to dress themselves. If not, they may be handicapped and embarrassed at school.

We help a child to learn to dress himself by giving him plenty of time, because he will take longer. If he tires before the end, help him unobtrusively. Let his routine be the same every day. Do not allow dressing after breakfast one morning and insist it be before breakfast the next morning. Arrange clothing so that the child gets the feeling of order: "First the sweater, now the leggings, now the cap, now the mittens." A colored stitching will identify the front and outside of the underwear for the child. Praise the child's accomplishments, however trivial they seem. Do not criticize or deride early efforts. He needs pride in himself.

Choice of Clothes

When selecting children's clothes, look for features that encourage selfdressing, such as wide elastic waistbands, clothes of one general style, front openings rather than back openings, and fasteners of the same type. Flat, round, nonslippery buttons the size of a nickel or a quarter are the easiest for little hands to manage. Clothes that are simple to manage at the toilet will make independence come sooner. Some toilet accidents could be prevented if the trousers of little boys were comfortably loose and did not press on their genitals.

Comfortable clothing for children is very important. The child's movements should not be hampered or his skin chafed. Raglan or kimono-type sleeves are preferable to "set-in" sleeves. The shoulder width should span the back and chest, so there is no straining. If the shirt is too large, the shoulder seams will not stay in place. Elastic at sleeve, waist, and legbands should go only part of the way around and never be so tight that it leaves red marks. The neckline should be low enough in front that it does not rub or choke, closely fit in back so it will not ride up, and not be so large as to slip off the shoulders. The hips and crotch should allow bending, stooping, sitting, and reaching without discomfort. The trousers and sleeves should not be too tight or too long. Separate skirts or trousers need to be suspended from the shoulders by straps that are crossed or fastened to prevent slipping or by built-up jumper tops.

Adults must remember that the child cannot use safety pins, and needle and thread. He cannot make or even suggest an alteration that would make his clothes more comfortable.

Clothing fads are often poor choices. Soft-soled ballerina slippers make it painful for a little girl to jump or climb the rungs of the gym set. Cowboy boots may prevent freedom of movement.

In winter, a child needs only enough clothing to prevent chilling. Two lightweight garments are better than one heavyweight garment. Some woolen sweaters may make a child's skin itch. Wash-and-wear fabrics, which require little or no ironing, are a boon for the mother.

Clothing should not be purchased so large that the child looks and feels awkward. These features allow for growth: side seams that can be let out, adjustable shoulder straps, tucks in skirts, folds under the waistline, deep hems, and extra-long skirts and blouses.

A shoe that is too large is just as uncomfortable as one that is too small. Both shoes and stockings should be checked often for size. Shoes should be one-fourth inch broader and one-half inch longer than the outline of a child's foot drawn on paper while he is standing. The heel of the shoe should fit snugly. Soles should be firm, flat, and moderately flexible. Illfitting shoes and stockings may injure or deform a child's feet.

Other Learnings

The three-year-old is beginning to understand time, size, space, and shape. He speaks in short sentences, which keep getting longer. He is curious about people and things. He asks many questions. In his expanding world, his father is beginning to be very important to him.

He can differentiate between a boy and a girl and will probably ask questions regarding sex differences. He should be given simple, reassuring answers on his level of understanding.

When the three-year-old asks where the new baby came from, it is usually enough to say, "The baby grew inside his mother." Detailed, factual information about the birth process would overwhelm a little child.

Children ask the same questions about sex and babies in different ways as they grow older. In answering their questions, and in conversations about birth that come up naturally, you gradually add to the child's knowledge.

The three-year-old likes excursions, and a trip to the supermarket or shopping center will be exciting to him.

The three-year-old enjoys helping with household tasks, such as running errands, dusting, or picking up things. He probably can put away his toys. Helping to feed the family pet will encourage gentleness and kindness in a child.

Play Activities and Toys

The three-year-old likes to be with other children and can play fairly well with one or two. He now says "we" and can wait his turn. He takes part in simple games and activities where no skill is required. He is boastful and is likely to tell other children what to do. His social development is progressing but is still incomplete.

He uses toys to *do* things. He likes the push-and-pull toys that he can fill and that will carry things. The wagon that he fills with toy farm animals or the dump truck that dumps sand are favorites. He wants to build with blocks of different sizes, and he notices letters of the alphabet.

The child needs many things to help his play of imitating adults and of "make-believe." Both boys and girls like dolls, dishes, cowboy guns, miniature automobiles, and toy spaceships. Pretending to be somebody else or an animal is very common.

The three-year-old likes to mess with finger paints, to mold with clay or mud, and to draw with crayon or pencil. He may be able to fit together a simple puzzle.

He likes stories and nursery rhymes. The repetition and sounds appeal to him, even though he may not understand all the words. He may show some sense of simple rhythm. He still likes simple stories and pictures of familiar things. However, he prefers seasonal stories, not the one-situation story of the two-year-old. Since he has an interest in "things that go," he likes to look at and talk about pictures of airplanes, boats, cars, and trains.

Questions for Discussion

1. Evaluate current styles in children's clothing. Which styles are poor choices?
2. What are suitable bedtime stories for three-year-olds?
3. Does the nursery school for two- and three-year-olds need separate toilet facilities for boys and girls?
4. What preparations for the cross-country automobile trip might enable the preschool child to sleep better?

Additional Readings

Blake, Florence G., and others. *Nursing Care of Children.* 8th ed., pp. 454–473. Philadelphia: J. B. Lippincott Company, 1970.
Child Training Leaflets by Department of National Health and Welfare, Ottawa, Canada (reprinted by Indiana State Board of Health, Indianapolis). *Sleeping, Bed-Wetting.*
How to Tell Your Child About Sex. New York: Public Affairs Pamphlet No. 149, 1949.
Hurlock, Elizabeth. *Child Development.* 4th ed., "Interest in Clothes," pp. 634–639. New York: McGraw-Hill Book Company, Inc., 1964.
Langford, Louise M. *Guidance of the Young Child.* "Clothing and the Preschooler," pp. 170–172. New York: John Wiley & Sons, Inc., 1960.
Scott, Lou Peveto. *Programmed Instruction and Review for Practical and Vocational Nurses.* Vol. 2: *Clinical and Community Nursing,* pp. 258–261. New York: The Macmillan Company, 1968.

Recommended Audiovisual Aids

FILM

Child Care and Development (17 min., McGraw-Hill, B&W, 1951)
    Good health habits are established early, and this film shows how establishing them is managed by one couple with four children. It explores the importance of and ways to provide good meals, meaningful play and exercise, sleep, proper clothing, and learning habits of cleanliness. It stresses that there are many good ways of bringing up children.

CHAPTER 9 / **THE FOUR-YEAR-OLD**

The four-year-old will talk to you, the strange nurse, and his running conversation may give you the impression that he is more adult and grown-up than he actually is. He will probably show more fear of physical pain and make a bigger fuss over "shots" than the two-year-old. His fears are related to his increased concern to keep his body from harm, his new awareness of sex, and his big imagination. He does not yet distinguish between make-believe and reality.

Although the four-year-old can tolerate separation from his parents better than the two- or three-year-old, he can turn any action or conversation that he does not understand into something horrible and frightening.

"We are going to take the leg cast off," may mean to the four-year-old, "take off the leg." He may wonder, "Is that the knife to cut your ears off if you cry?"

The nurse must be very careful to avoid any statement that the four-year-old can misinterpret. Talk to *him* and tell him gently what will happen and why. Let him ask you questions. At home, he continually asks, "Why? Why?" He wants to know, "Who am I? Am I different?" He may fear that what is happening to him in the hospital will make him different forever.

The four-year-old child is active, noisy, stormy, and experimental. He runs, jumps, and climbs with more grace and ease than the three-year-old. He bends an elbow as he "pitches" the ball.

Personal Habits

Since this is a period of more rapid growth, the four-year-old generally has a good appetite. He likes to eat with the rest of the family and feeds himself neatly. He can dress and undress himself if his clothes are simple. He may need help with overshoes and shoelaces. He can go to the toilet without help and rarely has a daytime "accident." He washes and dries his face (except for the ears) without help.

The four-year-old can get himself ready for bed. He still sleeps about 11 to 12 hours and needs an afternoon rest. A gradual change in his schedule prepares him for kindergarten the following year. If he objects to the afternoon nap, he should know that he does not have to sleep, but may just rest with a book or toy. Often he falls asleep, but, if not, being alone and quiet is sufficient.

Increasing Independence

The four-year-old's world is widening, and he needs more independence. He may be resentful if held too tightly within bounds. He may run away from home. With certain areas definitely restricted, he should be "on his own" within that area. He is thrilled with, and profits from, an occasional overnight separation from his family.

Often the four-year-old begins to use words that adults do not like. He picks up swear words or terms related to sex. If he gets a distinct reaction, this is fun, and he will repeat the words. The less attention given to the shocking language, the more quickly it disappears. If silence is impossible, try to say calmly, "We don't say that," or "That is enough," and substitute a ridiculously funny word. The four-year-old likes to be silly; so appeal to his funnybone with acceptable words.

Temper Tantrums

The four-year-old now fights with words. In a fit of rage, he may shout, "I hate you," or "You make me so mad."

The defiance and the temper tantrums of the four-year-old may be more exasperating to parents than the temper outbursts of the two-year-old. "He should know better," they reason. Parents may question their discipline methods, unless they realize that the new outbursts are indications of new growth.

Discipline

Learning to live by society's rules, to make wise decisions, to think of other people's feelings — these take a long time for the little child. If adults remember the true goals of discipline, the problems with the four-year-old will seem less difficult.

Ways of guiding children have changed through the years, but not as drastically as some poeple believe. Sound research did not support the permissive view that the child should never hear the word "no" or that his sense of security would be disturbed if he were denied anything.

A child's sense of security depends on firm, consistent discipline, but discipline that is fair, reasonable, and understood.

Today, in reaction to excessive permissiveness, we find some people returning to the horsewhip, rule-by-force approach. One director of a country child guidance clinic reported that many children with disturbed behavior were reacting to unhappy family relationships or harsh and excessive punishments: "There is too much whipping of children with belts in our county. Any parent who claims he has to resort to belt whipping to make a child behave has failed in discipline."

The child is not a miniature adult. We cannot reasonably expect him to be seen and not heard. Somewhere between the overly permissive view and the dictatorial, punitive approach lies a happy medium for discipline.

Discipline and Punishment

The terms "discipline" and "punishment" are not the same. One goal of discipline is to teach the child to make the right decisions for himself. In theory, punishment is needed only when discipline has failed. Realistically, sometimes it is necessary to show a child that he has behaved badly.

Punishment should not be an outlet for the adult. When possible, let the consequences of the child's act serve as the punishment. If Judy throws her glass of milk on the floor in a fit of temper, see that Judy helps to clean up the mess. Then she will realize her emotional outburst caused extra work. At least, let the punishment "fit the crime."

When a child has misbehaved, make it clear that you disapprove of the action, not the child. Children need to know that their parents love them regardless of what happens. The young patient also needs to know that his nurse accepts him regardless of what happens. However, when a child insists on doing dangerous things, swift, immediate punishment may be necessary.

The nurse must avoid corporal punishment. You do not want to force your will on the child only because you have the advantage of size and strength. He may become so upset that he loses all connection between the misdemeanor and the punishment. You definitely jeopardize the relationship between you, the nurse, and the little patient. Slapping a child usually makes his behavior worse.

Threats of punishment are ineffective, as children learn to disregard them as "just talk." They may associate punishment with fear of being caught, not with the wrong act. Some children are unduly frightened by threats. Enough fearsome things may happen in the hospital without additional threats.

Helps to Good Behavior

Serious behavior problems usually do not develop if the child has a happy home, with regular hours for sleep and meals, a good place to play, and companions and materials to keep him busy and to have fun with. The hospital situation is not completely different; the same principles apply.

A good relationship between the child and the adult implies mutual respect, affection, appreciation, and interest. If the child knows you are genuinely interested in him, he will accept more easily the rules and decisions, even if he does not always understand them. Do not give complicated explanations beyond the ability of the child to understand. Avoid lengthy rules that he could not possibly remember. If you know what to expect of children at different ages, you will know what he is ready to learn and what he is able to remember. Let him make decisions when possible: "Do you want a popsicle or a fudge bar?"

Be consistent in what is allowed. If one nurse permits the children to do what another nurse forbids, the children will soon learn to take advantage. Or if the nurse is lax one day and strict the next, children become confused.

Expecting good behavior often brings it about. Praising a child for good behavior is more effective than punishing him for misbehavior.

Discipline should be impersonal. A clear definition of rules can help the nurse to say, "We do it this way at our hospital," not, "Do it because I say so."

Firmness with kindness wins a child's cooperation, whereas harsh, angry words build up resentment and bitterness. The nurse's tone of voice is important. The nurse who asks or requests a child to "sit still" will get better results than the nurse who orders or commands. Also, if you make suggestions in the positive form, the child may heed an occasional "don't." Use the phrase, "let's play." Avoid saying, "bad girl," "bad boy," "obey," "must," and so forth.

Giving bribes for good behavior implies that the child has a choice, either to behave or to misbehave. Suppose that you offer Timmy a stick of chewing gum to go to the physical-therapy department for treatment. The next day he may decide the gum is not worth the effort. Or he may become a shrewd bargainer — now he wants two sticks of chewing gum. Timmy has missed the point that the treatments will help him get better.

The nurse who enjoys children, who can laugh, have fun, and yet be firm, will get along well with her young patients — even the independent four-year-old.

Age of Make-Believe

The four-year-old is likely to be boastful and to tell "tall tales." Only a thin line separates fact from fantasy. He is confused by television shows. How much is real? How much is make-believe?

The pretending of the three-year-old continues. He may have an imaginary companion, or he may imagine that he is someone else. Actually, such imagination does no harm unless the child continues to withdraw within himself.

It does somewhat impede his other problem — that of learning to tell the truth. Sometimes he tells what he wishes were true, instead of what really happened. Or he may think that his version is more interesting.

The Four-Year-Old

Companions and Play Activities

Understanding the play activities of the healthy four-year-old will help you to keep the hospitalized child happy.

The four-year-old craves being with other children. Adults cannot substitute satisfactorily for playmates. He has special friends of his own age with whom he likes to play hide-and-seek, tag, jump-the-rope, hopscotch, and marbles.

In this age of "make believe I am the mother, make believe you are the father," children need many props to imitate adult life. Both boys and girls like to act out the daily homemaking activities. They really use the toy carpet sweeper, the vacuum cleaner, the cooking set, and the ironing board. Little girls love to "dress up." The doll is likely to be taken through the whole range of the child's own experiences — bathed, fed, dressed, undressed, and put to bed. Clothes for the doll and doll accessories become more important as the child is more concerned with realistic detail.

Doctor and nurse kits, the fireman's and the postman's hats are all used for dramatic play. At this age children like farm sets with farm animals, barn, tractor, wagon, trucks, and fences. They enjoy the miniature racetrack and the filling station.

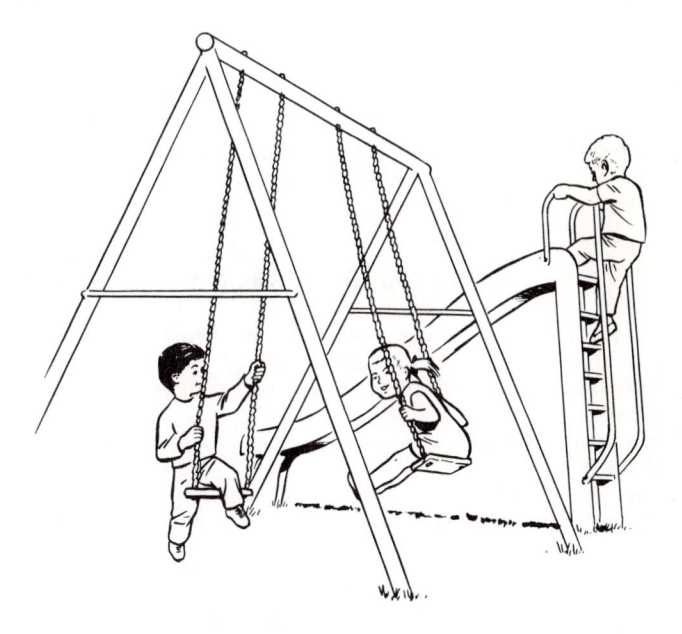

Figure 10. *The four-year-old needs playmates. Active play helps to release energy and develop muscles.*

Interest in store play requires scales, play money, a billfold or purse, containers for the shelves, and, of course, a cash register.

To encourage muscular development and to help release energy, the four-year-old needs equipment like swings, climbing bars, rope ladders, and a gym set. He (she) likes the wagon, scooter, doll carriage, tricycle, and wheelbarrow. The group of children may use a hoop or tire to roll, a wading pool, or a sled.

The four-year-old needs toys for construction, toys for special interest skills, or the so-called "educational toys." (Any toy that a child really uses is educational.) These include easy construction sets, puzzles with several pieces and shapes, lots of blocks for large buildings, interlocking blocks, hammer-and-peg boards, counting frames, magnets, musical instruments, and simple games. He likes simple carpentry tools — hammer, nails, saw, and pliers that he can actually use, and a strong, sturdy workbench.

The four-year-old needs "raw" materials for creative self-expression. Clay, paints, chalk, paper, crayons, sand, water — even mud — all are materials he can use as he wishes. He can shape and express his own ideas. Unhampered play space is essential for the full use of the materials. A coloring book is less desirable for the four-year-old than a plain pad of paper because the ideas have already been given shape. Also, the four-year-old cannot yet keep within the lines as he colors.

Because the four-year-old is fascinated by the fantasy world, he likes stories of fantasy. He may like stories of animals who act like people. Great favorites are "The Three Bears," "The Fox and the Little Hen," and "Peter Rabbit." The horror of *Grimm's Fairy Tales* may shock adults, but children seem to enjoy a threat to security while remaining personally secure.

Questions for Discussion

1. What are legitimate or reasonable ways of giving the four-year-old more independence than he had when he was three?
2. What are ways of handling discipline or behavior problems in the pediatrics ward?
3. What helps the four-year-old to begin to distinguish between make-believe and reality?
4. Does your community have a nursery school offering preschool education? What are the goals of preschool education?

Additional Readings

Child Training Leaflets by Department of National Health and Welfare, Ottawa, Canada (reprinted by Indiana State Board of Health, Indianapolis). *Discipline, Destruction, Obedience, Temper.*

The Four-Year-Old

Hartley, Ruth E., and Robert Goldenson. *Complete Book of Children's Play.* Rev. ed. New York: Thomas Y. Crowell Company, 1963.
Hurlock, Elizabeth. *Child Development.* 4th ed. Chap. 15, "Play and Playthings"; Chap. 16, "The Child's Companions." New York: McGraw-Hill Book Company, Inc., 1964.
Your Child from One to Six. Washington, D.C.: U.S. Department of Health, Education, and Welfare, Children's Bureau Publication No. 30. Rev. 1967.

Recommended Audiovisual Aids

FILMSTRIP

Discipline (43 frames, International Film Bureau, Color)
A filmstrip with captions and accompanying manual. By using animated drawings, it compares poor discipline (spanking, too much permissiveness) with principles of good discipline (love, guidance, firmness with affection, positive actions and attitudes).

FILM

Frustrating Four's and Fascinating Five's (22 min., McGraw-Hill, Color, 1952)
A film that would be a useful guide to parents, teachers, and nurses of four- and five-year-olds. Points with humor to the kind of behavior to be expected and indicates how to assist the child to grow and develop normally.

CHAPTER 10 / **THE FIVE-YEAR-OLD**

Hospitalization may not be as traumatic for the five-year-old as for younger children, but he requires gentle, "kid-glove" handling to protect him from emotional injury. Understanding what the five-year-old is like will help you, the nurse, to cope with his emotions as skillfully as his illness.

The physical development of the five-year-old consolidates the gains he was making as a four-year-old. He can hop, skip, turn somersaults, and handle with ease his sled, wagon, and bicycle. He learns to kick a football and to roller-skate.

He can look after his personal needs fairly well. He washes and dresses himself, goes to the toilet alone, and goes to bed regularly, according to the hands on the clock. He still needs a rest period, if not a nap, during the day and ten hours of sleep at night. Some children need more. He shows fatigue by fidgeting and restlessness, not tears.

The five-year-old is more dependable, stable, and reliable than the four-year-old. He has learned to do what is expected of him at home. He likes to help his mother and father with the home chores. He may sometimes forget a regularly assigned task but usually does it quickly when reminded. He likes to hammer, to paint, and to help wash the family car. He likes to run errands and may be trusted with small sums of money for definite purchases. He cannot yet make change, but he is learning numbers and their meanings. When asked his age the day after his fifth birthday, he may answer, "I am now five and one-half."

The five-year-old learns to print simple words of three or four letters and to print his own name. (The letters may mean nothing to him out of context.) He is interested in a week as a unit of time. He is also interested in relatives and is beginning to understand about cousins, aunts, and uncles.

The five-year-old speaks in complete sentences, fairly clearly. Many children enter school at six lacking the ability to pronounce certain sounds, not the ability to think clearly. When the five-year-old asks a question, he is serious and wants a thoughtful answer.

He can distinguish more reliably between reality and make-believe. Sometimes, an imaginary companion is still his friend, but real companions are more important to him.

The five-year-old is usually aware of the rights and feelings of others. He has increased respect for authority, and he understands rules.

Because of these, the five-year-old can be trusted to move freely in his own immediate neighborhood and to play unsupervised in the backyards of his companions. If he goes to kindergarten, he should be able to get there unattended.

Ready for School

The five-year-old is usually eager for school and, with the right guidance at home, willing to learn to be independent. These will be assets to him in his school world if:

1. He is interested in the world outside his home.
2. He can get along without his parents for short intervals.
3. He can safely cross streets and obey traffic lights.
4. He listens to instructions and follows directions.
5. He puts things back where they belong.
6. He can dress himself.
7. He can look after his possessions, including outdoor wraps.
8. He goes to the toilet unassisted and washes his hands thoroughly afterward.
9. He washes his hands before eating.

Health Examinations and Inoculations

Every child should have a preschool health examination. The physician will check the child's height, weight, posture, vision, and hearing. Many a beginner's problems in school can be traced to faulty vision and hearing.

Most parents agree that a periodic health examination is worth the time and trouble it requires. A child should be taken to the doctor's office or a well-baby clinic (child health conference) at least once a year.

If the child meets the doctor when he is well, he will more readily accept him as a friend. The doctor can learn what the child is like socially, emotionally, and intellectually. At regular visits, the doctor can be on the alert for symptoms of difficulties.

Inoculations against disease usually begin in the baby's first year. Most doctors combine inoculations for diphtheria, whooping cough, tetanus, and poliomyelitis with a series of three shots. Smallpox vaccination follows. Because the effects of inoculation gradually weaken, booster shots are necessary for continued protection. This probably means that the four-year-old needs further protection against diphtheria, whooping cough, and tetanus (often in a combined shot). At five or six years of age, the smallpox vaccination is repeated. Booster shots of polio vaccine may be needed at more frequent intervals.

Many states have health laws that require parental statement of inoculations for all new first grade pupils. The public health nurse assigned to the school carefully notes which youngsters have incomplete or no records and follows through with either a visit or phone call. Efforts are made to ensure that the child receives the inoculations as soon as possible. Immunization of children against disease may well be a community's sturdiest foundation for good health.

Child Safety

Many accidents happen to children around the age of five to six. Just at the time when parents hope the youngster understands the safety rules they have emphasized since toddler days, the child's world expands. The five-year-old has many chances for accidents. He is more agile, can get around better, and has access to matches, poisons, electricity, and machines. Also within range of the five-year-old are streets, roads, creeks, ditches, and neighbors. Vigilance is still needed. He is also likely to act out emotional conflicts. He frequently plays with older children and, in competition, overextends the safety boundaries he should remember.

For children aged 1 to 14 years, accidents claim more lives than the four leading diseases combined. Boys have more accidents than girls. The accident rate reaches a peak in the second year and remains relatively high throughout the preschool years.

There are many reasons for preschool accidents. Young children lack experience and knowledge. They do not recognize danger, and they cannot move away from it. This may partly account for the fire victims and the frequency of burn accidents. Homes are planned and built for adults. In order for the child to see what is on top of the table, he has to climb a chair or pull off the tablecloth.

As a student nurse you will see many children who have been accident victims. When you see their pain and suffering, the crippling and disfiguration for life, you realize clearly how important it is to prevent accidents.

Accidents that occur most frequently to children are motor-vehicle accidents, fires and burns, falls, contact with glass or sharp objects, drownings, and poisonings.

We cannot give the child a "shot" to prevent accidents, as we can inoculate him against diphtheria. The key lies with (1) a hazard-free environment and (2) education of the child.

Safety Education

A child must be taught to do safely all that he wants to do and is capable of doing. When he leaves home for school, he should be able to deal with the ordinary activities of his life.

A child learns safe habits from examples set by parents or older family members, through supervised and planned experience, and, least effectively, by command. Constantly shouting, "Stop that. Don't touch. You are bad," is not education.

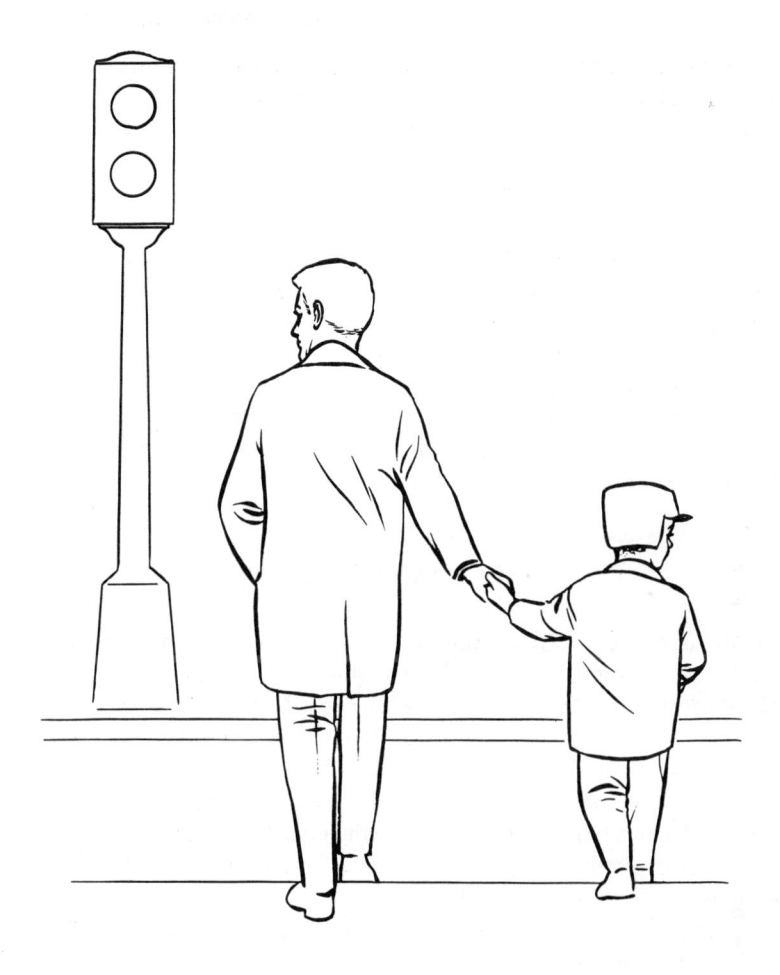

Figure 11. *He learns to cross safely more quickly if parents have always stopped and looked before stepping into the street.*

Children are great imitators, and adults who practice safe habits are helping the child to form safe habits. A child notices when his parents put away tools and equipment, pick up clothing dropped on the floor, or immediately clean up a spilled liquid. If the mother uses a chair as a stepladder to reach the jar on the top shelf, her son thinks it is all right for him to climb on chairs too. Adults and children drink from soft-drink bottles, hence putting refuse, cigarette ashes, or poisonous liquids in bottles may be dangerous. Keeping the stairs free from clutter is also a good practice.

    The child must be shown the difference between safe and unsafe practices. When he needs to climb, show him the right way. Teach him how to play in water. A five-year-old can learn to swim and may amaze adults with his skill, ability, and willingness to follow directions.

Planned Experiments

Perhaps the child will have to touch the warm coffeepot to realize the danger of touching the hot stove. If a child persists in tasting anything and everything, leave a mustard jar open within his reach. After this he may be less eager to taste an unknown liquid that could be kerosene or bleach. Also, perhaps he will believe what his mother said: "Don't taste until you ask Mother." Little fingers poked into an egg beater may help him to understand that one must not poke fingers into the blades of the lawn mower. Let the child make the decision at the intersection. Is this the time to cross the street? Is it safe?

Satisfy the Child's Curiosity

If the child's curiosity is satisfied, he may be less likely to experiment with the unknown. Children are naturally curious about matches and fire. Some mothers permit the child to blow out the match after the adult has lighted a cigarette. A school child might light his father's cigar. Let the youngster watch when the parents burn leaves or trash. He will learn the safe way if he sees the trash burned in a covered container, and if the adult stays with the fire while it is burning and leaves only after the fire is extinguished. Of course, matches and the cigarette lighter are kept out of his reach, but if he knows what they are, he may turn his attention to something else.

Children like to cut paper; so they should be provided with blunt-tipped, metal scissors or with plastic scissors.

Safe Environment

The alert nurse and the alert parent constantly watch for hazards that can result in accidents.

The yard, the living room, and the kitchen are where most home accidents occur.

Many ordinary household products can be poisonous to children. Aspirin is a leading child killer. Kerosene and gasoline are often stored in soft-drink bottles. Household products that can cause serious injury include liquid furniture polishes and waxes; laundry bleaches; ammonia; dry-cleaning fluids; and pesticides, such as rat and mouse killers, insect sprays, and weed killers. Also in the home may be charcoal and cigarette lighter fluids; sewer drain cleaners;

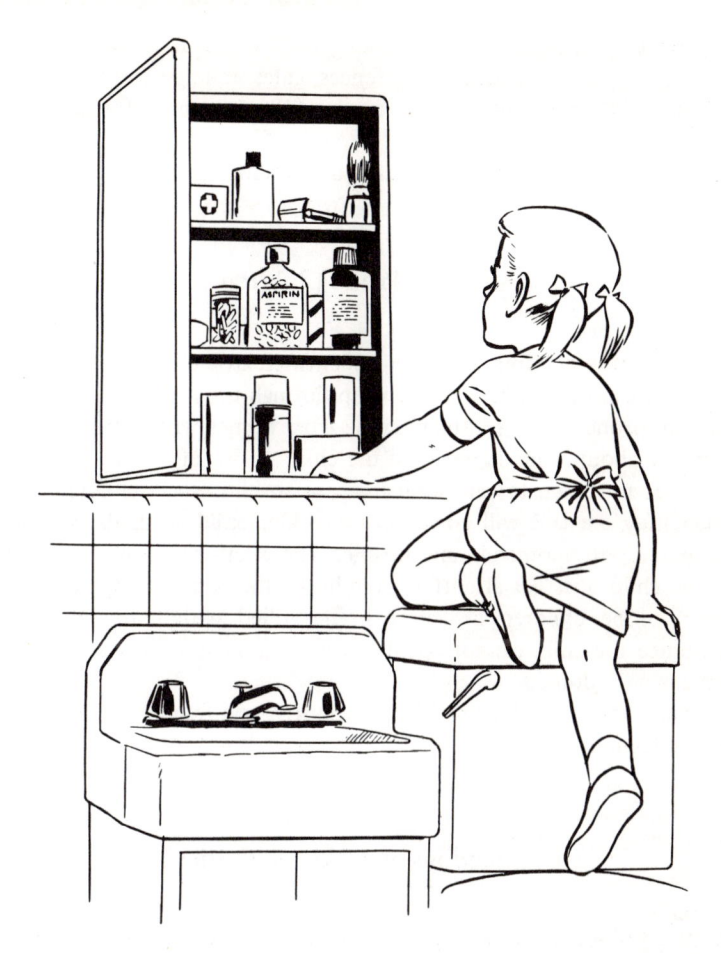

Figure 12. *Many items in the home medicine cabinet can be dangerous for the child.*

chrome cleaners, and automobile antifreeze solutions. All these products should be stored safely out of the reach of small children.

Consumer laws now require that poisonous substances be labeled as to content and that the antidote be given on the label. Therefore, leave a product in the labeled bottle. If an accident does occur, aid can then be given more quickly and effectively.

The child's clothing should be free from strings or belts that can strangle or trip him. Check clothing for flammable materials.

Electrical and gas appliances should be in good condition. Keep pots and pans placed on the stove so that the child cannot grab the handles. Play areas away from the kitchen, laundry, and heating rooms will help. Store sharp knives, tools, and sewing equipment where young children cannot reach them. Place guards in front of the fireplace. Keep fences, gates, railings, and screens in good repair. The child's play yard should be carefully inspected for any potential hazards.

With thought and care, many childhood accidents can be prevented.

Accident-Prone Children

Accident-prone children are usually identified around the ages of six, seven, and eight. The causes have been building up through the years.

Accident-prone children usually come from homes where the parents show little concern about what happens to the child. In his efforts to get attention, the child does not seem to care what happens to him. Some children try to act older than they are and will compete with older children in dangerous feats. Some children are resentful and hostile. The accidents may be intentional because the child does get attention from his mother when he is injured. Homes of accident-prone children are often homes filled with hate, rejection, and violence. Since the child cannot openly express his hostile feelings, the accident may be his way of doing so.

The child who has a feeling of love, security, and freedom within limits has reasons to safeguard his person.

Companions and Play Activities

The five-year-old is ready for cooperative play. He likes to play with other children, even though fighting is not uncommon.

He enjoys simple, competitive games that require taking turns, observing rules, and attaining goals — games such as dominoes, Uncle Wiggly, tiddlywinks, or tenpins. He likes group projects such as building houses, garages, and racetracks. He likes his own special friends; at this age, girls prefer playing with girls, boys with boys.

Sometimes this is called the age of achievement. The five-year-old prefers to play with other children, but he can amuse himself. He likes to cut, paste, and draw pictures. The little girl enjoys all types of dolls, and large wardrobes for the doll are important. She likes to "dress up," as does the four-year-old.

Little boys like boxing gloves, the train that runs, the helicopter that moves, and, of course, a two-wheeled bicycle. The mechanical train may satisfy the child who wants a train on tracks but who is not ready for the complex electric train.

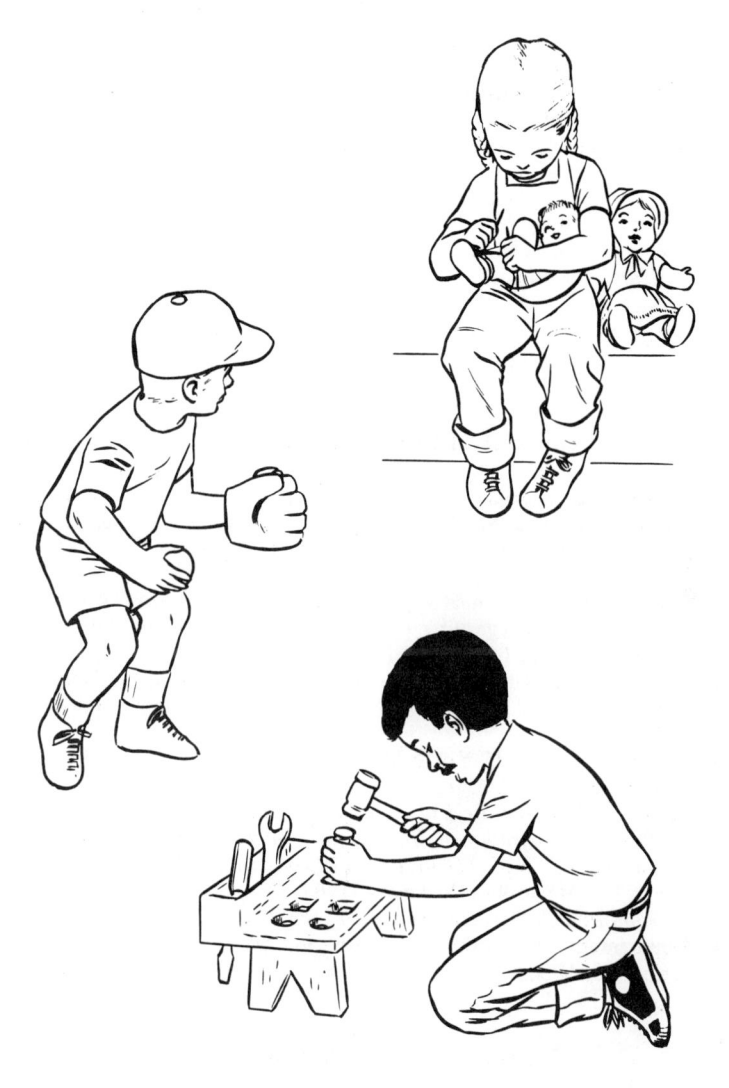

Figure 13. *The five-year-old's range of activities is unlimited.*

Boys like to build. The construction sets should have many pieces. The boy who learns to hammer, saw, and plane will make interesting objects.

Since interest in words, figures, and numbers develops about this time, the child will find good use for a blackboard and chalk or whiteboard and crayons. He may show skill with some artistic media that he formerly experimented with.

The five-year-old has a strong interest in imaginative stories of a simple type, especially stories in which children have imaginary adventures.

Questions for Discussion

1. Bring to the class newspaper clippings of child accidents. What could have prevented the accidents?
2. Tour a lounge or kitchen (food laboratory) in your school quarters to spot hazards for preschool children. What bottles or boxes would need to be placed out of the range of small children?
3. What are the health laws in your state regarding inoculations of schoolchildren?
4. Let one member of the class report on the orientation of first-graders by the schools in your community. Do the children visit school before they enroll?

Additional Readings

American Automobile Association. Traffic Engineering and Safety Department, Washington, D.C. 20006. Many pamphlets including: *The Safest Route to School; School Safety Patrols; The Young Pedestrian; Your Child and Traffic.*

Insurance companies, their health and safety divisions, print and distribute numerous pamphlets regarding child safety. For example, Liberty Mutual and Allstate Insurance have many leaflets available to their policyholders.

Kalafatich, Audrey, and Dorothy R. Meeks. *Maternal and Child Health.* Chap. 8, "The Preschool Child." Paterson, N.J.: Littlefield, Adams and Company, 1960.

National Safety Council, 425 North Michigan Avenue, Chicago, Illinois 60611. Many pamphlets available, including: *Child Safety in the Dangerous Years; Home Poisons; Kids Will Be Kids; Where Do Kids Play?*

Scott, Lou Peveto. *Programmed Instruction and Review for Practical and Vocational Nursing.* Vol. 2: *Clinical and Community Nursing,* pp. 262–263. New York: The Macmillan Company, 1968.

Selecting Automobile Safety Restraints for Small Children. Washington, D.C.: U.S. Department of Health, Education, and Welfare, Public Health Service Publication No. 1783.

Recommended Audiovisual Aids

FILMSTRIPS

Destructiveness (34 frames, International Film Bureau, Color)
Captions and manual. Using animated drawings, the filmstrip illustrates both innocent destructiveness and deliberate destructiveness, such as gang misdeeds. Suggestions are given on how to prevent each type of destructiveness.

Making Your Home Safe (41 frames, McGraw-Hill, Color)
This filmstrip emphasizes safety as an attitude rather than a set of rules. It shows pictures of all areas of the home and pinpoints needed safety measures.

The Five-Year-Old

FILM

The Giant Steps (15 min., U.S. Public Health Service, B&W, 1961)
 This film is very good for teaching child safety practices. It shows children learning safety at school and at home, and emphasizes that parents need to trust their children and to expect them to practice the safety lessons.

CHAPTER 11 / THE TODDLER, THE

PRESCHOOL CHILD, AND FOOD

Eating well helps your pediatric patient to recover, just as it helps other hospital patients. The nurse's role is complicated because the toddler is learning to eat different foods, is learning to feed himself, and is probably homesick. Food does not interest him. The number of foods that he likes may be limited. Getting him to eat anything may be an accomplishment, but the nurse should try to help him eat the food he needs and to continue his progress toward independence.

Food habits are established early in life, and children need skillful guidance to acquire good eating habits. The pediatric nurse needs to understand what food means to the child and how normal, healthy children learn to eat if she is to help the young patient to eat his food.

Meaning of Food to the Child

Eating is an emotional experience for children. To a little child, food means security, comfort, and love. To be fed is to be loved.

A child senses when his mother is concerned about his eating. Many mothers believe their success as a mother depends on her child's eating the food he is offered. The overanxious mother may encourage her child to eat because "this is good for you." Children should eat because they enjoy eating.

By refusing to eat, a child can assert independence, get attention, or make life exciting. Other children may overeat to win approval that is synonymous with love. Some children who eat continuously regard food as a substitute for the love, security, and satisfaction they get no other way.

The happy, healthy, active child usually has an eagerness for food and enjoys it. Because the young child shows such strong feelings of frustration or satisfaction about eating, we try to avoid severe conflicts over food. To insist that a child eat what he dislikes only invites trouble. Pleasant feeding experiences can give a child emotional satisfactions that help him in meeting other situations in life.

Pattern of Normal Eating

Most young children follow a general pattern for eating.

The infant gets used to a set routine and wants everything the same. He turns away because the new nipple is different. When he is between six months and a year old, he begins to mess with his food, poke it experimentally, and feel the texture. This preliminary step to self-feeding is as necessary as crawling is to walking. Too much interference sets up a roadblock on his way to healthy eating habits. When he wants to use a cup or spoon, let him try. If refused now, he may get the idea that this is your task, not his.

During the first year, growth is rapid, food needs are high, and the baby's appetite is good. He readily accepts a large quantity and variety of food.

During the second and third years, the growth rate slows. Food needs and intake diminish. He has less appetite. He also becomes fussy about food and expresses definite likes and dislikes. The color, form, and consistency of food are vitally important to him.

This is the time when a disturbingly large number of children develop feeding problems. Wise parents use every opportunity to encourage a toddler's interest in food and help him to establish good eating habits.

About the age of three and four, food "jags" are common. He may want applesauce every night for supper, then suddenly refuse it.

Sometimes at five or six, the appetite of infancy returns, but the child may be awkward, noisy, and critical.

This normal eating pattern varies with each child and with the emotional climate of each family. However, nothing but trouble comes from ignoring the general pattern or from trying to force a child out of his normal stage.

Appetite and Mealtime Atmosphere

The healthy child with regular hours for meals, wholesome activity, and sleep probably has a good appetite. If mealtime is a happy, unhurried time of good comradeship, he will look forward to meals. Correction for misbehavior, expecting perfect table manners, scolding, or nagging will all lessen his pleasure in eating and decrease his appetite.

Let the child "calm down" from active play before eating. Taking time to wash his hands may be part of the relaxing routine. Do not expect the frightened, angry, disappointed, or excited child to have interest in food. He may refuse violently. Handle emotionally disturbed children carefully. The memory of that meal may start a food prejudice. It may be best to allow him to miss a meal or to eat lightly.

Lack of appetite may be caused by overfatigue, approaching illness, or constipation. The child may be unhappy, worried, or poorly adjusted to his environment. When the appetite persistently lags, a physician should be consulted to rule out disease.

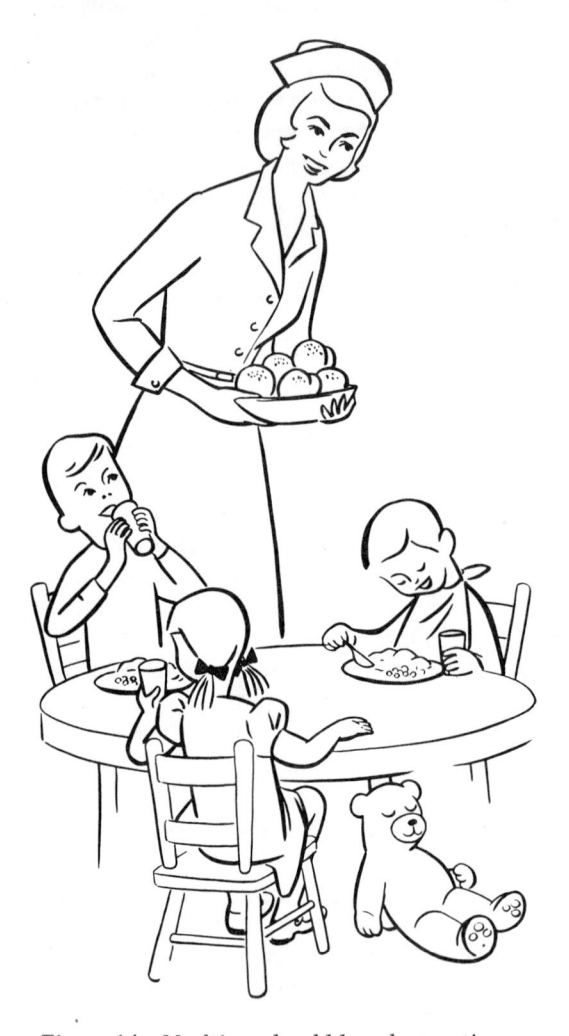

Figure 14. *Mealtime should be a happy time.*

Children's appetites normally fluctuate between very good and very poor. Children who are allowed to omit foods are less likely to develop lasting dislikes than if the food is forced on them. Feeding problems may result from tension at family meals, or the mealtime may be too long.

Chronic Vomiters

Feeding problems may become so critical that the child is hospitalized as a "chronic vomiter." That is, he vomits on all occasions, every time he tries to eat.

The treatment is most interesting. The child is put in a room near the nurse's station and is given a lot of love and attention by everyone who walks by him. Within two or three weeks, the child usually responds and begins to eat normally.

But the home situation has to be corrected, or the condition will return. Sometimes extreme friction or tension exists in the home, or the child may be rejected by his family. In some cases the child is placed in a foster home because the home situation cannot be improved.

Setting the Stage for Eating

Make mealtime comfortable for the child by providing a chair the right height for the surface on which glass and plate rest. Feet should touch the floor or a support.

Give the child eating utensils that he can handle easily. He will enjoy eating with a spoon or a fork suited to small hands, a cup or a glass that can be held securely, or a plate from which food can be scooped up easily. A divided plate is welcome. Soup is easy to drink from a mug.

Whether the child will eat with the family or alone should be weighed carefully. Eating is a sociable occasion, and children should learn to share this happy time. Yet adults have rights too. Also, perhaps the gathering of a large family provides too much excitement for the young child to concentrate on his food. He may not be able to sit still that long. Sometimes, one meal a day eaten with the family is a good compromise. The wise mother finds a legitimate excuse to permit the toddler to move about during mealtime.

Preparation and Serving of Food

The preschool child requires the same basic types of foods as the rest of the family, but the amount and the way the food is prepared may differ.

Children prefer simple meals of plain food served naturally. They have more taste buds than adults, even having taste buds in their cheeks. Mild-flavored foods are preferred to those that are salty, sour, or highly spiced. Strong-flavored vegetables are accepted better if served raw or with mild foods. With cooked cabbage, one might serve mild white potatoes and a lightly seasoned meat.

Children do not like food that is extremely hot or cold. The younger the child, the less he likes really hot food. He may prefer milk served room temperature rather than iced.

Take it for granted that the little child will eat, and serve his plate without consulting him. An older child may enjoy serving himself or be flattered to be able to choose between two vegetables. Avoid offering a large variety of dishes, as this encourages a child to be "choosy."

Encourage the child to feed himself. Let him eat in his own way, to a certain extent. A fruit dessert may be eaten along with the meal. Do not expect, or insist, that a child feed himself the entire meal when he is first learning self-feeding.

Always give the child small servings of food, a little less than you think he may want. If he wants more, he will ask.

Cut the food in bite-size pieces that are easily managed. Remove the tough connective tissue from liver, and cook the liver at a low temperature. Ground meats are easy to chew. Grapefruit is more welcome with the pulp removed from the tough part and served in bite-size pieces.

Finger foods are easily handled, particularly when the child is awkward at first in handling the fork and spoon. Meat, vegetables, and fruit may be offered as finger foods. The three-year-old, or older child, likes flowerlets of cauliflower or broccoli, sticks of carrots or celery, or leaves of lettuce that he can hold in his hand. Of course, all raw vegetables and fruits must be thoroughly washed.

Children are influenced by the color of food. They like pink ice cream and raspberry gelatin. They like contrasting textures in food. In every meal, strive to have one soft food, one chewy food, and one crisp food. Children like foods that require chewing but are discouraged if the entire meal is hard to chew.

Most children object to mixtures of food. They are suspicious of the next bite in a casserole mixture.

Children prefer moist meats and vegetables, not dry, hard, or gummy ones. They like foods thinner than those adults enjoy.

Encourage a child uninterested in food to help prepare some of the foods. One little boy who never ate vegetables was encouraged to plant his own vegetable patch. He ate every carrot that grew in his garden.

If a child does not like milk, serve him custards or puddings. A hidden fruit in the bottom of the custard is a surprise worth the effort. If we can look at food from the child's point of view, we will worry less, and we will worry *him* less.

Introducing a New Food

Since all new foods are introduced one by one, a child needs to begin early to get acquainted with a variety of foods. In addition to the previous ideas given, special consideration to the new food will help.

One teaspoon or one bite of a new food can be served at the beginning of the meal when the child is likely to be hungriest. Be certain he is in a good mood, not unhappy. Serve the new food along with a favorite food. Make no comment; do not urge him to eat the food. If he refuses, say nothing and serve it again later. Eventually, he will taste the food and eat it. Children are imitators. If the father refuses spinach, the son will also refuse it. Always serve new foods in small portions, one new food at a time. Do not pressure, nag, or force food.

Unsuitable Foods

Children can generally eat the same foods as adults with the exception of fried and greasy foods, rich pastries, an abundance of sweets, and highly seasoned foods. If the child fills his little stomach with too many sugars and sweet drinks, he will have neither space nor appetite for the essential foods. We cannot expect children to make wise food choices without our setting limits. Foods can be forbidden in such a way that the child is not resentful, but proud. "My mother won't let me eat that," says the three-year old.

The child under two should not be allowed such things as peanuts, the outer part of corn kernels, or popcorn. If the child chokes, hard fragments can be drawn into the lungs.

Eating Between Meals

The active, growing child needs a lot of food, but his stomach is small and cannot hold much food at one time. A nutritious snack at midmorning or midafternoon will add to the basic four food groups and will prevent him from becoming overhungry, tired, or cross. Children eat better if they are not ravenously hungry, just as they sleep better if they are not completely exhausted.

Some children, however, munch all day on cookies, potato chips, candy, or crackers with soft drinks to wash them down. They rarely eat a wholesome meal, and this is not good. Frequent nibbling also creates mouth conditions which encourage tooth decay.

At the same time each day, the child can be offered one or two of the following: fruit juice, raw vegetables such as carrot or celery strips, toast, sherbet, or plain crackers spread lightly with peanut butter or cottage cheese. If a child has a small appetite, give him skim milk rather than whole milk, milk rather than ice cream, or a fruit juice. These contain less fat, and the child is less likely to feel full at mealtime. The snack should help the appetite, not hinder it.

We should be reasonable in our expectations of little children. After all, do adults confine eating to three meals a day? Think of the popularity of the morning coffee break in America or the afternoon tea in England. Children are imitators.

Preschool Child's Meals at the Hospital

Aides from the diet department of the hospital bring meals to the pediatric floor, but usually nursing service has the responsibility of seeing that the little patients are fed. The nurses know the children by name, can get the right food to the right child, and should be able to use their knowledge of the child to help him eat well.

Pediatric nurses know they should not urge food on the child or insist that he eat food he does not want — unless the doctor specifically says to do so. All too often the child vomits the food that is urged on him.

Authorities on child feeding say:

> Don't urge food on a child whose appetite hasn't returned to normal. If you press food on him when it is still somewhat repulsive to him, you can quickly start a feeding problem which may take months to cure. If a convalescent child is not fussed with, his appetite will, when the disease is out of his system, return not just to normal, but to above normal, to make up for what he has missed.[1]

It helps the little patient to eat if mealtime is as homelike as possible. His environment is so new and different that eating may be difficult. To eliminate one tiny, minor difference may bring results.

The child who is permitted out of bed should be allowed to eat at a table. In a modern children's hospital, each room has a low table for use at mealtime. A family member, the nurse, or another child at the table will encourage the youngster to eat. If a poor eater sits between two good eaters, he may mimic them. A plastic tablecloth, vivid napkins, and artificial flowers lend a pleasant atmosphere.

For the child who has to stay in bed, it is doubly important to make mealtime happy and pleasant. He will feel more important if the food can be brought around on a hot serving table and he can see what is available. Soft music, gaily colored trays, and individual tray cloths will help, but the key to success is the attitude of the staff. Children respond quickly to a relaxed, friendly, "let's have fun" attitude.

Any device that can be worked out to interest children in food is worthwhile. Recently at one large hospital, a food tray was wrapped as a gift — more or less as a joke — and delivered to the pediatric ward. The

---

[1] Benjamin Spock and Miriam E. Lowenberg, *Feeding Your Baby and Child* (New York: Pocket Books, 1956), p. 191.

excitement it created led to gift wrapping of other food trays and more foods being consumed.

As a student nurse, regard the pediatric ward as a challenge — a challenge to adapt your knowledge of food and children to helping the young patient eat.

Questions for Discussion

1. Plan menus for a two-year-old child, a three-year-old, and a four-year-old.
2. What nutritious in-between-meal snacks might accompany these menus?
3. What desirable, and undesirable, practices of feeding children have you observed in private homes? In the hospital?
4. What can parents do when children crave (or demand) too many sweet foods?

Additional Readings

McEnery, E. T., and Margaret Jane Suydam. *Feeding Little Folks*. Chicago: National Dairy Council, 1966.

Scott, Lou Peveto. *Programmed Instruction and Review for Practical and Vocational Nursing*. Vol. 2; *Clinical and Community Nursing*, pp. 264–266. New York: The Macmillan Company, 1968.

Spock, Benjamin. *Baby and Child Care*. Rev. ed., pp. 295–307, 435–449. New York: Pocket Books, 1968.

Spock, Benjamin, and Miriam Lowenberg. *Feeding Your Baby and Child*. New York: Pocket Books, 1956.

Your Child from One to Six. Washington, D.C.: U.S. Department of Health, Education, and Welfare, Children's Bureau Publication, No. 30. Rev. 1967.

Recommended Audiovisual Aids

FILMSTRIPS

Feeding Habits (33 frames, International Film Bureau, Color)
Captions and manual. Animated drawings depict the "do's" and "don'ts" in establishing good feeding habits. It illustrates a corrective program for children who have developed poor eating habits.

How Food Is Digested (59 frames, McGraw-Hill, Color, 1948)
With photographs and cartoons, the filmstrip shows the process of digestion, illustrating the anatomy of digestive organs, enzyme action on specific foods, absorption and use of food materials in the body, elimination of undigested foods, and prevention of constipation and digestive tract disturbances. Timely and appropriate.

Nutrients in Food (57 frames, McGraw-Hill, Color, 1948)
>The filmstrip explains the use of each nutrient in the body and what nutrients are contained in various foods.

Serving Meals Attractively (40 frames, McGraw-Hill, Color)
>Pertains to selection of high quality, fresh foods; proper storage of foods; and proper cooking of foods. Illustrates the value of color contrast in foods and how to cook foods to preserve their appearance. Helpful to basic understanding of preparing good meals for both children and adults.

FILM

Food as Children See It (20 min., General Mills, Color, 1952)
>Timeless explanation that adults should try to see food as children do, as outlined by Dr. Miriam Lowenberg, child nutritionist. Good illustrations that show common child-feeding problems and suggested solutions, planning good meals for children, preparing food that the child can eat, and helping children learn to eat new foods.

CHAPTER 12 / **FEARS, HOSPITALIZATION, AND THE YOUNG CHILD**

A hospital stay can be an agonizing, frightening experience to the young child.

James Robertson theorizes that the distress of every newly admitted young patient is too painful for the doctor and nurse to tolerate. They cannot let themselves be affected repeatedly; hence they force themselves to become less sensitive so that they can care for the children.[1]

Perhaps you will have to do this. As an inexperienced student nurse in the pediatric ward, you will see the little child brought in and left with total strangers. But the child needs medical help. He may die or be handicapped for life if he does not have the benefits of modern medical knowledge. If you — the nurse who is probably closest to him — understand little children, if you know why he is afraid, you will be more likely to support him, reassure him, alleviate his fears, and possibly help him to be less disturbed when he returns home.

Some fears of young children are instinctive, normal fears of a dangerous physical situation. Other fears are learned or acquired through unpleasant environment or unfortunate incidents.

Hospitalization is particularly difficult because the situation has many elements of normal fears for little children.

Normal Fears and Anxiety Fears

A *normal* fear is reasonable fear of a truly dangerous situation. When face to face with growing danger, it would be abnormal *not* to be afraid.

An *anxiety* fear is an unreasonable, sometimes more intense, fear based on the dread of a danger that does not actually exist. It is a fear inside oneself, a deep, inner feeling of helplessness. The person who suffers from this kind of fear may feel upset or worried without knowing why. Chronic or long-continued anxiety is harmful to the child — as a child and as the adult he will become. It is important to treat all signs of anxiety seriously.

---

[1] James Robertson, *Young Children in Hospitals* (New York: Basic Books, 1958), p. 18.

The causes of normal fears are fairly well established. Infants and small children up to about the age of two are commonly afraid of falling or loss of support; of loud, unexpected noises; of sudden movements, especially when combined with noise; and of strange, unfamiliar objects, persons, or situations.[2]

Beginning at two or three, the little child fears being left alone, particularly in a strange place or in the dark. He fears pain and injury, as well as the people and objects associated with pain, such as doctors, nurses, medical instruments, and hospitals. He may fear animals that jump, wiggle, and make noises. He fears strange people who are different or crippled. He does not understand death; hence he fears it. Most important, he fears being deserted by his parents. These are normal, understandable fears.

Separation from Parents

Not only is his greatest fear that of being deserted by his parents, but their absence makes everything else more difficult to bear. A small child can take many things in his stride when his parents are near. When they are absent, the same things can be terrifying to him. He has learned from experience that unpleasant things can happen when his mother and father are away, and that he is safe when they are present. This is a normal response to a normal fear.

Hospitalization

When the child goes to the hospital, the situation has three elements of normal fear: pain, new surroundings, and absence of parents.

Think how the little child must feel. He leaves his familiar home, which seems to revolve around him. He goes into a totally new, strange place where the rooms are big, the floors are different, and the bed is not like his bed. All these people in white uniforms are strangers to him. He will probably get an injection that hurts or have surgery that leaves him in pain. He wonders: "What are all these strange objects? Why the masks? This awful bracelet on my arm is a mark. Will it always be there? Why can't I go home?" And (most important), "Where is Mommy?"

He is ill or facing a new, unknown (hence terrifying) situation and his mother is not there. The four- or five-year-old may be able to understand that his mother will be back, but not the two- or three-year-old. The two-year-old thinks, "If Mother is not here, she does not love me any more." This is desertion, jail, and punishment all in one. The child is used to his father coming and going, but mother is always supposed to be there.

[2] Nina Ridenour and Isabel Johnson, *Some Special Problems of Young Children* (New York: National Association for Mental Health, 1947), pp. 62–63.

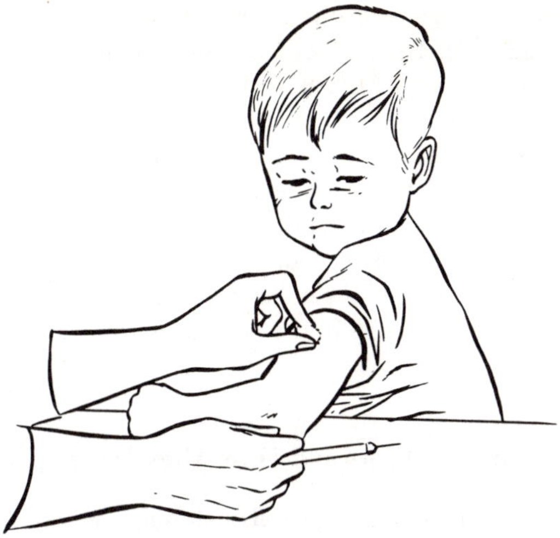

Figure 15. *Fear of pain is normal.*

Furthermore, the two-year-old cannot verbalize and cannot communicate his feelings. We adults talk when we are hurt, and this seems to help. But the child who cannot express himself becomes more frustrated and helpless.

After Hospitalization

If this temporary separation from his mother does no harm, how does one account for the personality change and the behavior problems that erupt when the child returns to his home? Dr. Florence Erickson[3] said that 33 out of 38 mothers reported that they "had an awful time when the child came home from the hospital. He was mean, sassy, sucked his thumb, or wet his pants." If the mother punished him, the child said, "I was right. She doesn't love me any more." Other forms of insecurity behavior appeared, such as nightmares, temper tantrums, clinging, hostility, and aggressiveness against the mother. Sometimes, emotional aftermaths have been known to appear even later in life.

Pediatric nurses have explained this regressive behavior by saying that all patients, adults and children, regress when ill. They are dependent. During convalescence, these barriers go down slowly as the person adjusts to the outside world again.

Yet studies show that when the mother is present during hospitalization, a relatively small amount of disturbed behavior results on the return home.[4]

---

[3] Florence Erickson, speaking on "Application of Growth and Development to Nursing" at Indiana University Medical Center, April 26, 1962, adapted remarks.
[4] A. D. Hunt and R. E. Trussell, "They Let Parents Help in Children's Care," *The Modern Hospital* (Sept. 1955).

If the mother has been with the child, the transition from hospital to the home will be undramatic. The mother is realistic and informed about the child's illness, the kind of child he is, his diet, and the care he will require. She feels she is able to continue his care.

As a child grows older, his ability to withstand separation from his parents increases. After the age of five, he is less likely to suffer harm from a hospital stay. A child of six or seven understands time and that "Mother will be back," as well as the reason for the absence of his parents. If wisely handled, many children who go to the hospital have no harmful emotional effects.

Careful handling of the child in the hospital helps to prevent anxiety fears from developing.

Anxiety Fears and How They Develop

Anxiety fears begin when a child feels unloved. The love of his parents, or of the adults caring for him, is the most important thing in his small world. When he is unsure of this love, his basic security is gone, and everything happening to him is potentially dangerous. He is filled with anxiety.

Even at home with parents who are completely devoted to him, many things can happen that cause him to fear the loss of their love. He may be hungry, or cold, or sick, or left alone for long hours, or suddenly taken care of by strangers. In many ways, he can be frustrated, deprived, or kept from receiving the reassurance of his parents' love. For instance, if a new baby arrives, the older child is jealous. He would like to hurt the baby and to hurt the parents too, but he dare not express his feelings because they might love him still less.

When we understand how anxiety develops, we see how a hospital stay could be the beginning of anxiety fears.

The anxious child has extra problems. Because everything is dangerous to him, he cannot take in his stride the normal, frightening experiences of childhood as can the better-adjusted child. The anxious child may react violently and be extremely hard to quiet. His fear may be entirely out of proportion to the thing causing it and may seem quite unrelated to it.

You will see evidences of anxiety fears in the pediatric ward. The anxious child may react to certain situations with greater violence than the adjusted child. He will probably be slow to adjust to hospital life. Experienced pediatric nurses believe that the child who can meet situations when well can adjust to hospital life.

The Frightened Child

Although we try, we cannot always prevent frightening experiences from occurring. As a student practical nurse, you may have a truly frightened child to care for. What do you do? He is not a naughty child; so scolding is not the answer.

Soothe and reassure him. If he will let you, take him in your arms. Talk to him gently, caress him, and let him feel your protection and your physical strength. He will not really understand what you are saying, so do not try to reason with him. But he will be reassured by your tone of voice and your physical presence. Never try to shock him out of his fears with threats of what may happen if he does not stop screaming. Do not shame the child with "You are too big for that," or "Only sissies are afraid." To the pediatric patient, you might be able to say truthfully, "Of course you are afraid. I would be too."

When he is a bit calm, when he is sure he is safe and protected, try to divert his attention.

Some people have the false idea that a child should be exposed immediately to the same frightening experience in order to prove the fear was groundless. A child frightened by a dog should not be forced to pat the dog so he will see that the dog does not bite. Later, *you* might pat the dog while the child watches. Wait until the child shows signs of wanting to get over his fears and help him in any way that you can. A child cannot be forced or reasoned into giving up a fear. He has to decide for himself.

To Conquer Fears

The child who has conquered normal childhood fears, or faced them squarely, has built up courage to meet the hospital situation.

The family at home can help the child to conquer fears with happy times. If a child is afraid of the dark at bedtime, his parents can strive to make bedtime a happy time. His father might spend a few minutes with him after the lights are out and let him have a flashlight to turn on or off. At the same time, the father can assure him that when he is older, he will not object to the dark. He does not have to be brave *now*.

If a child wants to talk about his fear, encourage him to express himself and to bring it out into the open. Sometimes playing games or acting out the fear helps.

Many fears can be prevented if one is on the alert for situations known to create fear. A young child might be frightened by the noise of a jet airplane if he is too close to it.

Sometimes it is possible to remove the object of fear, or to remove the child. For the one- or two-year-old, we try not to rely on language for warning. Instead of saying repeatedly, "It is hot," pick him up, deposit him in a safer spot, and direct his attention to a newer interest.

Building self-confidence in the small child helps to overcome fears. He needs to have fun with people and things, to know what to do in various situations, to plan with parents for a short visit away from home. Every new friend he makes and everything he learns to do for himself are helping him to become an independent little person who needs less reassurance from his parents.

The small child should be protected from the things that destroy confidence, such as criticism, repeated failure, too much competition, and neglect.

You, the nurse, hope the family have been careful about references to the hospital in normal conversation. Careless remarks can build up fear in the child's mind unconsciously.

To Prepare for the Hospital

A child under three really cannot be prepared for his hospital stay. He cannot understand what being without his mother means. As a nurse, however, you will be supposed to know what parents can do to prepare the young child for the hospital.

Their doctor will point the way for the family. For the planned hospitalization, the pediatrician should help them to choose a time when the child has the least stress in his life. If the child's personal world is upset by the arrival of a new baby, or if he is going through a phase of undue dependency on his mother, perhaps the scheduled operation can be postponed. Naturally, sudden illness leaves no choice.

The physician may give the family a cartoon booklet that will help familiarize the youngster with the hospital atmosphere. Some hospitals have slide talks or motion pictures to show the parents how to reduce fear in the children. Some of the booklets and movies designed for the children portray hospital equipment — X-ray machines and oxygen tents — as friendly cartoon characters whose job it is to help children get well fast. These are of more value to the older child than to the youngster under four years of age.

An unexpected dividend from the television medical programs is that children are familiar with doctors and nurses in white uniforms, the inside of hospital rooms, and hospital equipment. Unless the detailed television show has frightened them, they may associate "getting well" with the hospital.

The child feels more secure if he regards the doctor as his friend. Sometimes the child can actually visit the hospital prior to his admittance as a patient. It would be ideal if he could also meet the nurse and get to know her.

The doctor, and you, the nurse, must emphasize to the parents that they should tell the child truthfully, in a matter-of-fact manner, what will happen at the hospital. The amount of detail and information depends on the age of the child. They should avoid stressing details that will make him afraid, such as that he may have repeated injections or enemas. No question should be answered falsely, that is, if parents want their child to continue to believe them. He can be

Fears, Hospitalization, and the Young Child

told that some things will hurt, but he will be able to stand the pain, and later he will feel better.

Often the child is permitted to bring from home a favorite toy or blanket. If the mother also packs in the suitcase "clothes to wear home from the hospital," her morale may be bolstered at a sorely needed time. If parents can be calm and matter-of-fact, the youngster will be less apprehensive.

Acquaint the parents with the hospital visiting hours, so that they will be truthful with the child when they leave. Would you like to be the night nurse who is asked by a child at 2 A.M., "Please get my Mommy. She told me she would be downstairs." Perhaps this child sleeps right through the night at home, but at the hospital he wakens and wants his mother.

New Trends in Pediatrics

Progressive hospital administrators are constantly revising policies of handling children to eliminate old-fashioned practices that were unnecessarily harsh and disturbing to children. Drastic changes have taken place in many hospitals.

When a policy has been observed for many years, people tend to think, "This is the way it is done. It can be no other way." Change is difficult.

Dr. Milton Senn, director of the Child Study Center at Yale University, believes the training of nurses, doctors, and hospital administrators to be at the heart of the matter. In the foreword to Robertson's book, *Young Children in Hospitals*, Dr. Senn writes:

> Unless these people [doctors, nurses, and hospital administrators] ... develop insights into human behavior when they are in the formative periods of their professional lives, they will have difficulty later in renouncing the biases fostered by traditional practices.[5]

Dr. Senn might well be talking to you, the student practical nurse.

You are looking at the pediatric ward with a fresh, new viewpoint. Keep an open mind, and ask yourself "Why? Why?" when a child shows disturbed or problem behavior.

Why did it take three nurses and a doctor to change this four-year-old boy's clothes? Why did he object? Did he really have to change into hospital garments right then?

At random, these are improved hospital policies: There are relaxed visiting hours for parents. When the mother visits, she is encouraged to hold her child on her lap. When the child is admitted, only one resident physician sees him in the admitting room. The mother accompanies the child to his room and helps him to

---

[5] James Robertson, *Young Children in Hospitals* (New York: Basic Books, 1958), p. 18.

get acquainted. The nurse fills out the questionnaire, noting the child's expression for "bathroom," etc. No blood work, no "pricking," is done the first day. Team nursing reduces the number of strangers the child encounters. If a team of two nurses takes him through a series of tests, there is no longer a parade of strange technicians into his room. Everyone observes the precept "handle with care." Most important, the mother is regarded as part of the team to help her child to get well. At some hospitals, she can "room-in."

Work with the Mother

Regarding the child's mother as the enemy who handicaps her child's progress is wrong.

True, the child's mother may not understand that she can be a problem to the nurses. She does not have the information that the nurses have, and it is *her child* who is sick. Sometimes the child is more difficult to handle when his mother is in the room. He feels secure enough to express his feelings, and he lets the nurse know how he feels. If his mother is not there, he has the same feelings but perhaps not the courage to express them.

The nurses should take time to instruct the mother and teach her how to handle the child. The mother may be reluctant to do anything for her child because she feels inferior and inadequate. The efficient nurse who handles her child so well may appear in her eyes to be a rival for the child's affection.

With a short hospitalization, not every mother is capable and calm enough to assist the nurses. But many mothers are, and it would be unreasonable to exclude every mother because some cannot adjust.

The child's mother can learn many things from observing the care given to children in the hospital. The kind of food served to the children or the cleanliness routines followed may be new to her. A far greater carry-over into the home is possible if the mother is included as part of the team to help the child recover.

In hospitals where parents help to care for the child, the nurse's role is that of mother supplement, not mother substitute. Nurses who have made the change feel that the benefits are far-reaching.

One word of caution. Some doctors have noted that fewer nursing rounds are made when parents are visiting.[6]

Cues for the Nurse

As a student practical nurse, you do not decide hospital policies or make the rules. You follow orders. But you are responsible for your own attitude toward

---

[6] Florence Erickson, *Therapeutic Relationship of Nurse to Parents of a Sick Child* (Columbus, Ohio: Ross Laboratories, 1965).

the children and their parents, and this is the keynote to successful nursing care of young patients.

Let the child express rebellion. Many things are happening that he does not like. You can let him know that you understand and still insist that he take his medicine.

The quiet, docile child is not the goal in a pediatric ward. Normal behavior is *not* withdrawn and submissive. Actually, a nurse should feel complimented when a child fights back, expresses anger, or gripes.

Encourage the child to do as much as possible for himself. Let him help you. Let him see and handle the nursing equipment before it is used on him. Explain as much as you can to him. Remember that if explanations to a child are to be effective, they must be in terms of things that he can see, touch, or taste. After you have explained, carry out the procedure as soon as possible. Delays will make him apprehensive.

Warn the child of pain and how painful the procedure will be. When possible, avoid forceful handling of the child.

When he is brave, be generous with approval. A good nurse eternally gives reassurance to patients, but especially to the child.

You need an unhurried attitude with children. Give the impression, "This child is the most important person in the whole world."

To be a good pediatric nurse, you must have genuine acceptance and love for children. The child has uncanny perception. He may not understand all that is going on, but if you like him, he will know it. He will want to please you. He needs to be able to trust you.

Be patient with the child's mother. Help her, and let her help you whenever possible. The more she is involved in the care of her child, the better are the child's chances for a fast recovery and for fewer emotional problems when he returns home.

Questions for Discussion

1. Should there be limited or unlimited visiting hours in pediatric wards?
2. What are the regulations concerning visitors in the hospital where you train as a student nurse?
3. In your hospital, what is the attitude toward the child's mother? What provisions are made for her to stay overnight?
4. Give an illustration of a child who was able to overcome a fear. Was it easy?

Additional Readings

Berger, Knute, and others. *A Visit to the Doctor.* New York: Grosset & Dunlap, Inc., 1960.

Blake, Florence G., and others. *Nursing Care of Children.* 8th ed., pp. 444–454. Philadelphia: J. B. Lippincott Company, 1970.

Department of National Health and Welfare, Ottawa, Canada (reprinted by Indiana State Board of Health, Indianapolis). *Preparing Your Child for the Hospital.*

Dimock, Hedley C. *The Child in the Hospital.* Philadelphia: F. A. Davis Company, Publishers, 1960.

Jaeger, Margaret Ann. *Child Development and Nursing Care.* "Emotional Reactions," pp. 128–151. New York: The Macmillan Company, 1962.

Ridenour, Nina, and Isabel Johnson. *Some Special Problems of Young Children.* "When a Child Has Fears," p. 61–71. New York: National Association for Mental Health, Inc., 1947.

Robertson, James. *Hospitals and Children: A Parent's Eye View.* New York: International Universities Press, 1963.

Robertson, James. *Young Children in Hospitals.* New York: Basic Books, Inc., 1958.

Spock, Benjamin. *Baby and Child Care.* Rev. ed., pp. 462–469. New York: Pocket Books, Inc., 1968.

Spock, Benjamin, and Marion O. Lerrigo. *Caring for Your Disabled Child.* pp. 79–92. New York: The Macmillan Company, 1965.

Recommended Audiovisual Aids

FILMSTRIP

Fear (28 frames, International Film Bureau, Color)
   Filmstrip with captions and manual. Animated drawings depict normal fears of children, then show some common signs of deeper fears.

FILMS

Fears of Children (29 min., International Film Bureau, B&W)
   Excellent film showing how the normal fears of a five-year-old boy can be amplified and develop into anxiety fears by two factors: the father's desire for his son to show manliness, and the mother's instinct to coddle her child. Possible solutions are given.

Children in the Hospital (44 min., International Film Bureau, B&W)
   Films of children in Boston City Hospital that show their problems in adjusting to the hospital, particularly problems stemming from anxiety. It depicts the ranges of behavior in ages 4 to 8 in pediatric wards, problems such as symptoms of terror because the mother has left the child, and possible solutions, for example, encouraging the child to talk and to play out his fears. The film would be especially helpful if shown for orientation to pediatrics.

CHAPTER 13 / RECREATION FOR THE SICK

CHILD

Every child, well or sick, lives through play. Play to the child is everything that work, recreation, education, exploration, and self-expression are to the adult. Through play activities, a child learns about the world in which he lives. He gets rid of frustration, anger, and anxiety. He learns what is acceptable behavior and what is not acceptable. He learns how to get along with people.

A rich environment offers the child an abundance of playthings, a place to play, playmates, and freedom to use his toys as he wishes. These help a child to learn and to use the mental capacity with which he was born.

A poor environment with little opportunity to play, no playmates, and few toys will actually slow a child's learning. He will not progress as he could.

All children pass through the different stages of play. Some children remain longer at one stage than other children. A child with a history of illnesses might be expected to enjoy play typical of a child younger than his chronological years.

Problems of the Convalescent Child

The hospital- or home-confined child is deprived of the normal contacts with people and the daily activities that ordinarily help a child to learn. Parents and nurses should strive to make the convalescent child's play as meaningful as possible without tiring him. He needs his strength to get well.

As soon as the pain has gone, the sick child wants to play. It may be impossible for him to understand why he should be quiet, rest, or stay in bed. He may get bored, fussy, and irritable.

The alert, mischievous child may cause trouble and extra work at home and at the hospital. But remember, this is the way we want him to be. He should be mentally alert, eager for action, and maybe a bit hard to keep quiet. He is acting normal when he thinks for himself. We are the most concerned about the child who begins to "vegetate" in bed or wheelchair, a truly pitiful sight. Without recreation and activity, this can happen to the child with a long convalescence or with a chronic illness. It is especially easy for the child at home to sink gradually into this state.

The homebound, handicapped child desperately needs to see people other than his own family. The situation can get serious, sometimes even grim.

The nurse needs to be aware of these pitfalls and to be able to help families facing these problems.

Community Help

Many communities have organized ways of helping children confined to their homes. A home teacher is often available to help the school-age child keep up with his schoolwork. In some cities, a "lend-a-toy" agency has been established to lend toys to homebound children. If the child goes regularly to the rehabilitation center for treatment, he sees the outside world. He may suffer less than the child who is strictly confined to his home.

In New York City, the Handicapped Children's Home Service has voluntary recreation workers who make weekly calls on homebound children. The visitor brings supervised recreation and companionship into the home for both the child and his family.

Your own community may have a unique method of helping homebound children.

If you are fortunate enough to train as a student in a children's hospital, you can learn much by observing how recreation is handled.

A modern children's hospital has a playroom for ambulatory patients. The staff may be recreation workers, occupational therapists, nurses, or even nursery school teachers. These people know not only how to keep children active within limits, but also how to help them act out their feelings about hospitalization. Since children benefit the most from their play within range of a trusted adult, the staff should be constant.

Sometimes a "cheer guild" or organized volunteers will buy toys and give parties for the children.

However, some general-hospital staffs have neither paid nor volunteer workers who are responsible for the children's play program. This duty may fall onto the general-duty nurse, who may someday be you. The licensed practical nurse needs many resources at her fingertips.

Play Helps the Hospitalized Child

Appropriate play activities can help the child to cope with the tension, frustration, and anxieties he will likely experience in the hospital. His limited vocabulary does not allow him to find relief in words as many adults do; play can be his one form of expression.

For example, many children in hospitals will "take it out" on their dolls or teddy bears. Certainly it is better to turn aggressive feelings toward the dolls

Recreation for the Sick Child 119

than toward self-destruction. It is still better if the children have play materials that promote more constructive play, and fewer guilt feelings. Doll clothes, doll beds and blankets, and bowls of water for washing and bathing — all engage the youngsters in play activities. Often children in hospitals play "Nurse and Doctor" instead of "Mother and Father" as they do at home. With old stethoscopes, bandages, and used plastic syringes with needles removed, they can "play out" traumatic episodes, carrying out on the doll the traumatic experiences they must endure.

Types of Activity for the Sick Child

JUST WATCHING

A child's first activity after pain has ceased must be very simple. He may be fascinated to watch movements of a balloon attached to a light fixture, paper mobiles hung on a miniature clothesline, an old-fashioned hourglass, or goldfish in an aquarium.

Other suggestions are a magnifying glass and a tray of small objects that can be enlarged — buttons, rice grains, or tiny flowers; a pocket mirror "to catch the sunlight"; after dark, a miniature flashlight; and an easily handled record player with a supply of records.

Holiday and seasonal decorations may interest him — the Christmas tree and wreaths, jack-o'-lanterns, spring flowers, or autumn leaves.

ATTENTION SPAN

The convalescent child's attention span is usually shorter than when he feels well. He may turn frequently from one activity to another; hence he will need a greater variety of playthings. Many toys will be enjoyed for a short time only, but he should have some activities that promote a longer attention span. The child may be intrigued enough with a picture puzzle to want to complete it. Simple puzzles can be made from a picture postcard or any favorite picture mounted on cardboard.

SIMPLE ACTIVITIES

While recuperating, a child enjoys activities that are easier than those he normally undertakes. When he feels under par, his abilities are under par, too.

Some children like to string beads or to sort the buttons in mother's button box. Shell macaroons, dyed, are easy and fun to string. Sewing cards with big holes and large cords are easy to handle, and the child gets amazing results without much effort. Making a paper chain from the kit is simple. Paper folding has endless possibilities. Show the child how to fold an accordion-pleated fan; a model plane; or a boat with figures in it. By cutting, it is easy to fold dolls or animals.

Choose materials that are light and easy to handle. The convalescent child has no extra energy; so avoid heavy or bulky materials. Remember that children like clear, bright colors. Handling pretty fabrics with interesting textures gives pleasure to children as well as adults.

GIFTS

Illness tends to make us self-centered. If the sick child makes a gift for someone else, he is turning his attention outward and thinking of others.

A child might decorate boxes of all sizes and shapes, such as hatboxes or matchboxes to serve as pillboxes. He may enjoy making bookmarks as gifts.

STUDY OF TOY SELECTION

A university hospital study revealed the following toys to be especially valuable for the sick-in-bed child:

> A small, unpainted, washable wooden train with tracks and blocks; building blocks of plastic, rubber or wood; two or three small cars with blocks for a garage and street; small animals with blocks for barn and fences; interlocking figures of wood or plastic; magic blackboards and slates; picture and storybooks; colored trees, cones, and towers that can be taken apart and put back together; push-button marionettes and puppets; pounding sets; and a xylophone.[1]

Also recommended were the various "let's-make-it" kits and activity kits, such as doll-washing kits, baking outfits, tea party sets, dress-up kits for cowboys and Indians, paper chain kits, paper doll kits, airplane kits, and numerous others. Some preschool children would find certain kits too advanced; other children would not. The family and the nurse should be realistic about the child's ability. If he attempts a task too difficult for him, he will become discouraged.

Most hospital occupational therapists avoid toys and games that have several essential parts. The loss of one part may ruin the child's pleasure in the toy and cause undue fretting. The nurse usually does not have time to hunt for the lost piece.

CREATIVE ACTIVITIES

To stimulate thinking along imaginative avenues, let the child have materials that he can use to mold, draw, or paint as he wishes. Chalk and a small

---

[1] University Hospital School of the University of Michigan, Ann Arbor, as reported by Mildred H. Walton, "Toys and the Hospital Nurse" (New York: American Toy Institute.)

Recreation for the Sick Child

blackboard, crayons and paper can be a source of endless activity. Younger children enjoy temporary art work. If the design is not just what the child wishes, he can quickly and easily dismantle or erase it, then try again. Mosaic games, pegboards, wax and clay modeling, or blackboard work can be changed at will. Youngsters who wish their work to be lasting will enjoy finger painting, spatter painting, and crayoning. Crayons for small children should be the jumbo crayons. The younger the child, the bigger the crayon he needs.

Children love to "mess," so provide for "messy play," which can also be a good antidote to the unnatural state of cleanliness and order around the hospitalized child. Fingerpaints, sand, water, and clay or dough are excellent play material. Furthermore, play with these materials gives the child a legitimate outlet for the destructive feelings of anger, resentment, and frustration inherent in the hospital situation.

Finger paints should be used on shiny-surfaced papers, such as white shelf paper. Of course, safeguard the child's clothes and surroundings with a huge apron and lots of newspaper.

Make your own finger paints following these directions: Cream 1 cup of starch and ½ cup of cold water. Add 1½ cups of boiling water and ½ cup of soap flakes, then 1 tablespoon of glycerine. When the mixture is cool, add food-coloring tablets. Keep the mixture in tightly closed bottles to retard spoiling.

Hang the child's completed finger painting in a conspicuous place or plan to use it to cover a wastebasket or to wrap gift packages.

To make your own watercolor paints, dissolve shavings from crayons in nonflammable cleaning fluid or soak colored crepe paper in water.

Thin water paint and raw vegetables can be used for a kind of block printing. Cut the vegetables crosswise or lengthwise, dip in paint, and press firmly on paper or cloth. Carrots, potatoes, green peppers, and onions make pretty designs.

Both boys and girls like modeling clay, commercial or homemade. Give the child a tray on which to work and toothpicks or pipe cleaners to form arms and legs on the clay figures.

DRAMATIC AND IMITATIVE PLAY

Children are great imitators, and until they reach the age of five, there is little real dramatic play. Their play is mainly imitation of what they see and hear.

The toy telephone encourages quiet dramatic or imitative play. The mother or nurse can enter into the play. Dreaded medicines are not as terrifying if the child "receives a call" that treatment is on the way. Toy telephones can also be used by one child to talk to another child.

Dolls can be real comfort, for they furnish companionship for the isolated

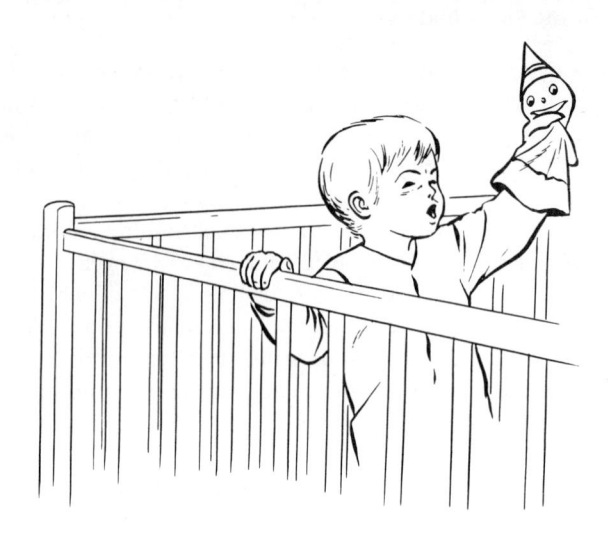

Figure 16. *The hand puppet can help a child to talk about his fear, and to act out aggressive or hostile feelings.*

child. As the child is able to move about, the doll accessories encourage quiet play – the dollhouse and furniture, the doll bed, and the doll carriage.

Children like to play "make-believe," and it helps them to relax. One student nurse told of the enjoyment she and her young son had with the imaginary "hide-and-seek" game they played while he was recuperating. "For two days, I couldn't guess where he was hiding. Finally, he told me. He imagined that he was hiding on the tip of my nose."

The nurse who enters into the imaginary play of children takes on the character of a playmate, and she may receive greater cooperation when treatment time comes. Also, this imaginative play demands very little extra time of the nurse because it takes place while she works.

Hand puppets help when the child is undergoing a trying experience, such as changing bandages. Let the child make the puppet do what the nurse suggests as she works.

TOWARD SOCIALIZATION

Social development progresses slowly when children are well; so we can anticipate that the development will be slower when a child's contacts and activities are limited.

Some toys and activities need to be shared. The five-year-olds can learn to play "old maid" or similar games. Younger children can share a set of toy dishes. A wagon can transport several toys. Social consciousness really begins with the school-age child.

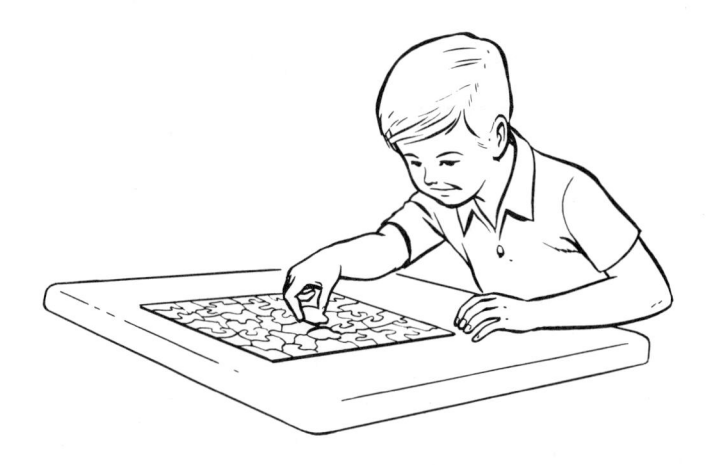

Figure 17. *Completing a jigsaw puzzle gives the child a sense of achievement and self-confidence.*

Most toys, however, are used alone. Avoid giving the child a game or toy he cannot enjoy alone.

SHARING FAMILY LIFE

With a little thought from the others, the child convalescing at home can feel that he is part of the family. In many little ways, he might help with the housework. He might fold paper napkins so that they are ready to use; wax the dustpan; or polish the silver. Organizing mother's button box may be more recreational than useful, but it is intriguing to some children. If the convalescent can keep up with the school and play activities of his healthy brothers and sisters, he may be more interested in other people and less self-centered.

Storybooks and the Little Patient

Storybooks, useful in helping to keep a youngster quiet, also help him to develop into an interesting individual.

In many ways, stories and poetry help a child to learn. He learns principles that are more impressive in story form than when presented bluntly. He learns new words and he increases his vocabulary. Good stories will also stimulate his imagination and spur his curiosity, both essential if the child is to use his intelligence to the fullest capacity.

Storybooks can help the hospitalized child to keep pace with events occurring in the world outside. Remember how quickly the word "sputnik" was added to our vocabularies? The right story can help children to keep abreast of such events.

SELECTION OF THE STORY

Careful selection of the story is important.

Does the story have action? Does it have a good ending? Does it promote ideals of good conduct? Does the story appeal to the child's imagination or sense of beauty? Is the story short enough to hold the child's interest? Would the story frighten or disturb the child? Does the subject of the story interest him? Is the story suited to the child's age level?

The characters in the story should be tolerant toward persons of a different race or religion and sympathetic toward handicapped people. The storybook policeman should be the mythical child's friend, just as we want the child to regard the policeman on the corner as his friend.

THE BOOK

Examine the book before giving it to the sick child.

Is the book light enough and small enough to hold easily? (Little children like little books.) Is the book printed in large, clear type? Does it have simple illustrations with action or story interest? Are the cover, the paper, and the binding durable? (The book may be handled roughly.) Is the content of suitable length? (A thick book may discourage the child; a thin book may interest him more.)

INFLUENCE OF ILLNESS ON SELECTION

The sick child loves funny stories and humorous poetry. He chuckles over the ridiculous. The hospitalized child wants "happy-family" stories, with a mother, a father, a little boy or girl, where everything is *right*.

Avoid stories that frighten, such as the version of "Little Red Riding Hood" where the wolf eats the grandmother. Avoid books with weird illustrations, such as tree branches shaped like fingers. If a child is receiving medication, his dreaming may be affected, and he may become disturbed or frightened by such pictures.

Try not to cross the sick child. We can often humor him in his choice of a story more easily than in his desire for other things. One child wanted stories only about chickens. The story of "Chicken Little" delighted him. Later, after a good relationship was established with the nurse, she succeeded in switching the child's interest to stories about ducks.

Above all, keep the story simple. For the sick child, one picture mounted on stiff cardboard may be enough to amuse him.

THE STORY HOUR

The story hour can help to foster a good relationship between the nurse and her young patient, just as it helps parents to establish good parent-child

Recreation for the Sick Child

relationships. It seems to satisfy the child's need for special attention from the adult and assures him of affection.

Particularly can this be a confidence-building hour if the nurse permits the child to interrupt the story with questions. If she answers his questions seriously, the child begins to realize that he can bring his problems to the nurse.

Little children usually have a favorite story that they like to hear read again and again. It is like an old friend to the children. For a variation, let the child "read" the story to you.

Children like sound effects, particularly repetition, in stories and poems.

They like gay pictures with a story if the book is read to them. No pictures are needed for the story that is made up and told to them.

A story-telling hour in the pediatric ward of one hospital was genuine playtime, with the children acting out the stories.[2] One person assumed the role of the "story lady," and the little children soon looked forward to her regular visits. (She may be a nurse, a student nurse, or a nonprofessional person.)

The three-, four-, and five-year-olds clapped hands in rhythm as nursery rhymes were chanted. "Little Miss Muffet" was chanted faster and faster as the spider frightened her away, and the children howled with laughter. Then "Little Boy Blue" faded away to a mere whisper as he was found "fast asleep." This set up a deep conspiracy between the "story lady" and the little patients.

A small, burned patient, lying under a canopy to keep the sheet from touching his tender legs, was entranced with the idea that he was an Indian living in a tent. It made an excellent opening for the legend of Hiawatha, the Indian boy.

Questions for Discussion

1. Find out what is done for homebound children in your community.
2. What recreational activities have you observed in the pediatric wards of your hospital? What could be added? Who supervises the children's play?
3. Get acquainted with any volunteer agencies that may help with the entertainment of children at your hospital.
4. What activities have you found successful for entertaining the sick child at home?
5. Some member of your class might contact a children's librarian and ask her to bring to class a set of children's books. Evaluate the stories that might be especially good for the hospitalized child.

BOOKS

Hartley, Ruth E., and Robert M. Goldenson. *The Complete Book of Children's Play*. Rev. ed. Chap. 17, "The Doctor Prescribes the Play." New York: Thomas Y. Crowell Company, 1963.

---

[2] Ethel M. Reese, "The Story Lady Nurse," *Nursing World* (Oct. 1958), pp. 15–17.

Johnson, June. *Home Play for the Preschool Child*. New York: Harper and Brothers, 1957.
Johnson, June. *838 Ways to Amuse a Child*. New York: Harper and Brothers, 1960.
Johnson, Pauline. *Creating with Paper*. Seattle: University of Washington Press, 1958.
Spock, Benjamin, and Marion O. Lerrigo. *Caring for Your Disabled Child*, p. 185–210. New York: The Macmillan Company, 1965.

PERIODICALS

Child Life Magazine
1100 Waterway Boulevard
Indianapolis, Indiana 46202

Children's Digest
Published by Parents' Magazine Enterprise, Inc.
Subscription Office: Bergenfield, New Jersey 07621

Highlights for Children
2300 West Fifth Avenue
Columbus, Ohio

Ideas Unlimited
Shulman Graff, Inc.
5865 North Lincoln Avenue
Chicago 45, Illinois

Jack and Jill
Independence Square
Philadelphia, Pennsylvania 19106

McCall's Needlework and Crafts
230 Park Avenue
New York 17, New York

Pack-O-Fun
Park Ridge Hobby Shop
30 Main Street
Park Ridge, Illinois

Recommended Audiovisual Aids

FILMSTRIP

Toys and Activities for the Preschool Child (59 frames, J. C. Penney Co., Color; with record, about 18 min., 1969).
    This filmstrip contains many good photographs of a variety of children's toys and play activities. Commentary explains the basic purpose of toys, and that play is serious business to the child. Pictures could serve as a basis for a discussion of greater depth. This filmstrip with record may be most useful in introducing the study of play.

PART IV / *The Family in the Middle Years*

CHAPTER 14 / THE FAMILY WITH

SCHOOLCHILDREN

Family life when the children have advanced beyond the preschool age, but are still at home with the parents, has been described as the nicest time of all.

Often the family with elementary school children also has younger ones at home. A distinct line cannot be drawn between families with preschool children and families with schoolchildren. But the nurse should realize that family life changes as the children enter school.

The family with older children is drawn more into community life. We shall consider community life and community resources for families along with the school life for children.

Characteristics of Family Life

Home life changes when the children enter grade school and then high school. The household buzzes with activity in the morning, in the evening, and at noon if the children return for lunch. During other hours, life at home is fairly quiet.

For the mother, life is much less difficult physically without little children who require constant supervision. She has more time and more energy at her disposal. If she develops interests of her own now, it will be easier to let her children become independent when the time comes. Both parents are drawn into community life. The mother becomes active in the PTA or as a Boy Scout den mother. The father's services are needed to supervise or help equip the playground. The family becomes acquainted with the neighborhood and broadens its outlook.

Expenses continue to mount as children grow older. Their clothes and recreation cost as much as the adults'. They have school expenses. Expenses reach the highest peak with teenagers and with college students. Father's income is higher, but usually not enough to cover increased expenses. For this reason, many mothers seek outside employment when the children enter school. The extra income may be necessary for the family to maintain what they regard as a minimum standard of living. The children do not need to suffer from mother's absence from the home. Often youngsters benefit if they are allowed to assume appropriate responsibilities, to become more independent, and to feel that they are "part of the team." This implies adequate supervision of the children when mother is away before or after school.

Changes in Family Relationships

The children gradually become less dependent on their parents and more independent. The parents find that tactful guidance is more effective than strict commands.

Children need the companionship of their father. Often the majority of their schoolteachers are women. If the mother is the only guiding hand at home, the children are completely under feminine influence.

The parents may have opportunity for recreation as a couple now that the children spend time with their friends. We say "sometimes," because transportation can be a stumbling block. One father insisted that they find a home that was within walking distance of the school, the swimming pool, the golf course, and the motion picture theater. He said, "I don't want to spend all my time as a chauffeur."

But as the children acquire interests outside the home, the family can easily grow apart. Mutual interests need emphasis. Backyard barbecues, picnics in the park, and family vacations can be enjoyed by everyone. The increased popularity of camping trips may indicate that families are discovering the pleasures of outdoor living. A vacation in a state or national park may appeal to the entire family.

Influence of the School

The schools are assuming more and more responsibility for the total child. Certain areas formerly considered home responsibility are now taken over by the school. Sex education is given in some schools. Boys and girls get exercise in physical education classes. Home economics classes help girls to develop skills, knowledge, and healthy attitudes toward homemaking.

Because school guidance varies so greatly from community to community, the nurse should learn what is being done in her area. She may expect to find more guidance in city schools than in rural schools. Generally, only vocational guidance is attempted. The schools are seldom qualified to handle personality counseling with children. The trend is to bring more nonteachers into the program (psychologists and social workers) and to handle problems within the school system, not refer the child to someone on the outside.

Parents are often overwhelmed by the extent of the influence the school has upon their children.

Housing Needs of the Family

Greatest demands on the house are made at this time. There is much wear and tear on the house and its furnishings as children are in and out of each other's homes.

Living space is at a premium. Parents need space for their activities and their friends. Children need space for their interests.

Storage facilities are strained to the utmost. There must be place for the baseball equipment, the ice skates, the fishing tackle, the golf clubs, the family of dolls, and all the other items that children collect.

There is a great need for privacy. The child needs space to withdraw from the family. If each child cannot have his own room, he should have space for his own personal possessions — his own desk and his own drawer space.

The atmosphere of the home is extremely important.

Illness Disrupts Home Life

Illness in the home can completely disrupt the lives of schoolchildren. It is difficult for children to remain quiet. They like to play games, to watch television, to act silly, and to entertain their friends. It is a tragedy for the child if these are forbidden.

Also, illness can bring most unwelcome expenses. The nurse should realize how doubly difficult all of this is for the family.

Setting up a home sickroom withdraws a great amount of living space from use by the family. The home care of patients, as discussed later, may be especially difficult if the family has schoolchildren.

Questions for Discussion

1. Explain why illness would be doubly difficult for a mother or father with school-age or adolescent children.
2. What provisions can a family make to give privacy to school-age children?
3. What are the boy's organizations in your community that are supervised by men?
4. Name vacation places that you believe are particularly suited for the entire family.

Additional Readings

Duvall, Evelyn Millis. *Family Living*, pp. 339–341. New York: The Macmillan Company, 1961.

Guiding Children's Social Growth. Better Living Booklet. Chicago: Science Research Associates, Inc., 1951.

Hartley, Ruth E., and Robert M. Goldenson. *The Complete Book of Children's Play.* 2nd ed. Chap. 18, "Fun on the Town." New York: Thomas Y. Crowell Company, 1963.

Your Child from 6 to 12. Washington, D.C.: U.S. Department of Health, Education, and Welfare, Children's Bureau Publication No. 324. Rev. 1966.

Recommended Audiovisual Aids

FILMS

The Bright Side (23 min., International Film Bureau, B&W)
  The film depicts the worries of parenthood (child crying, finances, health problems) and the brighter side of parenthood, the satisfaction of bringing up children to be self-reliant.

Right from the Start (25 min., U.S. Public Health Service, Color)
  The setting shows a public health nurse getting children to a clinic for immunization and discovering a case of diphtheria. The film stresses the importance of early immunization and the need to provide children with love, security, and safety. The simple explanation of immunization would aid classes in communicable disease.

CHAPTER 15 / THE SIX- TO TWELVE-YEAR-OLD

The schoolchild is no longer completely dependent on his parents. He can take hospitalization in his stride if he is treated with thoughtfulness and kindness. He is curious about everything, and he asks a lot of questions. Many things can frighten him, but he will try to understand your explanations about the hospital and nursing procedures. He is accustomed to being away from his parents for short intervals, and he can understand that "Mother will be back."

Many people expect too much from a ten-year-old child. They believe that when a child can look after his own physical needs — dress himself, feed himself, bathe, go to and from school safely — he is an independent person. Among certain ethnic (racial) groups and in certain communities, parents do wonderfully well raising a child until he reaches the age of nine or ten. Then he is placed almost completely "on his own." He goes and comes as he pleases and is accountable to no one. Is it coincidental that among these same ethnic groups and same communities, the rates of juvenile delinquency and crime are high? Of course, many other factors are involved, as these are disorganized areas. But to expect a child of ten to make adult decisions wisely is expecting too much, too soon.

Physical Growth

Important development takes place during the school years, but the rate of growth is slow. The growth records charts (Figs. 18 and 19) can be used to follow a child's progress, which is more realistic than comparing his growth with his companions. The charts show reasonable normal ranges for height (tall, average, and short) and weight (heavy, average, and light). Growth rate varies with the individual child.

Healthy children are extremely active. They cannot sit quietly for any length of time. They play vigorously and wholeheartedly and then collapse with exhaustion. Rest is absolutely necessary. All of these typical traits have a physical basis. The nurse who understands these causes will be better able to help families carry out health rules and recommendations.

Muscle Development

A child's muscles are more delicate and less firmly attached than adult muscles. This means they are more awkward and less efficient. The child tires easily but recovers quickly. He needs frequent rest periods.

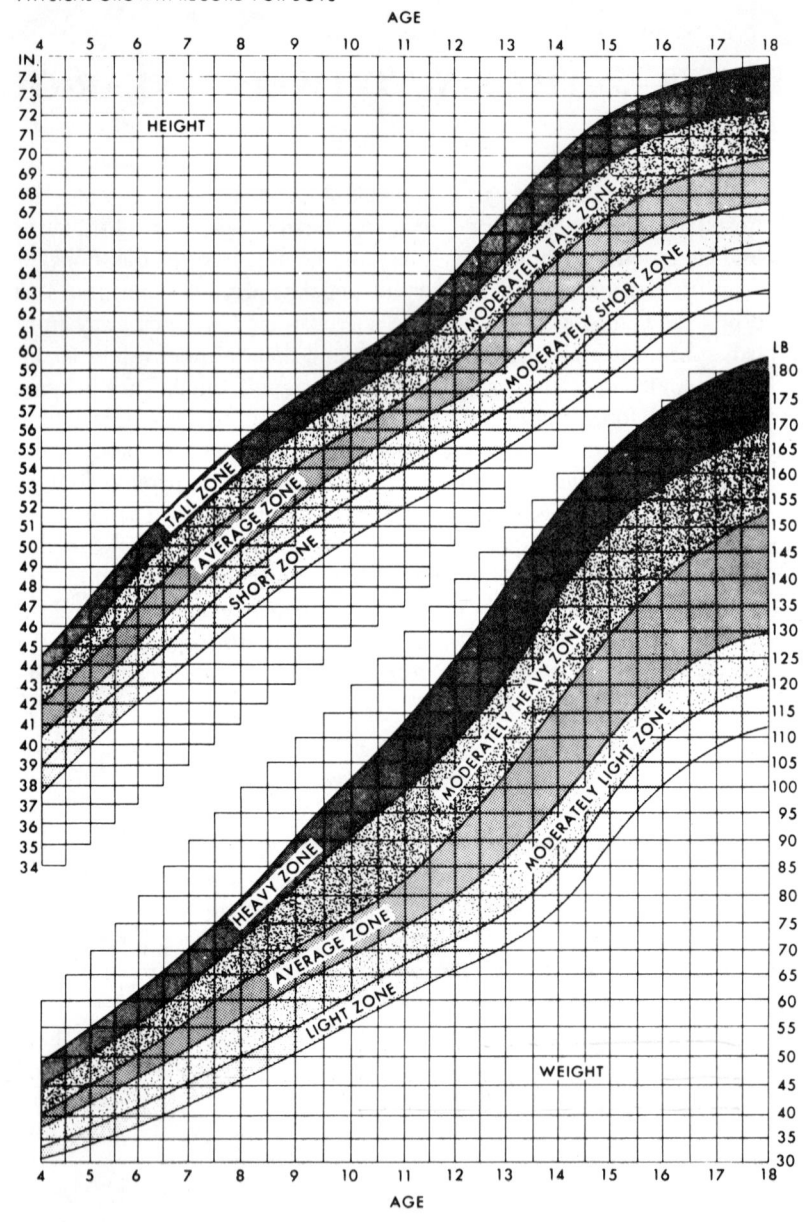

Figure 18. *Physical growth record for boys. (Adapted from* Today's Health, *December 1960 issue, published by the American Medical Association. Charts prepared by the Joint Committee on Health Problems in Education of the National Education Association and the American Medical Association, using data prepared by Howard Meredith, State University of Iowa.)*

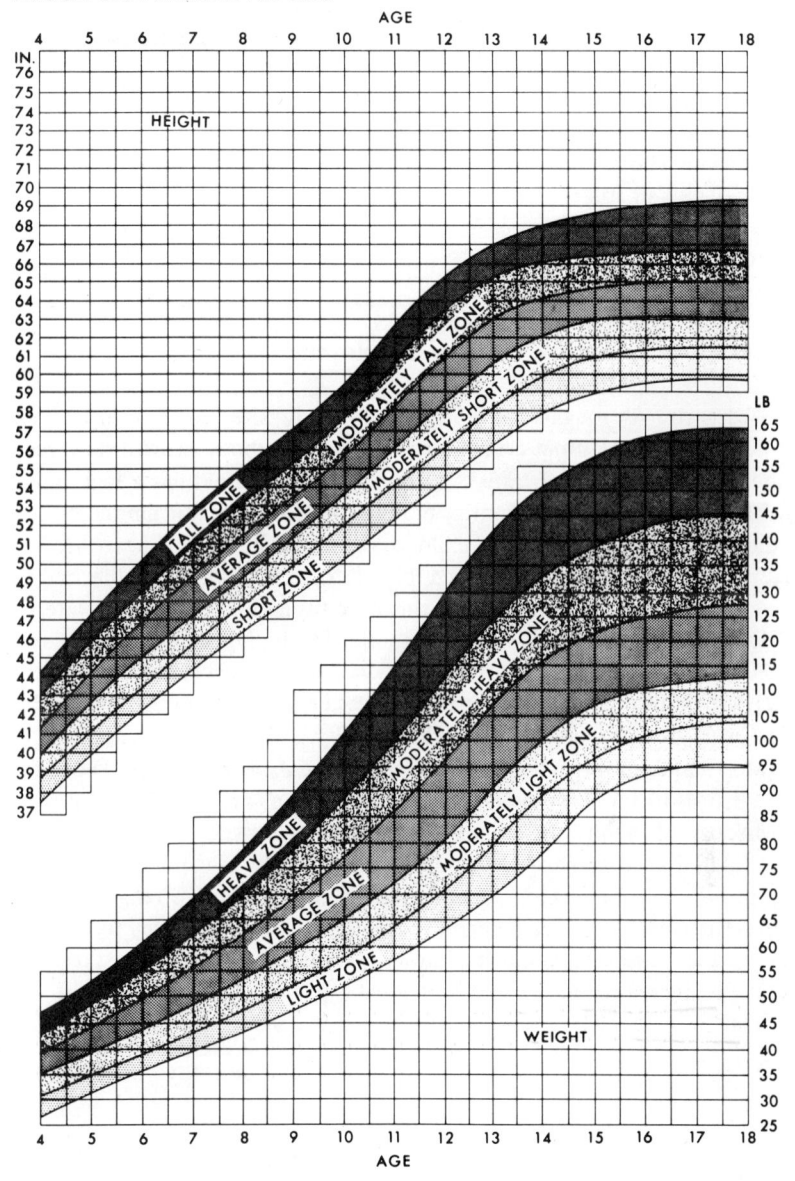

Figure 19. *Physical growth record for girls. (Adapted from* Today's Health, *December 1960 issue, published by the American Medical Association. Charts prepared by the Joint Committee on Health Problems in Education of the National Education Association and the American Medical Association, using data prepared by Howard Meredith, State University of Iowa.)*

To maintain any part of the body in a rigid position requires considerable muscle effort. The schoolchild cannot do this without strain and fatigue. He finds it difficult and tiring to sit quietly. Frequent change of activity is helpful in relieving muscle fatigue. Doubtlessly you know how tired you feel if you have to stand in one place for 30 minutes, or even 15 minutes. You are more tired than when moving about for 30 minutes. The same applies to the schoolchild. He tires from trying to sit still.

But there are other reasons why schoolchildren need to alternate rest and activity.

Organic Development

Heart size is roughly proportional to body size throughout life except during this period. During elementary school years, body growth rate is slightly greater than heart growth rate.[1] At rest, the young child has a high pulse and low blood pressure. The amount of blood expelled per beat is limited by the size of the heart. Hence, when the child is vigorously active, his heart has to beat very rapidly to supply the needed blood to various parts of the body. The circulatory system cannot maintain this pace for long; there must be alternation of rest with activity. This is essential to life. The body has built-in safeguards to protect it from overstrain. The child will rest when he gets out of breath, when he has a pain in the side, or when his muscles begin to cramp. As the child grows older, heart growth increases, as do the capacity and size of the lungs.

Most children rest when they are tired. The danger comes if (1) overfatigue and exhaustion lower body resistance to infection, or (2) the normal recovery processes are slowed to the extent that growth is arrested.

Children need activity and frequent rest periods. If children are not active, their muscles do not develop, and they do not have as much strength and energy. Exercise makes the skeletal muscles strong. Exercise also helps to develop the heart and the circulatory and respiratory systems. The healthy heart responds to exercise by increasing in size and functional capacity.

Thus we see that exercise is necessary if the schoolchild is to develop as he can and should. He needs both activity and rest.

Lack of Exercise

The soft, fat child and the weak, thin child are often uninterested in activity. They are not strong and vigorous; hence they do not enjoy strenuous play. Lack of activity hinders physical development. The child is less able, he

[1] American Association for Health, Physical Education, and Recreation, Department of N.E.A., *U.S. Children in Focus*, 1954 Yearbook, Washington, D.C., pp. 56–57.

may be somewhat shunned by playmates, and therefore he gets less practice. It is a vicious circle. These children tend to withdraw from active play unless they receive special attention. The nurse should realize the importance of helping the underweight child to gain, and the overweight child to lose, weight. Suggestions directed to eating habits are given later in this chapter.

Perfecting Skills

Muscular coordination of schoolchildren improves greatly as they practice and perfect skills that were only partly learned earlier.

They gain better control of the large muscles of the legs, arms, and back. They learn to ride a bicycle and to turn handsprings. Little girls like to play games that call for more precise muscular control, such as hopscotch, jacks, and jump-the-rope. Little boys learn to shoot a bow and arrow and to bounce a ball.

From six to nine years of age, interest in running games increases, while interest in toys decreases. At this age children like hide-and-seek, tag, baseball, basketball, "cops and robbers," and "spaceman."

Around the age of ten, the child's skill may astonish adults. The little girl wins three ice-skating trophies with her figure skating. Another girl can sew. The little boy builds a desk with his hammer, nails, saw, and plane. He can mow the lawn. The farm boy, who has always "tagged along" with his father, may drive the small farm tractor.

Competition from their own group of friends may encourage a child to do more practicing and to become more expert than any adult urging could.

Development of the small muscles, those in the hands and eyes, is more slow and uneven. Learning to write and to read requires very exact adjustments and coordination between hand and eye. The child is usually farsighted until the eighth year. The fine muscular coordination necessary for reading does not develop much before that time. The eye muscles often develop earlier in girls than in boys.

Because of the increase in the ability to use the fingers, later childhood is the time to begin playing a musical instrument.

Health Needs

Grade school years are healthy years, statisticians report. Even including accidents, death rates are lower between the ages of 5 and 14 than at any other time of life.[2] But many children do not enjoy optimum health, and great improvements can be made in health care during these years. The first year at

---

[2] *Accident Facts.* Chicago: National Safety Council, 1970 edition, p. 8.

school means exposure to colds, respiratory ills, and communicable diseases from schoolmates.

To be well-nourished, a child needs an orderly life balanced for sleep, exercise, fresh air, and good food. Malnutrition can result from an infection; from a lack of outdoor, active play; or from late hours, too little sleep, or poor sleeping conditions. The child may have poor eating habits, or too much attention may be given to his food habits.

His appetite may be dulled by stresses stemming from schoolwork, class competition, and trying to get along with many children.

Even though a child eats a variety of foods, his body has to operate efficiently for the food to be used.

Grade-school children can easily have so many activities to fill their day that they do not get enough rest or enough outdoor play. School, homework assignments, television, Cub Scouts or Camp Fire Girls, church choir, junior band, music lessons, Little League baseball — the list of activities for children is endless. In lower economic groups, activities may not be as well organized as in the middle or higher income groups, but children are busy.

Parents need to help the child to select his favorite activities and to eliminate the ones not as important to him. Less stimulation and fewer distractions may mean more playtime, better homework, and a happier child.

Schoolchildren need from 10 to 12 hours of sleep per night, varying with the child. Once the routine is established, the child realizes that he feels better with enough rest. One six-year-old informed her parents and older brother, "I don't care what the rest of you do this evening. I am going to bed. Tomorrow at school, I'm going to be teacher's helper, and I have to be on the ball." She went to bed.

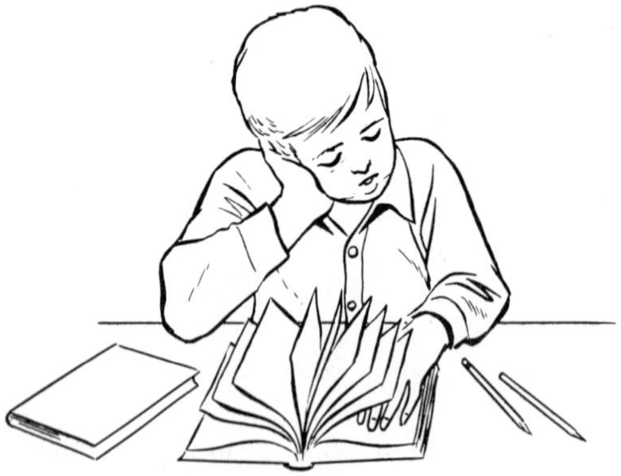

Figure 20. *The school-age child can "overdo" with too many outside interests, too many hours of watching television, too much homework.*

The Six- to Twelve-Year-Old

In your foods and nutrition class, you learn to plan well-balanced diets for every member of the family. Let us consider how to help the growing active child get the abundance of healthy foods he needs.

FOOD HABITS

Elementary school children are generally better fed than preschool children or adolescents.[3] They usually have good appetites. They like most foods with the possible exception of vegetables, which they often do not eat in sufficient amounts.

Eating problems may be caused by parents who are unduly concerned with good table manners and who expect adult behavior at mealtime. Children are usually in a hurry and do not like to take the time to eat a meal. It may help to require that they spend a certain length of time, say, 15 to 20 minutes, at the table.

Breakfast, especially, is likely to be skipped. Without a substantial breakfast, the schoolchild probably does not get the food his body needs.

Children will usually eat breakfast if other members of the family do, if breakfast is ready to eat, if the meal is appetizing, and if they have enough time to eat before going to school. This may mean assembling school clothes the night before and getting up a few minutes earlier. Not only should the child have time to eat breakfast, he needs time to go to the bathroom afterward. This is the natural time for the bowel movement.

Some children cannot eat breakfast even if they have enough time because they are afraid that they will be late to school. Parents and teachers need to cooperate on this. Generally, too much stress at school about being on time is not desirable in the first and second grades. A little later, the child may assume more responsibility for being punctual, but even then, he needs help from parents and teachers.

Group acceptance is extremely important to school children, and this extends to the food they eat. If they notice that their school chums look with disfavor at foods from a different cultural background, they may refuse to eat these foods at home, even though they are good. On the other hand, a youngster may be willing to try new foods within a group that he might not try alone. A good school lunch program may introduce new foods in a setting where the child is anxious to conform.

THE OVERWEIGHT CHILD

Many children are chubby during early and middle childhood, then become more slender as they become more muscular during adolescence. But not all

---

[3] Corinne Robinson, *Proudfit-Robinson's Normal and Therapeutic Nutrition*, 13th ed. (New York: The Macmillan Company, 1967), p. 369.

children lose the excess weight. Overweight or obese children tend to become overweight or obese adults. ("Overweight" describes the person who is 10 to 20 per cent heavier than the desirable weight for his age, height, and body build. He is "obese" if he carries 20 per cent or more extra weight.)

A group of adults who had been obese as children included five times as many obese people as did a group who had normal childhood weight. In one study conducted in England, 80 per cent of the overweight girls became overweight women.

We are not being fair to say of the fat child, "He will outgrow it," and to shrug off the matter as unimportant. Even if he does outgrow it in adolescence, obesity in childhood can be dangerous to emotional health and to personality growth. The fat child may be teased by his playmates, criticized by the adults in his world, and form an unhealthy opinion of himself. His schoolwork may suffer. As mentioned earlier, he may not get enough exercise to develop properly.

Preventing overweight in children is more successful than dieting. We really know very little about why some children cannot regulate the delicate balance between calorie intake and physical activity,[4] so undertake treatment with sympathy. The family doctor should examine the child to detect any possible physical difficulties. He may or may not recommend a reducing diet. Many people oppose a reducing diet for children because they need nutrients for proper growth. Frequently a diet only focuses attention on his weight. It may cause family arguments or encourage the child to eat hidden snacks.

Examining the child's life and the family's eating habits may offer clues. If the family's favorite foods are rich pastries, starchy vegetables, starchy main dishes, candy, and soft drinks, the child is probably eating too many calories. A balanced diet of the basic four food groups rarely provides too many calories. Of course, too many second helpings and "clean your plate" directives may cause weight gains. Some mothers offer sweets as a bribe for good behavior.

Perhaps the overweight child eats excessively because he is unhappy or worried. Sometimes he has formed the habit of turning to food in time of trouble. He may lack physical exercise and a variety of interests. The child who has fun doing things with other people has less time to think about food. It has been noted that very active children are seldom overweight, and that very overweight children are almost always inactive.

These statements should suggest to you, the nurse, how to support and to help the family with an overweight child.

Encourage the child to become more physically active, especially with outdoor play. The family should eat regular, well-balanced meals. Growing children need foods that are high in protein, moderate in fat, and low in carbohydrates. At mealtime, serve the overweight youngster smaller portions of

[4] Committee on Nutrition, American Academy of Pediatrics, "Obesity in Childhood," *Pediatrics*, Vol. 40 (Sept. 1967), p. 455.

The Six- to Twelve-Year-Old

food. If a reducing diet is necessary, make no comments; serve the food casually. Trim excess fat from meats. Offer lemon juice and vinegar in place of rich salad dressings. Do not attempt to prevent a child from eating snacks, but steer him away from those high in calories. A bowl of fresh fruit on the kitchen table or a supply of raw carrots, celery sticks, and radishes in the refrigerator provide tempting, low-calorie snacks. It helps to tell the child what he *can* eat, not what he cannot eat.

Above all, the overweight child needs to feel accepted and loved by his family, as he is. Some children can lose weight; some cannot. You, the nurse, should strive to help the family realize that a happy, outgoing child (although overweight) can become a well-adjusted adult.

THE UNDERWEIGHT CHILD

The underweight child is especially susceptible to childhood diseases. Communicable diseases reduce the appetite as well as increase the body's need for nutrients.

Gaining weight may not be easy. The first step should be a thorough health examination to rule out physical difficulties. Next, a careful look at the child's life may disclose a source of trouble. Sometimes extreme unhappiness or worry will destroy the appetite. Or he may have too many stimulating activities.

The underweight child simply cannot eat larger quantities of food, but he can eat more of the concentrated foods. He might have cream on his cereal instead of top milk, a milkshake, not soda, and an extra pat of butter. However, he still should have vegetables and fruits.

The nurse can help the family to realize that the underweight child needs more rest, more quiet play, and fewer hours of active play.

DENTAL CARE

Dental care is exceedingly important during these years when the second set of teeth, the permanent teeth, is forming. The first permanent teeth are called the "six-year molars" because they appear during the sixth year. They are especially subject to decay and need careful watching. During any period of rapid bone growth, cavities can develop surprisingly fast. The child should see his dentist twice a year.

The dentist will also examine the child's teeth for crookedness, or malocclusion (upper and lower teeth that do not come together properly). Because the child's jaw has not yet calcified, corrective work with braces may be started. Orthodontia is a long process, often painful and expensive, but worthwhile if the child feels his appearance for the rest of his life will be improved.

EYE AND EAR TESTS

Most elementary schools give massive "screening" tests for vision and hearing. If more detailed examinations are indicated, parents are expected to proceed from there.

The routine eye examinations may disclose only obvious eye defects. The child may not be aware of his visual problem. An observant nurse may detect such symptoms as frequent sties and bloodshot eyes, inability to see from a distance, squinting, holding a book close to the face, or tipping the head at odd angles when working. Eyeglasses are so attractively designed now that no stigma need be attached to wearing them.

The nurse should be alert for hearing difficulties in children. The child and his parents may not realize that he does not hear as well as other children. Ear problems detected early can often be arrested, if not cured. Left alone, the condition usually progresses, and deafness results. Impaired hearing greatly handicaps a child's learning at school. Many slow learners have been found to be hard-of-hearing. If the teacher and family know the child has limited hearing, he can be taught lip reading. His seat in the classroom can be moved to the front, where he can see the teacher's lips more clearly. In many ways, he can be helped to learn to get along with his handicap.

Conditions that can lead to ear trouble include the common cold, diseases such as measles that are associated with ear infections, and infections of the tonsils and adenoids.

Social and Emotional Development

SIX THROUGH NINE

Starting to school means entering a totally new world for the six-year-old. He learns many things. He has to learn to get along with others of his own age. He learns to regard his teacher as the authority and to observe the school rules. He acquires certain fundamental social skills. These adjustments may appear minor to adults, but they are vitally important in the youngster's progress toward maturity.

In the first years at school the child usually has one or two special friends. Usually boys play with boys, girls play with girls, but not necessarily so. The nine-year-old has learned a great deal about getting along at school and with his friends. He knows what is expected of him, although he may not always do it.

Discipline for the schoolchild means a few rules, well defined, in terms that he understands. He should know that he is to go straight home from school. He has a certain time to go to bed each night. He knows how long he is to practice music lessons and how much television he may watch.

Children need some limits set for them and then, within those limits, to have freedom to exercise their own judgment. Youngsters are more comfortable with limits set. It is too heavy a burden for them to decide everything. As the child grows older, he should have more and more responsibility for his own decisions.

THE PREADOLESCENT—TEN THROUGH TWELVE

To trust a preadolescent does not mean to leave him entirely to his own devices. It is not a sign of lack of trust if parents insist that an adult be present at boy-girl parties. It is not a sign of lack of confidence for parents to know that a trustworthy adult accompanies the girls on a weekend camping trip. Parents show confidence by acknowledging their child's right to have privacy, to have some secrecy, to choose his own friends, and, to some extent, to choose his own groups.

The gang or club is extremely important to the preadolescent. The 10-, 11-, and 12-year-olds grow toward greater independence by stronger association with those of their own age. Usually the 10-to-12-year-olds favor small groups of

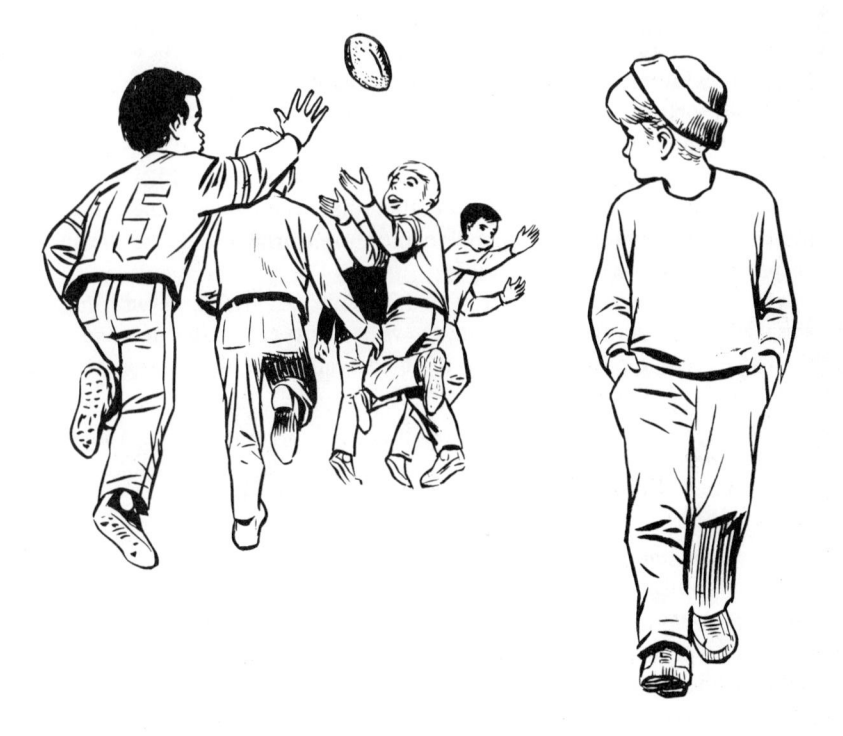

Figure 21. *The gang or club is extremely important to the preadolescent.*

three to six, not more than a year apart in age. Children are fiercely loyal, but not always kind. They do not hesitate to "cut down to size" with blunt criticism. The club members manage their own affairs, demanding that all members stand on their own feet. This encourages less dependence on parents and more self-reliance. Parents who do not understand that this is a sign of growth may feel hurt and unappreciated. If they show hurt feelings, tension between the two generations may arise.

Actually, the group or club sets its own code. Soon the members discover that some rules are necessary if the entire time together is not to be spent quarreling. Group life forces them to sort out, judge, sharpen, and put into words the principles they learned from their parents. Gradually, they incorporate their parents' standards into their own life.[5]

Through group life, the preadolescent improves his techniques of getting along with others. If he does this, his relationships during adolescence will be less strained.

Sometimes during the preteens, boy-girl parties are not successful. Each sex seems to regard the other with scorn or suspicion. They tend to draw apart, as though to gather strength for the years ahead. But they enjoy talking *about* each other.[6]

Youngsters are maturing earlier today. Some preteen girls are eager for dates, party clothes, and dances, which ordinarily accompany the adolescent years. But unfortunately, community pressure and overanxious mothers can rush girls into the dating stage before they are actually ready for it.

Usually the preteen girl is trying to form a clear picture of herself as a girl. The preteen boy is trying to assume the role of the masculine hero. With members of their own sex, each may feel more comfortable and find the answers to unspoken questions.

Left to their own devices, boys and girls are usually happy with informal parties, with ice skating or swimming, with backyard barbecues and "gang affairs." They will probably be content to wait until the middle teens for coupled dating.

Encouraging Learnings–Hobbies–Play

The schoolchild is interested in everything. He observes constantly and asks questions continually. He wants to know how things work and why.

As mentioned previously, through play the child perfects skills. He learns to play games. He participates in sports. He takes up hobbies. He may be getting acquainted with a musical instrument. It may be a collection of agates, or

---

[5] *Your Children and Their Gangs* (Washington, D.C.: U.S. Department of Health, Education, and Welfare, Children's Bureau Publication No. 384, 1960), p. 13.
[6] Ibid.

seashells, or model planes. Taking real pictures with a real camera is exciting. The fashion dolls are popular with girls.

Hobbies are likely to be short-lived. If parents do not realize that this is typical, they may think that their youngster lacks perseverance. The curriculum of a junior high school is directed toward acquainting the student with a wide variety of subjects and interests. In the seventh and eighth grades, each child may have an introduction to dramatics, music, the arts, sports, home economics or machine shop, and the crafts. After these brief contacts, he can make a better selection of the studies he wants to pursue further in high school.

The age of exploring and discovering also is apparent in life outside of school. In addition to participating in games and sports, the preteen likes to make things. It is the ideal time to introduce him to handicrafts and to the joys and satisfactions of a creative hobby. When the turmoil of adolescence comes, children hesitate to launch into a new activity. Then comes the first job or college. If the preadolescent does not discover the possible values of handicraft hobbies, the chances are that he will not do so for many years, if he ever does.

The 9-to-12-year-old can be a marvelous traveler. He is enthusiastic, energetic, and keenly alert. The tourist's favorite of the West Coast, San Francisco, can be most fascinating when viewed through the eyes of a red-haired, freckle-faced nine-year-old. He thrills to everything: the magnificent Golden Gate Bridge, the beautiful San Francisco Bay, the antique cable cars, the quaint, winding streets, the seals on the Seal Rocks near the Cliff House, the giant redwood trees of Muir Woods, Alcatraz Island, Chinatown, and Fisherman's Wharf. Years later, his friends may doubt his story, but he really did hear Tony Bennett sing in person.

Every city and every locality have places of interest for the family with schoolchildren. There are museums and art galleries, or perhaps an international airport, a maple syrup refinery, botanical gardens, or the docks with ocean-going vessels. Family excursions can be both wholesome fun and educational experiences. Parents who make the effort to show their children the sights usually find that they profit with continued growth.

Illness and the Hospital

The nurse who gives genuine thought to the needs of her school-age patient will be rewarded with cooperation and with the feeling of a job well done.

The preadolescent wants privacy. An 11-year-old will be painfully embarrassed to use the bedpan in the open ward. The nurse should respect his feelings. Always draw the curtain around the child's bed.

Tension and anxiety can be an obstacle to the schoolchild's recovery, as with any patient. The nurse should orient him to hospital procedures, functions, and the workers and their duties.

Remember, we said that the schoolchild is interested in everything and learns continually. He will continue learning inside the hospital if the nurse takes time to help him. Explain the equipment, routines, and, above all, the nursing procedures. The older child is capable of understanding why certain procedures are done. He may be proud to learn a few medical terms. Think of the fun he can have impressing his schoolmates by spouting technical terms.

But, of course, he needs continual reassurance, and he will regress. He may not act very grown up at times. His feelings toward his illness are extremely important. The younger child may think that his illness is a punishment for disobedience or some childish offense. Frequently, children blame their parents.

Sometimes your young patient has to "blow off steam." He may have just been informed that another operation is necessary, or that he cannot go home the next day as he had hoped. An adult finds negative news hard to take in his stride; so a child particularly needs help to develop inner control.

The child may be helped by meeting others with a similar disability. Practicing some skills may build up his self-confidence. Eventually he can begin to think about others and to think less about his own troubles.

Diversions

Their wide range of interests offers an ample selection of diversional activities for schoolchildren. Although the right diversion can help the child immeasurably, the wrong activity will discourage him.

Many communities provide for the continuing of schoolwork for the shut-in child. This may involve regular visits from a "home teacher" or school by telephone. The children's hospital typically has a schoolroom where ambulatory patients are taken for their classwork. The teacher realizes that a convalescent child may not have enough energy to maintain his grade level, but any progress that the child can make is worthwhile. How the child feels about himself is very important.

Some of the projects listed in Chapter 13, "Recreation for the Sick Child," are adaptable for many six-, seven-, and eight-year-olds. Some of the projects described are appropriate for an alert five-year-old.

Some activities enjoyed by schoolchildren include the following:

FINGER PAINTING

Clay modeling and papier mache sculptoring (particularly for making puppet heads; puppetry can become an intriguing hobby of long duration).

Spatter painting (*Equipment:* bright construction paper, a stencil design or leaf specimen, an old toothbrush, wire screening, and colored ink or white shoe polish. *Procedure:* Place design, or leaf specimen, on the paper. Hold wire

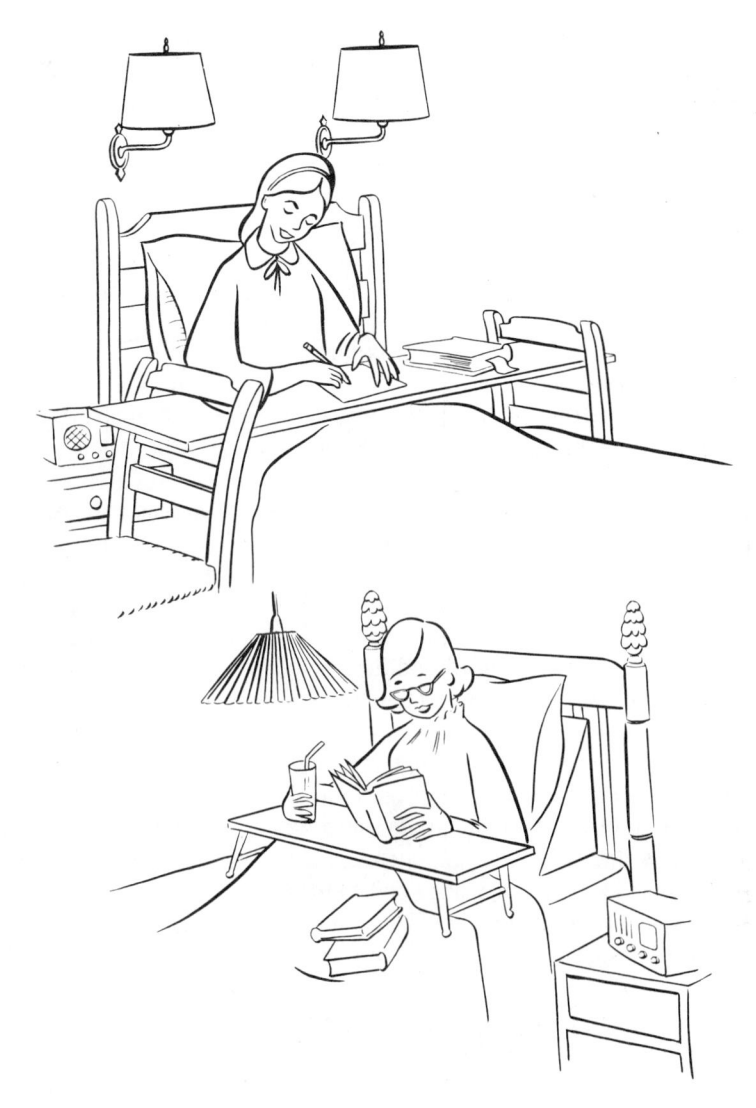

Figure 22. *Bed tables for meals or diversion.*

screening over paper 8 to 10 inches away. Dip toothbrush in ink and lightly brush over screen. Continue until desired color is obtained, then remove stencil.)

Roller Prints (*Equipment:* Leaf specimen, oil paint, sheet of paper, and old newspaper. *Procedure:* Apply oil paint to underside of leaf. Place leaf on paper and press between two newspapers, then remove leaf.)

The ozalid print (*Equipment:* Leaf specimen, or other design, sensitized paper and ammonia in a shallow container. *Procedure:* Place leaf specimen or

147

other design on the sensitized paper. Expose to bright sunlight for a few minutes. Place in the container of ammonia until desired color is obtained, then remove.)

Prints such as described here may be matted, framed, and hung, giving the youngster the satisfaction of having others see his work. Craft work practiced by Girl Scouts, Boy Scouts, Camp Fire Girls, and 4-H Clubs has countless possibilities for the convalescing youngster.

Many adult hobbies can be simplified for children. A girl who has watched her grandmother knit may want to learn the basic knit and purl stitches. Little fingers can crochet with thick rug yarns.

The convalescing child needs the companionship of other children. In the hospital, he is usually placed in a two- or four-bed room. Often a full-time staff person assumes the responsibility of supervising group recreation. However, this responsibility may fall to you, the practical nurse, and this will challenge all your ingenuity and resourcefulness.

Games have a magic appeal to children. The convalescing child may participate and benefit from certain games just as healthy children do.

Dominoes and card tricks give children practice with numbers. Spelling and vocabularies are improved with word games such as anagrams, Scrabble, and crossword puzzles. A child has to reason as he plays checkers, chess, or games like "20 Questions." If physical conditions will allow, action games (musical chairs, balloon blow, and shoe scramble) help children to release tension. Learning takes place when games are played that involve famous persons or geography. (Who can name the most state capitals? What person is associated with the telephone? The airplane?) Charades help to bring the timid child out of his shell. Because this is play, the youngster does not realize that he is learning. Almost any game increases alterness, encourages obedience to rules or principles, and provides practice in fair play and good sportsmanship.[7]

The home-confined youngster needs the companionship of other children, too. Playing games can help to make the visits of other children enjoyable for both the sick child and his guest. Large groups of children should not be invited, as this may be too exciting. When one or two children are guests, games such as jacks, monopoly, or Uncle Wiggly can be lots of fun.

Children at the hospital and at home will enjoy television shows. Programs need to be selected carefully, however, for an overstimulating program may be as damaging to certain patients as too much physical activity. The weekly radio and television schedules might be mounted on cardboard for safe handling.

In the home, the nurse or mother can place a bulletin board near the foot of the child's bed and surprise him with a new picture each day. She can also post medicine-taking time. A schoolchild may be more cooperative and develop

---

[7] Ruth B. Hartley, "What Games Can Do for Your Children," in *The Complete Book of Children's Play*, rev. ed. (New York: Crowell, 1963), pp. 235–238.

independence if he makes his own daily schedule, listing the time for taking medicines, meals, activity, and rest.

Helping with household tasks may give the schoolchild a feeling of belonging and of being necessary. But do not insult him with "busy work," and do show appreciation for work completed.

He might help to prepare fruits or vegetables, such as stemming fresh strawberries or stringing green beans. The ten-year-old girl might sew on buttons or do simple mending. A boy might like to clean old playing cards with spirits of camphor or repair tips of shoelaces by dipping them into clear nail polish.

The schoolchild might keep a shopping list for the family. He might plan menus, organize and bring up-to-date the family telephone and address book, or become the family weather prophet. A girl might help with the grooming of younger children, such as combing little sister's long hair.

If the youngster makes a real contribution to family life, the others may be less likely to be overprotective and oversympathetic.

Books for schoolchildren relate closely to their schoolwork. But in choosing stories, the nurse should remember certain basic trends.

The six- and seven-year-olds usually like stories about animals, birds, trees, flowers, and fish. They like *Reddy the Fox, Mrs. Quack, Peter Rabbit, Uncle Wiggly.*

The eight- and nine-year-olds lose interest in the story world of ducks, foxes, and rabbits. They glory in letting their imaginations expand. They like fairy tales, stories of the lands of elves, pixies, sleeping princesses, and bewitched toads. Their sense of fancy develops with their sense of adventure. They like stories about children who live in other lands, such as *Pretty One of China* and *Pedro of Old Mexico.*

Beginning about the age of nine or ten, boys like one kind of story, girls like another.

The boy wants fact. He likes stories about real boys, about Boy Scouts, boys in the North Woods, boys exploring caves — boys doing any exciting, adventuresome thing with which he possibly identifies himself. Stories of school life and school activities are important.

Girls begin to like fanciful stories and gentle romances. A girl may ask for an orphan story, "A book to make me cry." It is at nine, and for several years after, that most girls read *Little Women.*

Questions for Discussion

1. The aggressive youngster often receives more attention and disciplinary measures than the quiet child. Do we need to be concerned about the withdrawn, "model" child? What should the nurse do when she observes extreme secludedness in a child?

2. What are the safety precautions to be stressed for schoolchildren?

3. How can parents give their children experience in handling money?
4. What recreational facilities are available for schoolchildren in your hospital?

Additional Readings

Accidents and Children. Washington, D.C.: Department of Health, Education, and Welfare, Children's Bureau Publication No. 48, 1963.
Blake, Florence G., and F. Howell Wright. *Essentials of Pediatric Nursing.* 7th ed. Chaps. 25–28. Philadelphia: J. B. Lippincott Company, 1963.
Erickson, Florence. "When 6- to 12-Year-Olds Are Ill," *Nursing Outlook* 13:7 (July 1965), 48.
Jaeger, Margaret Ann. *Child Development and Nursing Care.* Chap. 4. New York: The Macmillan Company, 1962.
Marlow, Dorothy, and Gladys Sellew. *Text of Pediatric Nursing.* 2nd ed. Chaps. 21, 22, 23. Philadelphia: W. B. Saunders Company, 1965.
Rasmussen, Sandra. *Foundations of Practical and Vocational Nursing.* Chap. 45. New York: The Macmillan Company, 1967.
Scott, Lou Peveto. *Programmed Instruction and Review for Practical and Vocational Nurses,* pp. 266–285. New York: The Macmillan Company, 1968.
Smith, Christine Spahn. *Maternal–Child Nursing.* Chap. 8. Philadelphia: W. B. Saunders Company, 1963.
Thompson, Eleanor D. *Pediatrics for Practical Nurses.* Chaps. 13–14. Philadelphia: W. B. Saunders Company, 1965.
Your Child from 6 to 12. Washington, D.C.: U.S. Department of Health, Education, and Welfare, Children's Bureau Publication No. 324, 1966.
Your Children and Their Gangs. Washington, D.C.: U.S. Department of Health, Education, and Welfare, Children's Bureau Publication No. 384, 1960.
Your Child's Progress in School. Columbus, Ohio: Ross Laboratories, 1962.

Recommended Audiovisual Aids

FILMS

If These Were Your Children Parts I & II (49 min., Metropolitan Life Insurance Company, B&W)

Part I: This film shows how the emotional health of schoolage children can be improved. The action takes place in the classroom, and poses the question, "What lies behind their behavior?" Specific examples show that the child's behavior is influenced by his family life.

Part II: In the follow-up film, the physician in charge of the child guidance clinic stresses that the behavior of the child be interpreted properly. Specific cases are depicted. The film points out that the schoolteacher needs the help of the parents. Guidelines are given for evaluating and observing the behavior of children.

The Six- to Twelve-Year-Old

Frightened Child (19 min., International Film Bureau, B&W)

Janie, 11 years old, is accident prone. Her mother is dead: her father is a Navy officer, frequently away from home, so Janie has been living with her aunt, who dislikes men. Janie's father seeks help from a social agency, and Janie is placed in a suitable foster home. The film shows Janie's difficulty in relating to her foster father. When she is finally convinced that the foster father cares for her, she begins to develop a more positive attitude toward her own father.

The Hickory Stick (28 min., International Film Bureau, B&W)

This film on discipline shows how a good teacher maintains discipline in the classroom. It would be good for anyone who has the responsibility for the care of children. The problems of many children are shown, and correct ways of handling the problems.

FILMSTRIPS

How Shall I Tell My Young Child About Sex? (42 frames, International Film Bureau, Color)

With animated drawings, the filmstrip shows anatomy and physiology of male and female organs. It emphasizes the advantages of teaching this information in childhood and shows that sound attitudes toward sex can be developed with a healthy outlook on life. This would help the practical nurse to know how to advise parents on teaching about sex.

Shyness (37 frames, International Film Bureau, B&W)

The filmstrip supplements the film of the same name. It explains that preschool children are normally shy when in unfamiliar situations. If they fail to adjust, they will remain shy in their school years. This filmstrip would help the practical nurse who has a "shy" young patient.

CHAPTER 16 / **THE ADOLESCENT**

Your adolescent patient is a unique individual. If he is sent to the pediatric ward, he is insulted to be classified as a "baby." Yet he is unhappy among the adults. Imagine the effect on a teenage girl of listening to mature women discussing female problems or the distress of a teenage boy assigned to a bed between an alcoholic patient and a senile man. From another angle, the teenager's noisy enthusiasm or his transistor radio may annoy adults who yearn for quiet.

One possible solution is a teenage ward, where rules can be adapted to the special world of the teenager.

What is adolescence? Why is the adolescent a unique person? What is his special world? How does illness affect him?

Definition of Adolescence

Adolescence means to grow to maturity. Webster defines adolescence as "The state or process of growing up; *also*: the period of life from puberty to majority terminating legally at the age of majority."[1]

In less civilized societies, puberty — sexual maturity — marks the beginning of adult life. Today, puberty marks the beginning of adolescence, the in-between years, usually stretching from 12 to 20. Youth may be physically mature but not yet ready for full membership in the adult world. Much growing, developing, and adjusting take place during adolescence.

Teenage Problems Publicized

Every period of life, every change, calls for adjustments. It may be said that there are four important milestones on the road to maturity. The first milestone is passed when the baby learns to walk and he can investigate the world "on his own." The second major milestone comes when the six-year-old enters school, leaves his sheltered home and begins adjusting to the outside world. In adolescence greater freedom is achieved. The last important big step to maturity is leaving home for a job or marriage.

All these steps require major adjustments, yet the most attention and criticism are centered on the teen years.

---

[1] *Webster's Seventh New Collegiate Dictionary* (Springfield, Mass.: G. & C. Merriam Company, 1967), p. 12.

Apparently, the adult generation has always regarded young people as hopeless. Here is what Socrates wrote 2350 years ago:

> The children now love luxury; they show disrespect for elders and love chatter in place of exercise. Children are tyrants, not the servants of their households. They no longer rise when their elders enter the room. They contradict their parents, chatter before company, gobble up dainties at the table, cross their legs, and tyrannize over their teachers.

Ask an adult today to describe the slang, fads, songs and dances of his youth and his own father's opinion of the antics. If he is truthful, doubtless he will recall parental disapproval. The generation gap may appear glaringly wide today because the generations criticize each other so openly. In almost every aspect of life, differences are expressed and people speak out. This may be good mental hygiene, but it causes more open conflict between generations.

Some of the reasons for the publicity can be explained. Activities of teenagers are those that concern the public and bring him into the news. Delinquent acts of teenagers are more often front-page news than are successful science projects and community activities. Also, one group of teenagers can seem to be indicative of an entire community.

In one respect, adolescence may be regarded as a fairly new stage in the family life cycle. Not many years ago the teenager earned his living, married young, and immediately assumed responsibility for his family. Today increased schooling keeps the adolescent off the labor market. High school education is the rule, and large percentages of youth go to college. The tremendous increase in accumulated knowledge and the large number of technical occupations all require increased literacy and better training than formerly. A young man no longer follows his father's trade or business, with his father teaching him most of what he needs to know. Youth today are expected to be better educated than their parents. But the underlying motive is the desire to give children time to grow up, time to become individuals and acquire their own identity before they are burdened with the responsibilities of earning a living and of parenthood. The ideal is to give them time to learn to think creatively, thus to approach adult responsibilities and world problems with creative thinking.

Despite these factors we have reason to be concerned about the youth of today. In sheer numbers, more teens exist than ever before. The rate of juvenile delinquency has tripled since 1940, and continues to rise. The number of teenage, unwed mothers has increased. Two out of every five American children fail to finish high school. The high school dropout is a likely candidate for unemployment.

An urban, industrialized society poses many problems for youth. City life, as will be explored in a following chapter, particularly affects the adolescent. For example, young people cannot get by with roaming freely in their own neighborhoods, a privilege that today's adults may have had as youth in small town or rural communities.

Community mores may not reinforce parental discipline. Perhaps the parents' way of life was so different that they cannot set rules, and the young people make their own rules. Going to school outside one's own neighborhood means mingling with children of different backgrounds and different standards. This bringing together of many kinds of people in neighborhoods and schools has merits, but it increases hazards for teenagers. Some permissive parents set no limits, or give too much freedom too soon.

Choosing a vocation is not easy when one cannot be sure that this occupation will exist in five years, let alone a lifetime. Many schools are not realistically adjusting to the needs of the student who does not intend to go to college.

Yet the teen years do not have to be a time of frustration, indecision, and unhappiness. The teens can be happy years.

The teenager is adjusting to physical changes, getting acquainted with the opposite sex, learning to get along in his own world, confirming his religious beliefs, planning for a vocation, and establishing a moral code of behavior.

You will get along better with your teenage patient if you understand these physical changes, discern his health problems, and know what is important to him.

Social Acceptance

The teen years are primarily a time of social development and adjustments. To establish himself in his own society is overwhelmingly important to the adolescent, more important than anything else.

He wants to be with others of his own age group, his "peers," and he wants them to like him. The most admired person is not the famous television or movie star, but a popular member of his own group.

Adult opinions and standards are not as important now as those of his own age group. In manners and dress, he is completely conventional. Even though he acquires more responsibility for his own actions, he is not exactly sure of himself. He needs the support and approval of those his own age.

Parents must recede into the background, and this is difficult for them. The adolescent has to become independent of his home, but sometimes the process is a strain. Parents may also resent the fact that the child's devotion, which had been exclusively theirs, must now be shared with the clubs and crowds that are so dear to him. "The group becomes a bridge for the journey from childhood love for parents to the more mature relationships of adulthood which involve giving as well as receiving."[2]

[2] Nina Ridenour and Edith G. Nusser, *Your Children and Their Gangs* (Washington, D.C.: U.S. Department of Health, Education, and Welfare, Children's Bureau Publication No. 384, 1960), p. 9.

The Adolescent

Another essential task for the adolescent is to learn to get along with the opposite sex.

The unit of social life during adolescence is a small clique, the crowd, which has an equal number of boys and girls. Sometimes there are six to eight members, sometimes more. The age span may be as much as three or even five years.

The all-girl clubs and the all-boy clubs of the preteens still serve a purpose. Endless conversations are held. What kind of boys do girls like? What kind of girls do boys really like?

Dating is the universal social activity, with dates in the early teens being mostly group affairs. A group of girls may plan a party and invite their heroes of the moment. A group of boys may plan an outing and invite the girls. The girls are usually invited as individuals, not as a group. Each boy draws support from the others.

In the middle and late teens, boy-and-girl relationships may develop into love affairs. Often they do not, but they have helped the young person to learn about other people. At the time, the romance is crucially important.

A girl seeks social approval with pretty clothes, an attractive, neat coiffure, and the latest makeup. She must be able to dance, to swim, to play a musical instrument, and to give parties in her home. Girls are more likely than boys to strive for good grades in school.

An adolescent boy gains stature by excelling in sports, driving the car, or earning his own money. His appearance is important to him too.

Among teenagers, the popular person has pep, energy, and good looks. Are these not based on good health? Here is real motivation for teenagers to follow good health rules. The nurse who sees how to relate these desires to good health habits can truly be effective in teaching good health to the teenager.

Physical Growth and Development

The adolescent is concerned about his social adjustment, perhaps not realizing that the rapidity and variety of physical changes complicate his adjustment. In a few short years the physical changes take him from a childish to a mature level. Much research has been done on adolescent development, and to learn all the details would be an exacting study. Let us consider the phases of development that most affect the youngster's social and emotional development, and what the adolescent needs to know to understand his growth.

Girls mature earlier than boys, an important factor in the teen social world. The tremendous gains in height and weight usually occur in girls between the ages of 11 and 13, and in boys between 13 and 15. The average boy grows 8 inches between the ages of 13 and 15½, and the average girl grows 3¼ inches between the ages of 11 and 13½. Although everyone expects it, the growth spurt of 4 inches during the peak growing year is still amazing to family, friends and, most of all, the boy himself.[3]

Maximum height may be reached as much as two years earlier than it was 50 or 60 years ago. Boys ordinarily reach their maximum height by the age of 18 or 19, instead of 21. Girls usually reach their mature height about the age of 17, whereas their grandmothers were probably still growing at 18 or 19.[4] Early maturing is presumably the result of more food and better medical care.[5]

Bones change in number, size, and composition from birth to maturity. While the skeleton may reach full size at 17 or 19, bone mineralization continues for several years, provided that the diet is good. This helps to ensure bones less liable to injury under physical stress, an advantage to the girl in preparation for motherhood.[6]

Puberty is the period when sexual maturity is reached and secondary sex characteristics appear. Changes normally occur in the following pattern:

> In girls, the order is enlargement of the breasts; appearance of straight, pigmented pubic hair; period of maximum growth; appearance of kinky pubic hair; first menstruation; and growth of axillary (underarm) hair.
> In boys, the order is beginning of growth of testes; first pubic hair (straight, pigmented); early voice changes; first ejaculation; kinky pubic hair; period of maximum growth; axillary hair; marked voice changes; and development of the beard.[7]

Other changes occur during adolescence. In girls, the pelvis widens, and the body gradually becomes more rounded. In boys, the neck and shoulders become somewhat thicker and broader. Part of the weight gain during the growth spurt is due to the growth of muscle tissues, especially in the shoulders, arms, and legs. The early-maturing boy has an advantage in high school athletics over the late-maturing boy. He enjoys greater esteem from both peers and adults, and this — combined with other factors — leads to better social and psychological adjustments.[8] The late-maturing boy is likely to be regarded and treated as immature by both adults and peers; both boys and girls who mature late are likely to be less self-confident, more dependent, and have poorer relations with their parents. Girls who enter puberty early may be temporarily isolated from

---

[3] Mollie S. Smart and Russell C. Smart, *Children: Development and Relationships* (New York: The Macmillan Company, 1967), p. 442.

[4] Boyd McCandless, *Children: Behavior and Development,* 2nd ed. (New York: Holt, Rinehart and Winston, 1967), p. 386.

[5] Luella Cole, *Psychology of Adolescence,* 6th ed. (New York: Holt, Rinehart and Winston, 1964), p. 32.

[6] Corinne Robinson, *Proudfit-Robinson's Normal and Therapeutic Nutrition*, 13th ed. (New York: The Macmillan Company, 1967) p. 359.

[7] Dorothy Rogers, *The Psychology of Adolescence* (New York: Appleton-Century-Crofts, Inc., 1962), p. 78.

[8] Paul Henry Mussen and Mary Cover Jones, "The Behavior-Inferred Motivations of Late- and Early-Maturing Boys," in *Studies in Adolescence*, ed. Robert E. Grinder (New York: The Macmillan Company, 1963), p. 446.

The Adolescent

their classmates, but research shows them to have more favorable self-concepts than late-maturing girls.[9]

Possibly the disadvantages from late maturing could be lessened with increased knowledge and understanding. Children vary widely in the time they begin the growth spurt, reach the peak, and finish. A late growth spurt lasts longer; therefore, late maturers tend to be taller than early maturers.[10]

The adolescent may be embarrassed because his face may assume asymmetrical or unbalanced proportions. The nose grows earlier than the rest of the face; the forehead increases in height and protrudes; and finally the chin develops, which balances the face.

Internal organs also change in proportion. During childhood a small heart pumps blood through relatively large arteries and veins, but during adolescence a large heart pumps blood through relatively small vessels. This condition may impose strain upon the heart of the rapidly growing boy.[11] Adolescent lungs usually are quite capable of handling any pressures put upon them. Although they have not yet reached adult volume, they develop in proportion to demands.[12]

The organs of digestion also undergo considerable growth. The stomach increases in length and capacity, causing a craving for food. When coupled with an increase in the food required by rapid growth, the result is a tremendous appetite for three or four years.[13]

Accepting and Understanding Physical Changes

The adolescent is painfully aware of his physical changes. He is likely to feel unsure of himself. If he understands these changes, his embarrassment may be less and he may worry less.

Suddenly, hands and arms, legs and feet are longer. He may tower over the mother he once looked up to. He is probably awkward and clumsy. The clumsiness is more noticeable when the adolescent is in a strange situation or does not know exactly what is expected of him. When participating in a familiar athletic contest or performing an accomplished skill, the adolescent has excellent coordination.

An attractive physical appearance is exceedingly important to the teenager. As the girl looks at herself in the mirror, she sees how she will look for the rest

---

[9] Mary Cover Jones and Paul Henry Mussen, "Self Conceptions, Motivations, and Interpersonal Attitudes of Early- and Late-Maturing Girls," in *Studies in Adolescence*, ed. Robert E. Grinder (New York: The Macmillan Company, 1963), pp. 454–456.

[10] Mollie S. Smart and Russell C. Smart, *Children: Development and Relationships* (New York: The Macmillan Company, 1967), pp. 443–444.

[11] Luella Cole, *Psychology of Adolescence*, 6th ed. (New York: Holt, Rinehart and Winston, 1964), p. 58.

[12] Luella Cole, op. cit., p. 61.

[13] Luella Cole, op cit., p. 61.

of her life. She studies her assets and her defects. She wonders, "How do I detract from a long neck?" "Do I look best in straight skirts or full skirts?"

Most adolescents are dissatisfied with something about their size or shape. They worry because they are too tall, too short, too thin, overweight, too underdeveloped, or too clumsy. An adolescent suffers if he thinks he is "different."

Boys and girls need help from adults to understand the changes that have taken place within their bodies and to acquire sensible attitudes toward them. Good sexual hygiene is necessary to keep normal boys and girls comfortable, contented, and well adjusted.[14]

Girls need information about menstruation before it begins. Advice from parents commonly comes late or is lacking altogether. Piecemeal information is often faulty or misleading or conveys a poor attitude with such terms as "the curse." Explanations should be given in relatively unscientific, but correct terms.

In your studies of body structure and personal health, you will learn enough to be able to give the teenage girl the information she needs. As a practical nurse you will be able to reassure the teenager that this is a normal process. Although she may feel low in spirits during these periods, she can still have a good time and enjoy life. She can learn to accept menstruation and to take it in her stride.

Boys need information about nocturnal emissions or the spontaneous release of semen. They may be anxious if ignorant of its significance. The average age for first ejaculation is 14½ years.[15]

Good Health Habits

The ideal of the teen world is "toughness," not general good health. A health program for teenagers can easily become a mechanical listing of do's and don't's. Adolescents need realistic guidance on their health problems.

The teenager looks to his doctor for sound advice. He may also ask the nurse serious questions. He should have factual answers. He may ask, "Why is smoking harmful?" "What are the effects of drinking?" "What is wrong with using marijuana or LSD?" You need to know enough to give him a helpful answer. Your studies of pharmacology and health should give you a good basis for explanations. Let us see how these relate to the teenager.

TEMPTATION TO EXPERIMENT

A teenager who experiences self-doubts and shyness in social situations may turn to alcohol to bolster his courage and gain self-confidence. He may not

---

[14] Luella Cole, op. cit., p. 90, adapted.
[15] Dorothy Rogers, *The Psychology of Adolescence* (New York: Appleton-Century-Crofts, 1962), p. 91.

The Adolescent

realize that he is resorting to a dangerous crutch, one that could impair his health and remove important self-restraints.

Some adolescents regard smoking and drinking as signs of being grown up. The teenager should be helped to understand that this decision is an adult privilege. Give him information on which to make his decision. After all, the teenager will eventually make his own choice.

The temptation to experiment may extend to the use of amphetamines, barbiturates, marijuana, and the hallucinogenic drugs such as LSD. The rising increase of drug usage among young people is a significant problem. Causes are numerous and individual. In some places, and to a degree, trying drugs is today's big dare, replacing drinking as proof that a youngster is not "chicken." Most drug takers indulge their taste as a group activity. It may be that in some areas, partying with drugs is beginning to compete with partying with liquor. Youngsters often commit acts bolstered by peer approval that they would not do alone. And remember, our society has become a "pill-popping" society. Adults take a pill for anything and everything. Small wonder that taking "pep pills" does not seem terribly wrong or illegal to some adolescents.

Effective solutions are elusive because too few facts are known. Much more scientific research is needed on the effect of drugs. Lack of knowledge is one reason to avoid using drugs. Nurses with a good basic knowledge of clinical drugs are in a unique position to help young people without resorting to education based completely on fear.

GOOD GROOMING

To be accepted in his world, the teenager needs to be well dressed and well groomed. Body odors are especially noticeable because dancing, dating, and sports involve frequent and close body contact. The teenager now has the full responsibility for his own grooming at a time when preventing body odors is especially difficult. Also, he may not yet have mastered all the skills of good grooming.

Puberty marks the development of functioning of the apocrine sweat glands, which are found in the areas of the body with significance for sex functions, such as breasts and genital areas. The characteristic odor is somewhat unpleasant. The girl should be told that apocrine glands are especially active during menstruation. She may be nervous and perspire more freely. During menstruation, she will need to take more baths, use a deodorant, and change underclothes frequently. The boy needs to know that he should always take a shower after strenuous exercise, and use a deodorant.

Many teenagers express their concern with pimples and blackheads, which occur mostly after puberty. The sebaceous glands are more active in producing oil at a time when the excretory glands have not increased proportionately, and drainage is poor. The normal discharge collects dirt and hardens, resulting in blackheads. Acne results when the blocked glands become infected. Acne may also be caused by imbalance between male and female hormones.

Parents owe it to their children to help prevent acne, as physical appearance has an emotional impact, and the face may become scarred for life. A physician's advice should be sought. Treatment varies, sometimes including ultraviolet treatments and/or increased vitamin A.

The nurse can safely recommend (1) extra cleanliness, such as washing the face several times daily with warm water and soap, rinsing carefully; (2) balanced diet, eliminating chocolate, highly concentrated sweets, and oily foods; and (3) squeezing out blackheads only after both face and hands are thoroughly washed.

FATIGUE AND POSTURE

Although the adolescent seems to have an unlimited source of energy, fatigue can be a problem. Strenuous exercise may damage a heart already weakened from some other cause. Since to be "tough" is important, an adolescent may try to prove that he can "take" anything. From the excitement of a competitive sport and through tremendous peer pressure, an adolescent can exhaust himself. He can push a normally adequate body past its critical level of endurance, with lifelong damage resulting. Often fatigue results from poorly planned routines. Both boys and girls may be caught in a social whirl and fail to get sufficient rest.

Good posture is more easily attained if the young person is proud of height. The father of one 13-year-old girl purposely pointed out to her, and made favorable comments about, tall, attractive women. The self-confidence of her shorter twin brother was bolstered by noting the successful men of the world who were short. The adolescent who can forget his body is more likely to have good posture than one who receives constant comment on his way of walking or sitting. Some authorities believe that it may be harmful to force erectness of the spine at a time when the backbones are not yet strong enough to support erectness. "No nagging" is often the best policy.

TEENAGE NUTRITION

The majority of today's teenagers are healthier, taller, and mentally sharper than their parents. These gains have resulted from good physical care and good nutrition from birth through childhood, actually beginning with the mother's good prenatal care. Adolescents today more closely fulfill their hereditary potential than previous generations.

Yet an examination of the status of teenage nutrition and food habits creates doubt that youth will carry this advantage throughout life. The picture may not be as bleak as presented in earlier studies based upon rigid interpreta-

The Adolescent

tions of the recommendations of the Foods and Nutrition Board of the National Research Council. The recommended dietary allowances have since been revised. One recent study of preadolescents and adolescents in northern Utah reported: "No real deficiencies occurred."[16] It is probable that the amount of malnutrition is related somewhat to economic status. Pockets of malnutrition exist, and cases of teenage malnutrition are found in the more comfortable levels of living.

One indication of the quality of nutrition is body weight. Visit a class of 30 high school students and you will likely notice that entirely too many students are overweight.

Research shows that too many adolescents are overweight, more girls than boys. More boys than girls are underweight. The degree of overweight or underweight increases with the age of the child.[17] Older children, more often than younger children, fall short of the recommended amounts of specific nutrients. The most neglected nutrients are iron and calcium, especially in girls, and then ascorbic acid and vitamin A. These lacks occur with inadequate intake of milk, fruit (especially citrus), and vegetables (especially the green leafy or deep yellow.)[18]

Adolescents need increased amounts of food nutrients to support the tremendous growth of new cells and new tissues, supply energy, strengthen resistance to disease, and repair and maintain body tissues. Basal metabolism is correspondingly high during the peak growing periods, and calorie needs are greater than at any other time in life. Recommended daily dietary allowances[19] are:

Boys, aged 12 to 14 — 2700 calories
aged 14 to 18 — 3000 calories
Girls, aged 12 to 14 — 2300 calories
aged 14 to 16 — 2400 calories
aged 16 to 18 — 2300 calories

Calorie requirements gradually decrease as growth slows.

The adolescent boy and girl require larger amounts of protein, calcium, and vitamin D than adults. Allowances for thiamine, riboflavin, and niacin are based on calorie requirements; hence boys will need more of the vitamin B group than girls or adults.

Adolescent girls urgently need a diet adequate in iron and protein. Because of menstruation, girls need these nutrients to form and regenerate red blood cells. Anemia develops frequently. The girl's diet should include all the basic foods, with special emphasis on high-iron foods such as liver, red meats, leafy green vegetables, and dried fruits.

---

[16] *Nutrition Abstract Review*, Vol. 36 (1967), p. 177.
[17] Corinne Robinson, op. cit., p. 362.
[18] Corinne Robinson, op. cit., p. 363.
[19] From the Foods and Nutrition Board, National Research Council, 1968.

Considering the food needs of adolescents, we recognize the dangers created by "crash diets," which are tempting to teenagers.

FOOD HABITS OF TEENAGERS

Teenagers eat frequently, with one-fourth of the total calorie intake coming from snacks. Eating frequently has not been shown to be harmful.[20] If the choice of snacks is good, the snack habit may be preferable to three meals a day. If the snack foods are mainly carbohydrates, as with girls, snacking can contribute to overweight. Boys tend to eat sandwiches and other protein-rich foods.

Breakfast is frequently missed, more often by girls than boys. Girls need ample time to dress in the morning. If they oversleep, breakfast is omitted. It may be that no one is there to prepare or to share breakfast. Lack of variety of foods available may discourage eating in the morning. Nothing is wrong with a bowl of soup, pizza, or hamburger for breakfast if the foods appeal to a teenager. Any protein-rich food that is eaten is better than a customary food that is not eaten.

Many children who had good food habits during elementary school years change their eating habits when they get into high school. They no longer drink milk, or drink insufficient amounts of milk. They take part in many activities that keep them away from home during meal hours. They may fail to participate in a school lunch program, and spend lunch money for poorly chosen snacks. (School lunch programs can be ill-prepared and unappetizing.) Many children prepare their own meals without adult guidance. Perhaps the habits of their friends are more influential than those of their families. Deciding what to eat, even though it is an unwise decision is one way of asserting independence.

Emotional stress has a negative effect on the body's use of nutrients. Emotional difficulties may come from a feeling of social inadequacies or pressures of schoolwork. Tension in the home caused by conflict between parent and child can contribute to emotional stress.

One reason that the teenage girl has the poorest diet of any age group is that she is afraid of being fat. Even the thin girl will not eat properly because she fears gaining weight. The California study showed that teenagers are extremely conscious of their figures.[21] More than 50 percent of the girls considered themselves obese, although measurements showed that only one-fourth were obese or somewhat obese. Boys were unhappy about underweight.

Studies pinpoint facts that might be helpful to know when one is working with the obese teenager. Calorie intake of overweight girls frequently is not as great as that of girls of normal weight; it is the activity of the overweight girls

---

[20] M. C. Hampton and others, "Caloric and Nutrient Intakes of Teenagers," *Journal of American Dietetic Association*, Vol. 50 (May 1967), p. 385.

[21] Corinne Robinson, op. cit., p. 372.

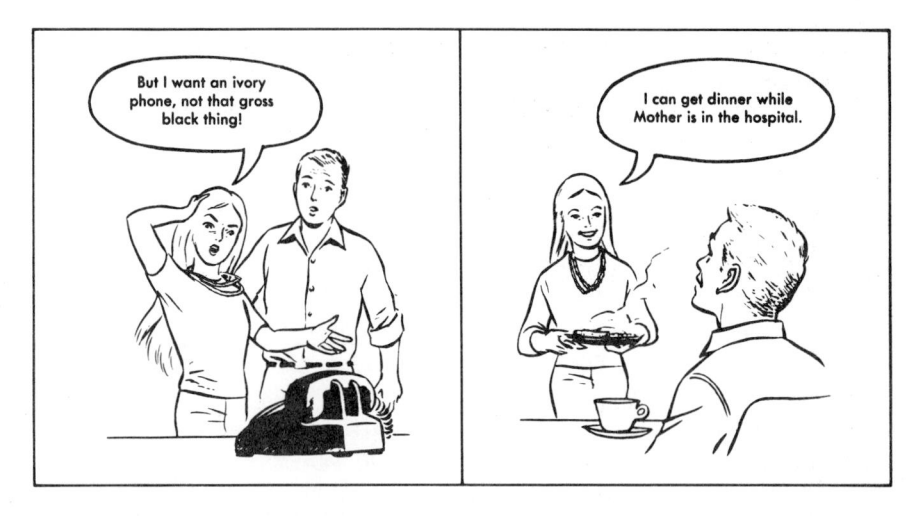

Figure 23. *Adults need to accept and adjust to the fact that the adolescent is sometimes a child, sometimes adult.*

that is likely to be less. The obese girl rarely takes part in active sports. She prefers to sit and watch television rather than exert herself physically.

Obese boys and girls tend to eat fewer fruits and vegetables than boys and girls of normal weight, and to eat less frequently, missing more meals.[22]

Food habits of adolescents might be questioned on the basis of three points: (1) Too many teenagers are obese, and overweight signifies less-than-perfect nutrition. (2) We have evidence of a lack of iron, and possibly calcium, ascorbic acid, and vitamin A. (3) Are teenage boys forming habits of eating huge quantities of food, habits that will not change when their demand for food is less? The thirty-year-old man who eats as much food as an active, growing teenage boy will surely gain weight.

Teenagers are Teachable

Teenage nutrition can be improved, as one study showed.[23] The teenagers with better eating habits were (1) those who had knowledge of nutrition and (2) those who had health problems or were concerned with health.

Boys who mentioned the basic four food groups in a questionnaire had the fewest nutrients that were below the recommended amounts.[24] Also, good

---

[22] M. C. Hampton and others, op. cit., p. 385.
[23] Ercell Eppright, "Challenge of Change to Nutrition." Paper presented at the 6th Conference on Human Nutrition held at Ohio State University, Columbus, March 9 and 10, 1962.
[24] M. C. Hampton and others, op. cit., p. 385.

family relations and good personal adjustments seemed to accompany good eating habits.

Your teenage patients are teachable where nutrition is concerned. The nurse who has a good knowledge of nutrition can accomplish much by emphasizing to the teenager that good nutrition promotes an attractive physical appearance and an abundance of pep and energy, both of which lead to popularity and friends.

The nurse should remember that those admired most by the teenager are members of his own age group. If influential teenagers can be persuaded to eat a well-balanced diet and consider it "the thing to do," others may follow their example. Appealing to the group may be more effective than appealing to the individual. However, behavior changes only when one discovers for himself that the belief of the group or group leader works for him.[25] For example, the youngster will most likely eat breakfast regularly when he notes that he truly feels better during the day if he has eaten in the morning.

You have still another approach to the teenage girl. Perhaps the unspoken dream of every girl is to have her own family of healthy children. The girl should know that there is evidence to show that the woman's nutritional state before she becomes pregnant influences the chances of the baby's being healthy at birth.

Teenage Mothers

The nurse should realize that motherhood for the teenage girl is not to be taken lightly. Parenthood creates added physiological stress for the teenage girl, whose body is still in the formative stage. At the baby's conception, she faces increased nutritional requirements both for preparation and growth of her own body and for development and subsequent feeding of her baby. Many young girls show the results of poor food habits, and some show malnutrition of long duration prior to childbearing. Malnourished teenagers are frequently poor obstetrical risks. Their babies may be born prematurely or have congenital defects. The baby may have an inadequate nutritional store to protect him during the birth process and physiological adaptation to independent living for the first few days and months of life. If young women are underweight or excessively overweight at the time of conception, they are prone to preeclampsia and other conditions that have permanently weakening effects.[26]

During your clinical experience in obstetrics, you will probably have a teenage patient. She may be quiet, shy, and hesitant to ask questions. She may show signs of fear or bewilderment during physical examinations, especially

---

[25] W. G. Bennis, K. D. Benne, and R. Chin, eds., *The Planning of Change-Readings in the Applied Behavioral Sciences* (New York: Holt, Rinehart and Winston, 1966).
[26] Evelyn B. Spindler, "Motivating Teen-Agers to Improve Nutrition," *J. Home Economics* (Jan. 1963), p. 30.

rectal and vaginal. If the nursing or medical personnel have time to explain to her what is happening and the reasons for the examinations and the nursing procedures, the young mother will be more likely to develop a feeling of trust in the medical team. Labor will be less difficult for her than for an older woman. This could be due to more flexible pelvic bones in the teenager, as well as to her having fewer fears.

After delivery of the baby and during the postpartum period, the teenage mother may give the impression that she is fully self-confident in caring for herself, her new baby, and her husband. But often the young mother is unsure of herself. She is eager for knowledge about babies and family life. Teenagers need help in becoming good parents, but the nurse should guard against being too motherly or too sympathetic or giving too much specific advice.

Delinquent Teenagers

Because nurses frequently contact the antisocial teenager, it is well to realize that juvenile delinquents are not all the same, nor does only one cause exist for delinquency. Three major types of delinquents can be distinguished.

The *subcultural delinquent* is a product of the inner-city and poverty area of large cities, where standards of value differ from those of the conventional middle class. Antisocial behaviors such as stealing, fighting, and sexual acting-out are not only acceptable but demanded by the teenager's peers – the street corner or neighborhood "gang." Delinquent behavior in the inner-city area may be due to the adolescent's need to conform, not to an emotional disturbance.

The *sociopathic type of delinquent* comes from the middle or upper class. The youngster has never learned to please anyone but himself, nor has he learned to accept the normal limitations set by society. In the normal person, this learning takes place in childhood and is reinforced by parental affection and discipline. The child learns to conform to please his parents and to avoid punishment. These techniques also help the growing child to deal with his own problems and anxieties, and to help him feel protected by powerful adult figures. The child who grows up without this adult attention remains fixed at a childish level of self-gratification. He knows the rules of the game but has never learned to abide by them. He gives free expression to his impulses, then rationalizes and blames others if he is apprehended or punished. He cannot relate affectionately to others because he has never experienced an affectionate relationship. The school authorities represent his parents; thus he usually has difficulty at school. The sociopathic delinquent characteristically does not experience anxiety, depression, or true guilt feelings.

The *neurotic type of delinquent* exhibits many of the same characteristics as the sociopathic type, but with a difference. The neurotic type experiences guilt about his behavior, or becomes depressed over his inability to control it. The

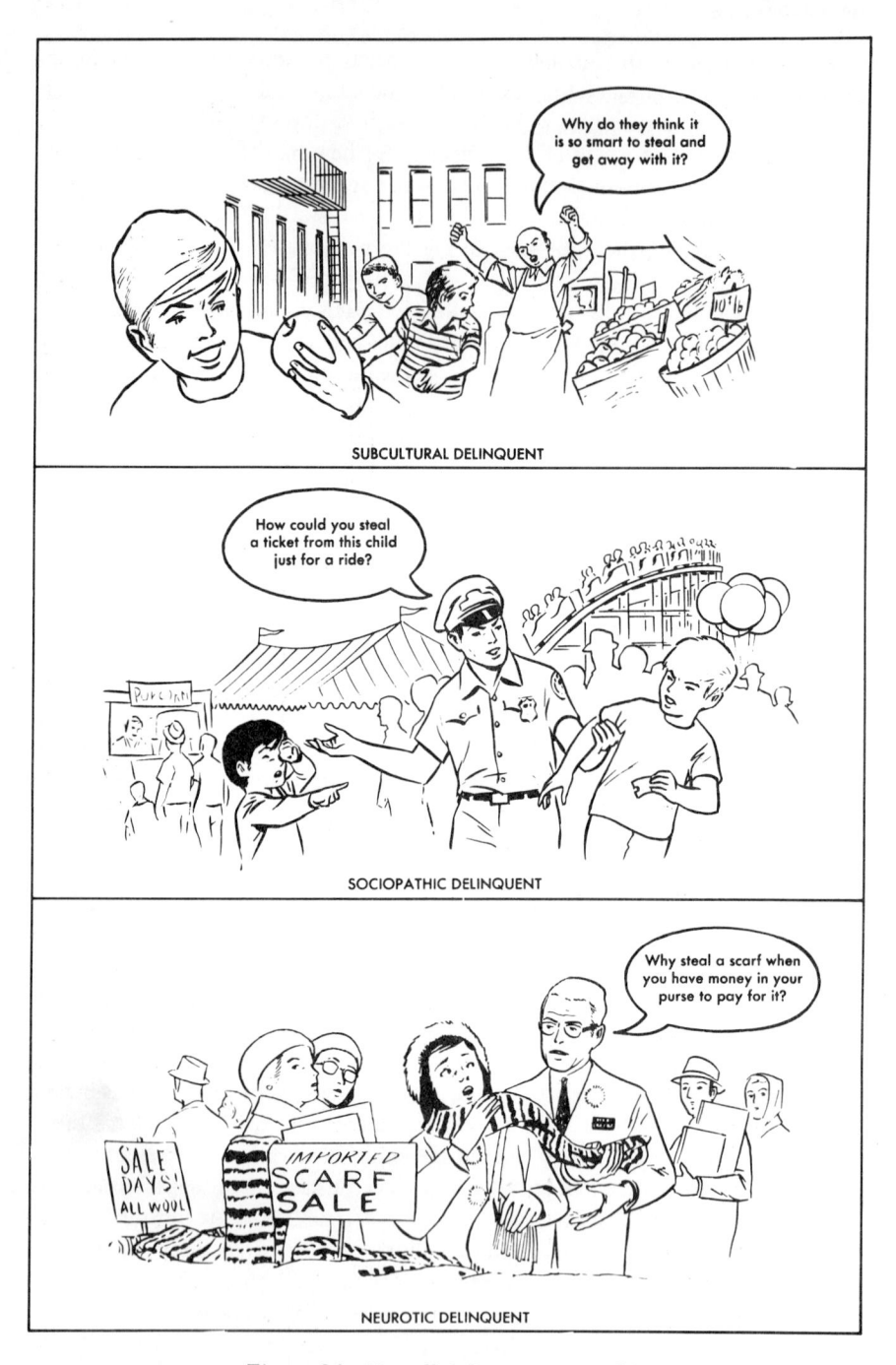

Figure 24. *Not all delinquents are alike.*

The Adolescent

causes may be exactly opposite. The sociopathic delinquent is likely to be the victim of too little parental attention; the neurotic may be a victim of too much. Harsh and/or inconsistent punishment may lead the growing child to reject social conformity as a way of rejecting his parents. The overprotected child may not have been permitted enough independence to develop self-esteem with which to deal with his problems. Acting-out is a way of proving to himself that he is not anxious, weak, or overly dependent. Or, the neurotic delinquent may be a product of both too much and too little. For example, too much control and too little affection may lead to sexual promiscuity in the teenage girl.

The basic causes of delinquent behavior come from misuse of discipline (punishment) and affection (reward) during the developmental years. Profound deviations from the normal in either case or in both cases may lead to delinquency.

Illness and the Teenager

The adolescent has a tendency to blame himself for illness or injury; children blame their parents, but teenagers blame themselves.[27]

Injuries are mainly a problem of the teenage boy. His activities are more hazardous than those of the girl. Also, girls are taught from infancy to be cautious.

Many injuries are related to instability. (The teenage boy is the most dangerous driver on the road.) An angry driver may seek a scapegoat on the road, and an accident is likely to occur. A person who feels inferior may run personal risks to prove himself superior, and it is understandable that many situations exist in which the teenage boy is made to feel inferior.

Since the teenager wants to conform, he fears anything that makes him different. Also, the hero is the physically strong and adept person. The boy is hauntingly afraid of being physically weak. In addition, he is desperately unhappy if he is away from the company of his friends, the only people with whom he feels comfortable at this time. He cannot bear to be "left out."

Ill health will affect the social development of the adolescent. Poor health tends to lead to a secluded, withdrawn life. A 14-year-old girl was injured while skating. She was confined to bed and then a wheelchair for the remainder of her high school days. She had visitors, but she was isolated from the social life of her friends. She did not have the chance to learn with the others how to dance, how to act on a date, how to converse about social trivia, and how to be at ease in a restaurant. After she recovered, she was shy and retiring for many years.

This is another example of the need for rehabilitation. Perhaps you are beginning to understand that rehabilitation involves every patient.

[27] Dorothy Rogers, *The Psychology of Adolescence* (New York: Appleton-Century-Crofts, 1962), p. 96.

Your Teenage Patient

The adolescent patient is extremely modest. He needs privacy, even more than the 11-year-old needs it. The nurse can help by not unnecessarily exposing the body during treatment time. Some embarrassment may be avoided if she explains carefully all the nursing procedures.

One student practical nurse told of helping her teenage daughter to get ready for a tonsillectomy. "Now, Terry," she explained, "here is the hospital gown. Put this on and take off your other clothes." The girl's eyes widened. "Oh no. He is going to operate on me up *here*," placing her hands on her throat. "My underwear stays on." It did, too.

Many times the teenage patient is very matter-of-fact. He wants to know specifically what is wrong and what is happening. You may be surprised by his store of knowledge.

The teenager is less dependent on his family than the younger child. But there are other problems for the nurse. The young student nurse – so very appealing in her fresh, immaculate uniform – can easily be the subject of a real "crush." What is she to do? To encourage the patient is the worst possible nursing ethics. Yet to be brusquely rude is wrong, too. After all, his high opinion of her is a compliment. The solution may be to maintain a friendly, but impersonal attitude. She can address him with his given name, not his nickname. A sense of humor helps. She can be efficient and businesslike without being oversentimental.

The teenager needs help from everyone to accept his illness. The nurse can help in many ways. Avoid being too authoritative. He will resent it from you as much as from his parents. Praise what you can praise honestly. Avoid belittling and derogatory remarks. Help the patient to look forward to the future.

Diversions for the Adolescent

Adolescent interests are guided by individual hobbies, just as is the case with adults. But remembering what the adolescent is like will help the nurse to suggest the appropriate adult hobbies.

The adolescent boy who is trying to act manly would be insulted by any suggestion of a feminine hobby. Boys are likely to be interested in building model cars or model airplanes.

One 13-year-old boy, who was very scientific-minded, was thrilled with a ready-to-assemble model of the prop-jet engine. He was learning the principles of jet power as he assembled the several hundred parts. The model was authentic because the engine manufacturer had given the specifications and $20,000 to the toy manufacturer to produce a reasonably priced, accurate model engine. The

The Adolescent

13-year-old was so enthusiastic he could scarcely bother to eat or sleep for three days until he had assembled the engine and flicked the switch, putting all the moving parts into motion.

Other ready-to-assemble kits are available that are educational. A plastic model of the human skeleton may even help a student nurse with her study of human anatomy.

Teenage girls are interested in clothes and personal appearance; so capitalize on this interest to suggest a hobby for them. One teenage girl became skillful in making lovely corsages of wood fiber. She returned to school in time for the spring style show that the sewing classes presented. Her dress was not finished, but she had a pretty corsage for the finished dresses of all the other girls. Adding correct accessories to homemade garments is extremely important; hence a lovely corsage to adorn each dress was a real contribution. This teenager had helped to make the style show a success.

The teenage boy who is a sports fan might enjoy making a scrapbook about his favorite baseball team. A miniature printing press might encourage another teenager to publish a newspaper. He could have fun with a local "gossip sheet."

Books suitable for the adolescent are probably those read by adults. Reading choices are guided by individual interests, hobbies, and school subjects. Today's libraries offer an excellent selection of career books, historical romances, biographies, stories of World War II, and of the astronauts.

The region of the country influences the type of stories that boys read. Boys living on the West Coast and on the East Coast like sea stories and navy stories. In Indianapolis, Indiana, home of the 500-mile automobile speedway, librarians have difficulty meeting requests for stories about automobiles and automobile racing. One hospital librarian finally subscribed to a "hot-rod" magazine to appease the demands of her teenage patients.

For some adolescent patients, suspense stories should be omitted. One cardiac teenager requested the Nancy Drew mystery stories, but the librarian tactfully substituted another book. A well-meaning relative, however, brought in one book of the series. The nurses attributed the relapse that followed to the girl's intense interest in the story.

Questions for Discussion

1. What provisions are made for adolescent patients in your hospital? Are they placed with pediatric patients?
2. What specific techniques can the nurse observe to help prevent embarrassment for the adolescent patient?
3. In many communities, too many teenagers leave high school before graduation. What can the nurse do about this as a responsible citizen?
4. What is being done to combat juvenile delinquency in your community?

Additional Readings

The Adolescent in Your Family Washington, D.C.: U.S. Department of Health, Education, and Welfare, Children's Bureau Publication No. 347. Rev. 1955.
Cole, Luella, and Irma Hall. *The Psychology of Adolescence*. 6th ed. New York: Holt, Rinehart and Winston, Inc., 1964.
Grinder, Robert E. ed. *Studies in Adolescence*. New York: The Macmillan Company, 1963.
Hasler, Doris, and Norman B. Hasler. *Personal, Home, and Community Health*. Chap. 5, "Feminine Hygiene"; Chap. 7, "Stimulants and Narcotics." New York: The Macmillan Company, 1967.
Jaeger, Margaret Ann. *Child Development and Nursing Care*. Chap. 5, "The Adolescent." New York: The Macmillan Company, 1962.
Kuhlen, Raymond G. *Psychology of Adolescent Development*. Part II, "Physical Growth and Development in Adolescence." New York: Harper and Brothers, 1952.
Mead, Margaret, and Ken Heyman. *The Family*, pp. 185–208. New York: The Macmillan Company, 1965.
Rasmussen, Sandra. *Foundations of Practical and Vocational Nursing*. Chap. 46, "The Adolescent." New York: The Macmillan Company, 1967.
Rogers, Dorothy. *Psychology of Adolescence*. New York: Appleton-Century-Crofts, Inc., 1962.
Smith, Christine Spahn. *Maternal-Child Nursing*. Chap. 9, "The Adolescent Years." Philadelphia: W. B. Saunders Company, 1963.
Your Children and Their Gangs. Washington, D.C.: U.S. Department of Health, Education, and Welfare, Children's Bureau Publication No. 384, 1960.

Recommended Audiovisual Aids

FILMS

Girl to Woman (18 min., Churchill Films, Color)
> This film is planned for teenage girls, but would help the practical nurse to understand adolescent growth and change. With animation, it shows male and female sex organs, fertilization, and general growth of embryo.

Boy to Man (16 min., Churchill Films, Color)
> This film shows actual photographs of vocal cords and skin changes. With animation, it shows the male and female sex organs; menstruation; ejaculation. It explains wet dreams (nocturnal emissions) and masturbation.

Boy with a Knife (18 min., Dudley Pictures Corporation, B&W)
> A teenage boy, rejected by his stepmother and let down by his father, is lonely and begins to misbehave. He carries a knife and gets into a fight. A group work specialist consults with father and with son. When the father

finally begins to stand up to the stepmother in defense of the boy, the boy's behavior begins to improve. This film shows how properly trained psychologists can help young people in trouble.

Howard (27 min., International Film Bureau, B&W)
Howard, a teenager, is caught between adult opinion and youthful enthusiasms. His part-time employer gives him sound advice on the value of thinking for himself rather than listening to conflicting opinions of parents, girl friend, and boy friend. The film would help the practical nursing student to see that one phase of maturity is being able to think and to make decisions for oneself.

The Teens (25 min., McGraw-Hill, B&W. Ages and Stages Series)
Normal teenagers are self-centered. This film is about three normal teenagers, and shows how parents can help them. It emphasizes the importance of good rules, but suggests that parents can sometimes permit rules to be broken. Teenagers need space to entertain.

Who Should Decide (11 min., Coronet, Color)
Teenage discipline is considered, both from parents' and children's viewpoints. The teenagers want to do more than they should. Finally, the family gets together and decides which decisions will be made by whom. The film gives no conclusive answers; hence it could stimulate classroom discussion.

FILMSTRIPS

Anxiety (39 frames, High School Guidance Filmstrip of the Month Club, Color)
This filmstrip explains causes of anxiety and suggests acceptable ways of handling it.

Dangers of Narcotics (47 frames, McGraw-Hill, Color)
The harmful effects of narcotics are illustrated. The explanation of stimulants and depressants and of legal and illegal use of narcotics would help the student nurse.

Frustration (40 frames, High School Guidance Filmstrip of the Month Club, Color)
The filmstrip explains what frustration is, what causes frustration, and ways to compensate for it.

Future in Hand (29 frames, Stanley-Bowmar Company, B&W)
Although planned for teenagers, the filmstrip would help younger practical nursing students. It explains that home life today is related to future life and poses such questions as teenagers' rights and the parents' rights.

Getting Along with Your Family (37 frames, Filmstrip of the Month Club, Color)

    The Green family is pictured — how they work and play together and try to understand and help each other. It would be good for teenagers to see, and also will help parents to know how teenagers feel about them.

How Shall I Tell My Child About Sex? (42 frames, International Film Bureau, Color)

    Animated drawings depict structure and function of reproductive organs, fertilization, pregnancy, and childbirth. Suggestions are made for developing healthy attitudes toward sex. It will help adults to know how this subject may be presented to teenagers.

Personal Problem Solving (40 frames, High School Guidance Filmstrip of the Month Club, Color)

    Common individual problems are illustrated, and advice given on how to solve them.

Sex: A Moral Dilemma for Teenagers, Part I and Part II (68 and 81 frames, Guidance Associates, Color. Two 12-inch, long-playing records, with counselor's guide)

    These filmstrips are designed to help open the lines of communication between adults and teenagers. Part I deals with the teenager's resentment at being forced to accept without question the morality standards of other generations. Part II explores the basic confusion about sex that exists for both young and older generations.

Shyness (40 frames, High School Guidance Filmstrip of the Month Club, Color)

    Two teenagers are depicted: one shy, one not. Causes are given for shyness and suggestions made on how to overcome feelings of inadequacy.

The Tuned-Out Generation, Part I and Part II (74 and 72 frames, Guidance Associates, Color. Two 12-inch, long-playing records; with teacher's manual, counselor's guide)

    These two filmstrips with accompanying records point out that the two generations (teenagers and parents) are not "tuned in" to each other. They are designed to stimulate discussion and deepen the concern of teenagers in communication between the older and younger generations.

Values for Teenagers: The Choice is Yours — Part I, Part II (Guidance Associates, Color. Two 12-inch, long-playing records. Running time: Part I — 18 min. Part II — $13\frac{1}{2}$ min.; with counselor's guide)

    Several genuine teenagers (not actors) speak on the pressure and problems that they face today. Adults could profit from these two filmstrips with records by gaining greater understanding of teenagers' problems.

The Adolescent

Your Fight Against Fear (40 frames, High School Guidance Filmstrip of the Month Club, Color)
    This filmstrip explains that a certain degree of fear is natural and normal, shows causes of fears, and offers suggestions that will help to conquer fears.

TRANSPARENCIES

Carlson, Nancy. Home Economics No. 19, *Fundamentals of Grooming.* 23 different transparencies. 3M Company, 3M Center, Visual Products Division, St. Paul Minnesota.

CHAPTER 17 / **THE YOUNG ADULT**

The young person establishing himself in the adult world represents an important phase in the family life cycle. This phase includes the dating period, engagement, and wedding. It means college, nurse's training, business preparation, or vocational school. It may include service in the armed forces, or an apprenticeship in a trade, or first position as secretary or clerk. This can be an exciting, challenging, dramatic, or troublesome phase. Unquestionably, expenses can be high.

If illness occurs, these matters (except financial) may seem less important and fade into the background. But even if no open discussions are held, the nurse should realize that the situation exists.

The parents are vitally concerned, but they may need to express opinions cautiously. Some parents rigidly insist on making the decisions. Other parents go to the opposite extreme and are never available for advice. The majority of parents recognize their children's rights to grow up and to make their own decisions. They do not wish to interfere or dominate. They want only to help if they can, but how to help may be baffling.

The Activists and the Dropout Generation

Enough young people today reject the established pattern of life to call attention to themselves. Those expressing extreme rebellion, the "hippies" or "flower children," and the activists or agitators are in the minority. The majority of young people continue trying to communicate with the rest of society and to plan for the future, but among them dissatisfaction exists. The generation gap is real.

Generally, our young people have had material wishes supplied immediately. They do not hesitate to use credit, to pay later for something that they want now. Youth in upper- and middle-class homes have never suffered real want. They have only read and heard about the depression during the 1930's; they did not experience those years.

Today's youth have been taught to think for themselves. They look critically at the world their parents helped to shape, and do not like what they see. They do not necessarily accept their parents' middle-class virtues and goals: hard work, sacrifice, self-improvement, getting ahead, financial success.

Some young people object to the many years of preparation required of the professions, years they call "prolonged adolescence." They want to become involved *now*.

The Young Adult

The "hippies" or "flower children" reject the established way of life by withdrawing from society. They want no part of it. Withdrawal is accomplished by different routes.

The most tragic ones are those who seek to escape through drugs. To "drop out" the LSD way can appear to be a painless way to escape temporarily into a bright and shiny world in which what really matters is what one is and wants to be. You may encounter in your nursing career young adults who have been physically harmed by using drugs.

The activists are an entirely different group, a small segment organized for the purpose of tearing down established society. This is also an attack on the institutions created by society. The nurse is not expected to know the solutions, but she can be a quieting element in her community if she recognizes an activist and lets the authorities know that she is alert to his method of operation. Administrators need the support of the public. The activists generate trouble by making demands on the administration of the institution, college, or high school. Whether this is granted or not, they demand something else and continue demanding with the hopes of destroying the school. Key words used by the agitators are "relevance," "involvement," "dissent," "amnesty," "open discussion" – all, individually, reasonable terms. True, established society is not perfect and has many weaknesses. But it is our way of life. Without organization, anarchy results. Nurses need to be aware of what is happening around and among them.

Choosing a Career

To many young people, adult life appears uncertain and without clear-cut goals. Choosing a career is further complicated by the changes in the technological world. Once qualified for a certain type of work, the worker must continually study to keep informed of new knowledge, new methods. Or, as mentioned in Chapter 16, he may face the possibility that his chosen occupation is becoming obsolete. The 17-year-old may wonder, "Why train for an occupation that may not exist ten years from now?"

Most families desire that the young person choose his own life work. Parents may be puzzled or disappointed when their son does not choose a career in business, or does not wish to follow the same profession as his father's. Career choices of today's brightest college students stem from the desire to help others, not to make the most money.

Choosing a vocation is tremendously important. If you are the student practical nurse who is newly graduated from high school, undoubtedly you have heard this many times. If you are the student with a background of working experience, you have firsthand knowledge of what it means to be suited for the job and to like your work.

To choose wisely the teenager needs to get information about occupations and to take self-inventory. In theory, a child may choose from among some 30,000 different kinds of occupations in the United States. Actually, his choice may be limited by his family status, race, religion, education, and locality. Yet his own preference and his own drive are significant. In self-inventory, the young person should realistically study his abilities, aptitudes, interests, health, and financial resources. His family, school counselors, and other interested people will help him to think through his situation. The final decision should really be his own.

Most high school girls today expect that homemaking will be their life work, and many girls do not prepare themselves for work outside the home. Yet the common practice today is for women to reenter the labor force after the age of 30, when their youngest child is in school. If the mother has no particular training, she can apply only for unskilled positions.

The young woman preparing for a nursing career will find that it has many advantages. She joins a profession that will always be in demand. It is like an insurance policy, to be cashed when an emergency arises. Her nursing skills and knowledge are not stored away in the guest closet when she becomes a full-time homemaker. The experience and knowledge of a nurse will enable her to be a better wife, mother, and homemaker. Like the home economist, the nurse shares the knowledge of her profession with her loved ones.

One of the saddest situations today in our country exists with regard to the young people who have dropped out of school without being prepared for an occupation. They are unemployed and unemployable. Today, a person has to have some skill to offer the employment world. Perhaps you learned this if you ever applied, untrained, for work in a hospital.

Young people are guided into careers in many ways, by many different people. You would receive varied answers if you were to ask your classmates, "Why did you choose to enroll in practical nursing? Who influenced you?" Many people choose practical nursing because they have known and respected a licensed practical nurse who was happy in her work. By your own actions as a student nurse and as a graduate practical nurse, you will encourage – or discourage – others from entering the field of practical nursing.

From School to Work

The act of getting a job seems to mark the emergence of the adult from childhood. We tend to regard earning a living as one indication of the mature person.

For parents a crucial milestone is reached when their children are on their own. They should feel successful when their youngster takes his responsible place in the working world, when their daughter creates a real home of her own.

The Young Adult

But they should also realize that transferring from school to work may bring acute problems. Many young people find it hard to leave the company of their friends, to adjust to the routine and tempo of steady employment, and to get used to the demands of work on their time and energy. Many young workers fail to adjust to authority and to their co-workers. This is a common cause of job dissatisfaction and change.

These problems may be duplicated in a practical nursing school with young students who have never worked or who have had few home responsibilities. One year is a short time to learn the duties of a nurse and the duties of a responsible adult.

From personal observation, the author believes that a class of practical nursing students composed of both inexperienced and mature students offers advantages to both groups. The older student who has managed work or family responsibilities can be a steadying hand to the young student making this important transition from school to work. But the young student has been in school recently and is probably more adept with study techniques. When people have been away from books and studying for years, discipline is needed to relearn habits of study and concentration. Students can cooperate and help each other in many ways.

Serious Choice of Life Partner

Not only is the young person seeking a place in the working world, he is also thinking about marriage. Many people — church people and lay people — believe that a casual attitude toward marriage is responsible for the appalling divorce rate and other evidences of family breakdown. Clergymen — Catholic, Protestant, and Jewish — offer premarital counseling emphasizing (1) careful choice of the marriage partner and (2) a willingness to work at marriage.

Unquestionably, marriage would be more stable if young people gave truly serious thought and consideration to the choice of a husband or wife. Sometimes they ponder more deeply about the purchase of a new car than about the decision to get married.

The young American wants to choose his own mate. The arranged marriage that still is made in some parts of Europe and the Orient is not popular in America. In fact, if parents offer liberal advice, regardless of how well meant, the young person is likely to decide the opposite of their suggestion.

How can parents help? The influence and help of the parents are probably already established by this time. By their own actions and conduct, parents have helped their children to establish moral codes of behavior and goals in life. Young people usually seek these same standards in a mate.

If the parents have a good marriage, the young person has a satisfactory model to copy. He realizes that one argument does not end a marriage if he has seen his parents disagree, discuss a problem, and work out a compromise solution. In a mentally healthy home, individuals face their problems realistically and cope with them in constructive ways. The young person who has seen his parents attempt to solve problems with escape, such as by drinking, may unconsciously imitate. A favorite defense of the young drug addict is, "Adults use alcohol as a crutch or an escape. Why should they condemn us for using drugs?" Some young people actually insist that drugs are less harmful than alcohol which has proved over the years to have harmful effects when imbibed in excess.

The young person has an advantage if his home has been a place of good understanding and of lack of serious conflict between parents and children. Also he is helped if his parents have raised him to think of others. For example, it is easy for an only child to grow up thinking first of himself.

A happy, friendly home aids children in becoming friendly teenagers and friendly adults. The friendly person is more likely to meet a variety of people and to select a suitable marriage partner. During dating and courtship, young people become acquainted with a variety of members of the opposite sex. This helps toward meeting and marrying a compatible person.

Engagement

Engagement should mean more than buying and wearing a ring. This period can be such a happy, gay whirlwind of showers, trousseau buying, and wedding plans that the true values of engagement are ignored.

During this time, the boy and girl learn to know each other better. They begin to learn what it means to be a couple. Before accepting an invitation to a Saturday night party, the girl consults her fiancé. The two are being accepted as a couple by the community, their friends, and their families. If Mary's friends do not accept her Johnny, she has to decide: "Do we make new friends?" She may give serious thought to the reasons for their objections.

A reasonably long engagement affords opportunity for differences to come to light and for conflicting opinions to rise.

The couple should discuss seriously any important differences. If their religions are different, what is their compromise? What kind of social activities do they both really enjoy? Will the wife work? What is the wife's role to be as far as entertaining socially for her husband's business? How will they handle the money? What are their real goals in life? An ambitious woman may not be compatible with an easygoing or an irresponsible husband. Do they both want children? How many? What do they consider the worthwhile things in life?

Competent premarital counseling will help to ensure that the young couple consider these and other adjustments to be made in marriage. A couple should be able to reach an agreement on most of these questions, to plan a workable budget, and to plan for their home together. Frequent quarrels, emotional explosions, general unhappiness during engagement — these are all danger signals of an unworkable marriage. A broken engagement is better than an unhappy marriage.

Today, marriages are held together by mutual attraction, companionship, affection, and common interests. Without these bonds, the chances are the couple will not continue to live together.

The approximate length of engagement varies greatly. Too short an engagement does not give the couple enough time to get to know each other. Short acquaintances and short engagements may predict marital unhappiness. A lengthy engagement encourages intimacy. One authority recommends a minimum of six months.[1]

Development Toward Maturity

The young person attempting to assume the status of the responsible adult needs "gentle guidance" by those with greater experience. Parents and counselors should strive to be patient and tolerant. Occasional lapses into adolescent or childish behavior are to be expected. Perhaps it is sufficient for parents to give reassurance now and then on important decisions. Young people need guidance in some great moral issues, but they do not want moralistic judgments.

Often a sympathetic adult outside the family circle can be a source of help. The capable, understanding nurse — by being just what she is, a good nurse — can be a beacon of inspiration to the young adult, struggling so hard to be grown up. Think for a moment of the people who have been a source of inspiration to you — a minister, priest, nun, or teacher. No doubt you were favorably impressed by the quality of person he (she) was — good, kind, understanding, unselfish, courageous. Similarly, a nurse can be a help to the young adults within her circle of acquaintances.

The individual is progressing toward maturity all through life; maturity is not a stage that is reached at one definite point. In fact, a definition of it is not easy to give. There is physical maturity, social maturity, emotional maturity, and spiritual maturity. Some people believe that emotional maturity is not attained until about the age of 35 and that spiritual maturity is reached even later.

One definition of emotional maturity or good mental health is: a state in which the individual lives in harmony with himself and with others. He can meet the stresses of life without abnormal emotional reactions. He has self-reliance and self-respect, and he accepts others as they are.

---

[1] Judson T. Landis and Mary G. Landis, *Personal Adjustment: Marriage and Family Living*, 4th ed. (Englewood Cliffs, N.J.: Prentice-Hall, 1966), pp. 144–145.

For many of us, these feelings are anchored in a belief in God. We are all part of His universal plan — the basic, intrinsic part, but still only one small segment. When we can keep this perspective, we do not regard great personal tragedies as the end of the world. Life goes on.

In the hospital, you will be in constant contact with people experiencing great personal tragedies. You need to be understanding, sympathetic, and helpful, yet able to exercise self-control. Nursing is no profession for the immature, unstable person.

The Single Adult

Not every person marries. Your patient may be one of the twelve and one-half million single adults in our country.[2] About nine out of ten people marry; about one out of ten does not.

We have been thinking about the patient as a family member. The family may include parents, grandparents, brothers and sisters, aunts and uncles, nieces and nephews — not necessarily husband, wife, and children. Many adults are completely alone, with no close family ties.

Some people remain single by choice. The man who travels widely in his work may postpone marriage. Certain people prefer to devote their lives to a career. Their work genuinely comes first in their lives, and they tolerate no mediocrity. Sometimes either a son or daughter may have the responsibility for invalid parents at the time when others their age are marrying. Thus there are many reasons why people do not marry. Most unmarried adults probably did not plan it that way — it just happened. Marriage is not a requirement today, but a choice.

The single person is not necessarily an unhappy, useless individual. Every person experiences disappointment at some time in his life. He has to accept and face reality. Happiness for most people means making the best of one's life. If the single person does this, he will enjoy the advantages that he has and not be unhappy about the things he does not have.

The single person learns to rely on himself. He is independent because he has to be. He may have built up inner sources of courage that can help him in times of illness.

The happy, single person is usually truly involved in a challenging career, with a goal to work toward and other people to think about. She (he) channels her time and energy into a cause that is greater than herself. It may be a worthwhile community project, in addition to her work.

Many mothers have said that the happiest time of their family life was when their children were still at home. This was the woman's busiest time, when she

---

[2] *U.S. News and World Report,* June 3, 1963, p. 44; figures from U.S. Census Bureau.

had so much to do for her husband and her children that she could not possibly think about herself.

The same could be true of the single person. Think of the woman with a full-time secretarial position who conducts, in her own home, a weekly class in religious instruction for underprivileged children. In the evenings, she helps adults learn to read via a shortened "literary" method. This dedicated, gracious woman is too busy living for other people to brood about herself. Yes, there can be many ways to live a fulfilled life.

Many single people cherish family ties and make concentrated efforts to keep in touch with nieces and nephews, cousins, aunts, and uncles. It might be difficult to say who enjoyed most the camping trip to the Canadian woods, north of Quebec City: the uncle (an experienced traveler and camper), his 12-year-old nephew, or the nephew's friend. They all had a marvelous time.

Of course, the single person needs to avoid being "married to her job." The nurse makes a career of giving unselfish, devoted care to her patients. But she needs other interests and hobbies to balance her life.

Perhaps society is maturing when it recognizes that many ways of living can be good.

Health Needs and the Effect of Illness

The young adult is probably at his peak of effectiveness, both physically and intellectually. He continues to increase in learning from experience and in exercising judgment, however. Optimum health is the goal: balanced meals, proper rest, regular exercise, and attention to minor symptoms — all contribute to optimum health.

Young women need to eat meals that provide enough iron; both young men and young women need to balance calorie intake with physical activity. Overeating leads to obesity, a significant health problem in the United States because it provokes the onset and increases the severity of many chronic diseases.

Our way of life tends to foster inactivity. We ride, not walk; we take the elevator, not the stairs; we are spectators, not participants. Unless a person chooses to eat spartan meals all his life, he should consciously plan for physical activity. Any physical activity requires calories, and it may also have a longer-term effect by raising the rate of metabolism while resting. Several studies have reported an increase of 20 percent or more in basal metabolic rate the day following heavy exercise.[3]

Young adults have accidents, but disability is rarer at this period of life than

---

[3] Robert B. Bradfield, "The Relative Importance of Physical Activity for the Overweight," *Nutrition News*, Vol. 31, No. 4 (Dec. 1968).

it ever will be again.[4] But when poor health does come, it is a severe blow. Illness is unexpected. It seriously disrupts the person's concept of himself. The man is not too far removed from the adolescent's overevaluation of physical strength. He must look upon himself as an invalid, not as a healthy young man. If he cannot earn his living and provide for his wife and family, he regards himself as a failure.

Illness brings problems for the young adult woman too. The single girl fears she will have no dates and no opportunity to marry. The young mother may feel she is failing in her job as a wife and mother.

Helping these people to accept prolonged illness or handicaps is a real challenge to the nurse. This is another example of the need for rehabilitation.

Questions for Discussion

1. What factors would an 18-year-old girl weigh before deciding to enroll in a one-year, two-year, three-year, or four-year nursing program? Where are the sources of information in your community?
2. Where is premarital counseling available in your community?
3. Review the skills and knowledge a practical nurse acquires that are used in managing a home and rearing a family.
4. Describe an unmarried adult you know who has a successful career or useful life.

Additional Readings

Duvall, Evelyn Millis. *Family Development.* 4th ed. Philadelphia: J. B. Lippincott Company, 1967.
Landis, Judson T., and Mary G. Landis. *Personal Adjustment: Marriage and Family Living.* 4th ed. Chap. 12, "Engagement." Englewood Cliffs, N.J.: Prentice-Hall, Inc., 1966.
Landis, Judson T., and Mary G. Landis. *Building a Successful Marriage.* 4th ed. Chap. 7, "Some Will Never Marry." Englewood Cliffs, N.J.: Prentice-Hall, Inc., 1963.

Recommended Audiovisual Aids

FILMSTRIPS

Seeing Double (29 frames, Stanley-Bowmar Company, B&W)
Questions on "going steady" are presented. The filmstrip considers the purpose of courtship. It poses questions on differences in social and

---

[4] Paul V. Lemkau, *Mental Hygiene in Public Health* (New York: McGraw-Hill, 1949), pp. 238–239.

The Young Adult

economic backgrounds and mixed marriages. The ending emphasizes that courtship should not be rushed.

What You Should Know Before Going to Work (Guidance Associates, Color. Two filmstrips with accompanying records, 14 and 15 min. each; counselor's guide)

The filmstrips illustrate the value of preparing for an occupation. They discuss the job interview and qualities needed for success on the job.

When Are We Ready for Marriage? (37 frames, Popular Science Filmstrip of the Month Club, Color)

The filmstrip shows the variety of practical matters to be considered to create a harmonious marriage, pointing out the disadvantages of early marriage. It would be good for teenagers or young adults considering marriage.

With This Ring (29 frames, Stanley-Bowmar Company, B&W)

The filmstrip consists of advice on engagement; meaning of the ring; value of good planning; and effect of maturity and immaturity on the success of marriage. It would be helpful to the nurse considering marriage, and to the nurse who needs to advise others or to understand her own marital problems.

CHAPTER 18 / **THE MATURE ADULT**

Your study of illness conditions, of medical-surgical nursing will be focused on the adult patient. You study symptoms, treatments, and rehabilitation of adults. Nursing interest frequently deviates from the adult and centers on the dependent group, the very young and the very old, because unless specific attention is given to their needs, they may be neglected.

So although much of the content of this book is concerned with children and elderly people, we must realize what illness means to the adult, the person from 35 to 60 years of age. These so-called middle-aged people are generally the established citizens, the ones who manage homes, businesses, government, and the care of the young and the old. Illness of the responsible adult quickly and drastically affects the lives of many others. In order to give the best possible care to the adult patient and consideration to his family, the nurse needs to be aware of the health needs, physical changes, and adjustments continually present in the 35- to 60-age group.

A big adjustment is required in the relatively new stage in the family life cycle that may be called "Rediscovery."

Rediscovery

Your patient may be the mature woman or man whose children are married, working, or at college — away from the family home.

Even 50 years ago, this period of the family life cycle was not likely to exist. People are marrying earlier today, having their children closer together, and living longer. Formerly, it was unusual for both parents to be living when the last child was married. Today, more than one out of four families are in this stage, sometimes called "The Empty Nest."

Usually, the struggle to earn a living has lessened. Although the group represents one-tenth of our total population, it gets one-fifth of our annual personal income. Business and professional people are at the height of their careers; the highest average incomes are found in the group aged 50 to 65.[1] This is the least debt-burdened of all age groups. The house mortgage is probably paid off, as well as the typical 20-year life insurance policy and educational debts. The wife has perfected her homemaking skills and manages a well-organized household. Both husband and wife may have more leisure time.

[1] *U.S. News and World Report,* January 6, 1969, p. 68. Source: U.S. Census Bureau.

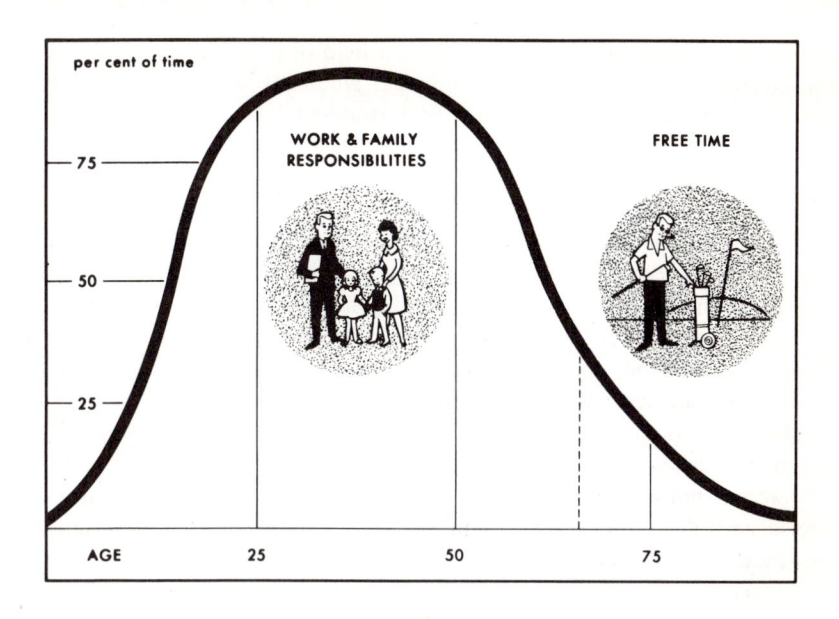

Figure 25. *Free time increases as children grow up. In preindustrial societies, most adults were engaged in making a living as long as they lived. Today, the middle-aged and older worker has more time free than he spends on the job. (1961 White House Conference on Aging,* Chart Book, Chart 62, Federal Council on Aging.)

This can be a second honeymoon for the couple if they have remained close through the years, continued to grow and mature with adjustable attitudes. Yet for those unable to accept changes and unable to continue growing, maturing, and developing, this can be an unhappy time.

WIFE'S PROBLEM

The wife whose whole interest has been her children and her home will find that her job is cut in half. She has much less work to do and much less influence in her children's lives. Since this drastic change in her life comes at the time her body is undergoing a physical change, she may feel frustrated, useless, even ill without apparent cause.

She needs a vital interest in life to replace her mothering role. A creative hobby, a new job, the presidency of her favorite club — something to be truly excited about will help her to keep from "meddling" in her grown children's lives or her husband's business. The wise woman has had interests through the years that will help her to let her children grow and go. If not, she needs new interests that will fill the second half of her life.

Sometimes the wife needs additional vocational training before volunteering her services or applying for work. Our own field of practical nursing has been enriched by numerous women of this age, women who are truly giving of themselves to others. In doing so, they find happiness.

HUSBAND'S PROBLEM

At this time in his life, the man must accept himself as he is — with his failures and his accomplishments. A young man in his twenties has visions of being president of the company, of owning his own business, of being truly successful. Now in his fifties he can see how far he can progress, and perhaps this does not equal his boyish dreams. With retirement around the corner at age 65, he must also realistically plan for the use of his leisure time.

The man's family, especially his wife, can be a source of comfort to him now. If he knows that she is truly proud of him and his status in life, he can better accept himself. But to remind him subtly or openly that someone else is more successful, to push and urge him forward, is dangerous. He cannot take the pressures that he once could.

STRENGTHENING THEIR MARRIAGE

After the children have left home, many couples realize they are almost strangers to each other. The husband may have devoted himself completely to his work, while the wife became so engrossed in the children that they have grown apart. With a real desire to do so, the husband and wife can reorganize their lives and make this a truly wonderful time. Any relationship needs to be nourished by developing more common interests as the years go by. Enriching the husband-wife relationship means cultivating new, shared experiences, keeping up with the times, and having something to talk about. Husband and wife need to make new friends, possibly more nonfamily contacts. Church activities, community affairs, politics, travel, refurnishing the home — all kinds of exciting adventures are available to the couple who will seek them.

Keeping up personal appearances will please the spouse and the children, in addition to helping maintain high morale and youthful attitudes.

Failure to strengthen their marriage and to establish worthy purposes for living can lead to many problems, such as divorce and alcoholism.

RELATIONSHIP WITH ADULT CHILDREN

Generally, parents with many outside interests have less difficulty untying apron strings and letting their children become mature and responsible adults than parents with no outside interests. Parents of teenagers realize that they need to replace gradually the dependent relationship with affection on a more man-to-man basis. Many in-law problems can be avoided if parents show they recognize their children as adults and wish the two generations to associate in mutually helpful ways.

Continuous emotional growth implies that the parents extend their love to include sons- and daughters-in-law, families of the in-laws, and grandchildren. But even more, love extends into a "big-hearted" interest in others and in humanity as a whole.

This advice is easy for the outsider to give, sometimes not so easy to follow. So have sympathy for your mature patient whose doctor cannot pinpoint the physical reason for his illness. The pain is real.

Alone Again

Many married couples are not privileged to have years together after their children are independent. Traumatic adjustments are required of the person bereft of a mate after 20 to 30 years of married life. Habits of living can be more entrenched than realized. Many widows and widowers find it helpful to continue their way of life, making no big changes for at least one year. Children, relatives, and friends can help, but the individual has to rebuild his own life. Unfair as it may seem, the widow may find that she is no longer a normal part of the circle of friends she and her husband had enjoyed as a couple. To make new friends and to find new interests may contribute the most to regaining personal strength.

Physical Changes

With the possible exception of menopause, physical changes in the adult occur so gradually that the person may be unaware of any change until faced with an emergency situation. The man who remains fairly active can continue his ordinary pace, but may not be able to exert tremendous lifting power should he attempt it. The woman continues her household work and social activities or outside employment, but she cannot stay up all night and then work the next day.

As the person gets older, body tissues change in composition to relatively more fat and less muscular tissue. It is estimated that the percentage of body weight that is fat would be:

man, aged 25 — 13.4 percent fat
aged 35 — 18.6 percent fat
aged 45 — 22.5 percent fat
aged 55 — 25 percent fat[2]

[2] Eva D. Wilson and others, *Principles of Nutrition,* 2nd ed. (New York: Wiley, 1965), p. 473.

Of course, the individual who exercises and uses his muscles retains his strength longer than the individual who does not. A professional golfer in his fifties has played excellent golf, winning in the first day of competition. But after the second or third consecutive day playing 36 holes of golf, the championship was won by a competitor in his twenties.

Similarly, the body organs of the middle-aged person are less able to cope with stress and strain that would have caused little difficulty in younger years.

Middle age is associated with bifocal glasses. In early adulthood the lens of the eyes begin to lose elasticity. In middle age the lens have lost enough elasticity that near vision recedes. In fact, if the change does not occur somewhere between the ages of 40 and 47, it could indicate that cataracts are forming. The nurse should know the importance of regular eye examinations. Not only does it become more difficult to focus on near objects, distant vision also begins to fade. Bifocal glasses help most individuals to see both near and far objects.

Hearing losses actually begin in the twenties, but may not be noticeable until the middle or late fifties. Research has not yet disclosed ways of preventing this almost universal loss in hearing. However, most adults are able to adjust and to compensate for minor hearing losses.

MENOPAUSE

Menopause is the time when menstruation stops, the ovaries cease to function, and a woman's reproductive power is ended. The physical symptoms are mainly due to estrogen deficiency — hot flushes, sweats, insomnia, and fatigue are among the most common. The aging process seems to accelerate — the skin wrinkles and becomes dry, the hair grays, the waistline widens, and the breasts sag.

More serious are the physical disabling consequences of severe estrogen deficiency: tendency to osteoporosis, making her fracture-prone; a negative balance leading to severe muscle weakness; and greater vulnerability to heart disease and hypertension.

Because menopause is a natural physiological occurrence, physicians formerly felt that treatment was unnecessary. This view is changing. Replacement therapy with estrogenic hormones can often prevent the usual consequences of estrogen deficiency when started early, and reverse the symptoms if started later. The estrogen level can be checked, and women with low estrogen levels can be treated as soon as the deficiency is discovered. Nurses are in a unique position to help clarify the concept that women do not always have to suffer the inconveniences and incapacities of menopause.

The nurse can be more effective if she realizes that for many women, menopause is as disturbing a transition as the onset of menstruation. The "change" may suddenly reveal the rapid passage of the years, the realization that

The Mature Adult

she can no longer have children, the fear that her sex life is ended. The latter is not substantiated, as numerous studies have shown that the loss of ovarian hormones has virtually no effect on sexual desire, sexual performance, or sexual response.

Superstitions are beginning to be replaced by a more calm, sensible, and practical approach to menopause. It is accepted that disturbing symptoms are intensified by excitement and nervous tension. Women today have more interests in life as they grow older, and less time to feel sorry for themselves. When accompanied by the "empty nest syndrome," as has been described, the situation is more difficult but not hopeless.

Even for the well-informed women, however, one visit to the doctor is recommended for the assurance that all is going well. Any unusual symptoms should be reported, as it is easy to blame the menopause for symptoms that, at another time, would be considered alarming.

Fewer emotional traumas accompany menopause today, but an increase in osteoporosis (bone thinning) among women past the age of 55 has been noted. It appears more prevalent among women who have had children, and who have had a calcium deficiency over a period of years. Most authorities attribute postmenopausal osteoporosis to withdrawal of estrogen, which interferes with normal protein metabolism. Lack of protein, in turn, prevents normal bone metabolism, and osteoporosis results. Treatment can arrest the condition, but not reverse the kyphosis (hunchback) that may have developed. Therapeutic routines suggested are as follows: (1) Encourage activity. (2) Maintain adequate protein, calcium, and vitamin intake, increasing the amount of vitamin D to 1000 I.U. daily.[3] (3) Prescribe androgen combined with estrogen.[4]

MALE CLIMACTERIC

There is debate as to whether men experience an abrupt change in the gonadal functions, or a counterpart of the menopause. It is known that men as well as women experience a lessening of sexual activity. The symptoms of poor memory, asocial behavior, loss of sex drive, and nervousness may respond to testosterone therapy.

OVERALL PICTURE IS OPTIMISTIC

The description of the physical changes that occur are not meant to present a gloomy picture of middle age. Innumerable adults maintain remarkably good health, a zest for living, and true interest in their professions and other people. You can cite many names of entertainment figures who effervesce vigor,

---

[3] Pregnant women need 400 I.U. of vitamin D daily; typical adult much less.
[4] Arthur J. Heather, *Manual of Care for the Disabled Patient* (New York: Macmillan, 1960), p. 72.

glamor, and joy of living. You also probably know intimately people who are living examples that this can be a wonderful and rewarding time of life. Most of these people live in the present with few regrets for the past, have plans for the future, observe healthy routines of living, and take time for periodic health examinations.

Periodic Health Consultation

Yearly physical examinations for everyone represent the ideal situation. After the fortieth birthday is reached, the ideal becomes the necessity. Regular health examinations, with thoughtful discussion between physician and patient, are essential to maintaining optimum health during middle age. It is also a significant preparation for a healthy older age. Most of the chronic diseases of the advancing years have their beginning in middle age. The symptoms are often disregarded because they are slight, not usually painful in the beginning, not accompanied by marked prostration, and do not cause fever. Recognizing early symptoms of chronic illness or degeneration makes possible intervention and treatment.

Many serious conditions may be avoided by early and timely removal of sources of infection. The person with diabetes can be taught how to prevent complications. Avoiding heavy strain may postpone coronary thrombosis. Proper attention to varicose veins may prevent serious complications, such as skin ulcers that are difficult to cure.

The health consultation serves to direct attention to possible breaks in the health of the person before such breaks occur. The purpose of the health consultation is to determine and measure the functional reserve capacity of the person under stress. If he knows how he may stand up under physical or mental exertion, he will be more likely to heed warnings against the careless use of his reserve physical strength.

During the health consultation, the physician takes a personal history to learn of family hereditary disease, any childhood or previous illnesses, accidents, operations, and present living habits. He conducts a thorough physical examination, with complete urinalysis and necessary X rays, blood work, and bacteriological tests. After diagnosis, the physician discusses his findings with the patient and recommends treatments necessary, proper nutrition, and general hygienic measures as related to exercise and habits. All these are designed to help the person to live wisely and well at his age level and in harmony with his environment.

Health Routines

Middle age can be a time of excesses and deficits: too much food; too much work without play; too much tobacco and alcohol; and lack of exercise, rest,

The Mature Adult

and freedom from strain. Increased work responsibilities and more demanding social life make it difficult for people to lighten the strain of living, and "to take it easy." But if more people recognized the importance, they might make the effort to find a healthy balance of work, rest, and recreation adapted to a slightly less able physical condition.

Moderation and consistency are the key words to health routines for the busy adult. He needs plenty of fresh air and exercise, but should avoid strenuous exertion that places undue stress on the circulatory system. After exercising, he should feel pleasantly tired, not exhausted. For this reason, he should leave for the young adult the highly competitive golf games, track sports, football, and boxing. Recommended are leisurely played golf, mild rowing, bicycling, walking, swimming, and pool. Calisthenics are excellent, but people are more likely to participate regularly if the exercise is a form of recreation, or "fun."

Exercise helps to develop good muscle tone, to maintain good posture, to prevent constipation, and to slow the appearance of osteoporosis. The adult can derive some of the same benefits that children derive from play, namely relief of tensions, anxiety, and pent-up emotions.

More rest is needed, but is not always easy to attain. Frequent rest periods can be the answer, and "catnaps" should be encouraged.

People of mature years need to cultivate habits of good mental hygiene, courage, self-control, and poise. Avoiding nervous strain brought on by worry, excessive excitement, and exhausting emotions help provide rest for the nervous system and the entire body.

Food Needs Change

People in the middle years should cut down on food intake, and be moderate in the use of fats (especially saturated fats), salt, condiments, and stimulants. Drinking plenty of liquids will help promote proper elimination. If milk is the liquid, the calcium deficiency might not be as extensive. Obesity and calcium deficiency are the two national nutritional problems in persons of middle years and older.[5]

The person at age 55 needs the protein, minerals, and vitamins that he needed at age 25, but in a diet supplying fewer calories. The vitamin B group are related to calorie needs, so he needs less riboflavin, thiamine, and niacin. After the menopause, women no longer need an additional supply of iron. The recommended amount is the same as that for men. Calcium needs are constant.

Energy needs are less after the years of early adulthood because of less activity and lowered basal metabolism caused by change in body composition and change in function of certain endocrine glands. The Foods and Nutrition

[5] G. A. Emerson, "Nutritional Status, USA," *Journal of Nutrition*, 91 (Suppl. 1), 1967, pp. 51–54.

Board of the National Research Council recommend reducing calories 5 per cent per decade between ages 35 and 55, and then reducing 8 per cent per decade between ages 55 and 75. For example, a woman whose ideal weight is 128 pounds might need 2000 calories daily at age 25; 1800 calories daily at age 45; and at age 65, 1500 calories per day.[6]

Calorie needs are always individual, related to the person's activity, health, status of nutrition, and general body build. But it is easy for a person to eat just a little more than he needs each day, and slowly gain weight. A gain of one pound a month amounts to a gain of 120 pounds in 10 years; gaining 5 pounds a year results in 50 extra pounds in 10 years. Ten years can pass very quickly! A person can gain one pound a month simply by eating every week two extra candy bars, a second piece of frosted cake, and drinking one extra cup of cocoa and a malted milk. This is above what he should have.

Use of Leisure Time

The use of leisure time influences to a great extent the amount of happiness or unhappiness of adults during the middle and later years of life. The person who learns to use wisely his leisure time while he is working can often adjust successfully to retirement. As the American working week gets shorter, more people are faced with the question of what to do when work is over. Not everyone can have stimulating daily work, but off-working hours can compensate for dull routines.

Free-time activities should offer a change from work. The person who sits at a desk most of the day will benefit from an outdoor sport. The person who exerts considerable physical energy may need extra rest and a quiet pastime to aid in relaxation. The floor duty nurse hardly needs to choose hiking as her recreation. But does not bowling involve seldom-used body muscles? She might also meet people outside the nursing profession.

Participating in active sports, as mentioned previously, strengthens health routines. Activities can also benefit the adult socially. Impersonal city life causes many people to be terribly lonely. They hunger for companionship. The great popularity of night school classes for adults indicates that an activity shared has more appeal than one practiced alone. It is more stimulating to learn typing, Spanish, or weaving in a class with others than at home alone.

Participating in community activities is a constructive use of leisure time. The volunteer groups in your hospital are helping sick people. Sometimes a sorority or church group "adopts" an old-age home, a convalescent center, or an institution for the handicapped. They visit, put on shows, give parties, and play games with the patients. A hobby can serve a useful purpose, although this is not necessary.

[6] Based on 1968 revision of RDA.

The Mature Adult

Leisure time used only to relax should not be discounted. We all need time to think, to browse, to do nothing, to "unwind." The schoolteacher who has a strenuous day of demonstrations and lectures to a roomful of lively teenagers needs quiet. Not every minute of the day has to be filled with purposeful activity. Each person needs to seek his own way of renewing his energy and refreshing his spirit. Someone else cannot prescribe this for him.

Diversions for the Adult Patient

Good mental health implies a balance of work, rest, and recreation. Everyone needs new experiences. To learn something new is exhilarating; to gradually gain control of a new game, a new skill, gives a feeling of personal satisfaction.

The bed patient and the convalescent also need a balance of work, rest, and play. Each day should furnish a new experience.

When a patient is first admitted to the hospital, perhaps this is the new experience. He will be adjusting to a new routine and to new surroundings. He may be having tests made, with a variety of technicians in and out of his room.

TABLE 2./PHYSICAL CONDITIONS LIMITING CHOICE OF DIVERSION

Limitation	Points to Consider	Suggested Activities
One hand	Is it the dominant hand (right or left)? A project easy to do with one hand. Avoid fine coordination that requires both hands. Can project be anchored or stabilized?	Number painting, crepe-paper woven plate, woodstick craft, loopers, weave-it, mosaic tile, leather lacing (stabilized), ceramics.
Limited strength for grasping	Use lightweight materials, easy to handle. Avoid heavy, bulky materials. Larger-sized pieces are easier to hold than tiny pieces. No strenuous activity possible.	Huck-towel weaving (Swedish embroidery), jewelry made from shells or sequins, rickrack earrings, flexible fabric clown, knitting, crocheting, leather lacing, mosaic work, braiding, wood-fiber flowers.
Poor eyesight	Use designs with bold patterns and definite, contrasting colors. No fine detail. Person needs to develop sense of touch and hearing. Place materials in same position each day. Small magnifying glass helps some people.	Knitting and crocheting (if already familiar), refinishing antique furniture, finger-painting a wastebasket design, basket weaving, making brooms, mosaic work using big pieces – crazy-patch design.

TABLE 2. (*Cont.*)

Limitation	Points to Consider	Suggested Activities
Diabetic	Avoid sharp tools or rough materials that might injure the skin. Eyesight may be poor. Muscles may be weak; so watch posture and do not let him become overfatigued.	Liquid embroidery, textile painting, stamp collections, pipe-cleaner art, felt craft, any needlework activity, almost any sedentary activity.
Cardiac	Complete bed rest may be ordered. No activity permitted.	Reading, holding lightweight small book, listening to music.
	Limited activities. Avoid activities that require extensive arm movements. No reaching. Work placed directly in front of person.	Huck embroidery with short thread; painting on small picture, potholder, liquid embroidery.
Hyperactive (nervous)	Needs to keep hands busy all the time. Relieves tension.	Knitting, crocheting, any activity that the patient enjoys.
Poor muscular coordination	Limited hand and eye coordination. Begin with activity that has large movements. Avoid activities requiring fine, detailed movements. Avoid fine design.	Jersey loop rug, scatter-type mosaic work with indefinite pattern, weaving with large looms, braided rugs, copper tooling with templates.
Bed patient	Lightweight materials. Patient must be in comfortable position. Prevent eyestrain. Furnish good lighting.	Cord knotting, embroidery, knitting, leatherwork, glove making, needlework, rug weaving and hooking, soft-toy making, potholders. Games: puzzles, card games, Scrabble, anagrams, chess.

It may be that the newly admitted hospital patient needs no diversion. Some people appreciate the opportunity to rest. But beginning with the second week and in the third week and the fourth week — the patient needs to do something besides look at the four walls or talk to the patient in the next bed. This is when diversions are important.

The type of nursing you do after graduation will influence the need for diversional activities among your patients. One graduate practical nurse told of much dissent among men patients in the ward where she was employed. But after she successfully maneuvered one man to start weaving and another to work on leather, the bickering ceased.

Nursing today comprises the total care of the patient. We regard him as a complete individual, and his emotional well-being influences his recovery. The mentally stimulated, the cheerful patient will have a better chance for recovery — other things being equal — than the depressed, unhappy, irritable, or anxious patient.

Questions for Discussion

1. Describe jobs, businesses, or careers that you know are being handled by mature women with grown children.
2. What areas of nursing are particularly suitable for the nurse between ages 40 and 60?
3. What community services are often rendered by men and women of this age?
4. Name particular projects, hobbies, etc., that a husband and wife might both enjoy, which could help to draw them closer together.
5. Why have the forties and fifties of a man commonly been referred to as "the dangerous years"?
6. What volunteer groups assist at your hospital? What are the goals for each group?
7. During your clinical experience, you will have contact with the physical therapy and the occupational therapy departments of your hospital. What other sources of diversional therapy do patients have?
8. Where are the arts and crafts supply houses and hobby shops in your community? Could a patient order supplies by phone or by mail?

Additional Readings

Hasler, Doris, and N. B. Hasler. *Personal, Home, and Community Health*. Chap. 3, "Routines for Healthful Living"; Chap. 5, "Feminine Hygiene"; Chap. 7, "Stimulants and Narcotics." New York: The Macmillan Company, 1967.

Rasmussen, Sandra. *Foundations of Practical and Vocational Nursing*. Chap. 48, "The Middle-Aged Adult." New York: The Macmillan Company, 1967.

Reynolds, Frank W., and Paul C. Barsam. *Adult Health*. Chap. 1, "Prevention of Chronic Disease." New York: The Macmillan Company, 1967.

Sharman, Albert. *The Middle Years, The Change of Life*. Baltimore: Williams and Wilkins Company, 1962.

Sinacore, John S. *Health: A Quality of Life*. Chap. 13, "Drugs in our Society." New York: The Macmillan Company, 1968.

Smith, Dorothy W., and Claudia D. Gipe. *Care of the Adult Patient*. 2nd ed., pp. 3–22. Philadelphia: J. B. Lippincott Company, 1966.

Today's Health Guide. Part II, Chap. 5, "Menopause"; Part IV, Chap. 4, "Obesity"; Part VI, "Recreation and Relaxation." Chicago: American Medical Association, 1965.

Recommended Audiovisual Aids

FILMS

The Critical Decades. (31 min., U.S. Public Health Service, Division of Chronic Diseases, B&W)

 The film compares the health habits of an overweight person with those of a man 100 years old. It stresses the detrimental effects of poor health habits, such as overeating, heavy smoking, alcoholism, lack of exercise, and overwork. It would help the nurse to understand that life patterns should be corrected in the 40's and 50's, as habits usually will not be changed in later years. The film also illustrates the value of learning to live with a disability.

Making Life Adjustments (20 min., McGraw-Hill, B&W)

 The role of the counselor is shown in this film about a college boy making poor grades because of pressure from his mother on his choice of a profession. After seeing the counselor, the boy makes his decision clear to his mother and clarifies a misunderstanding with his girl friend.

CHAPTER 19 / **THE NURSE, THE FAMILY,**

THE COMMUNITY

A thoughtful consideration of today's family must include study of the community and its subtle, but powerful, influence on the family.

The patient is influenced by his family. He has an obligation to his family, and he expects certain privileges and certain benefits.

The family is actually part of a larger family, the community. Therefore the family members are influenced by the kind of community in which they live. They expect certain privileges from their community, and they have an obligation to their community.

Communities today are predominantly urban (city). The 1960 census showed that 70 per cent of the people lived in urban areas on less than 2 per cent of the land. If present trends continue, by the year 2000 some 208 million people (71 per cent of the population) will live in cities and suburbs on 3 per cent of the land; 43 million people (14 per cent) will reside in smaller cities on 1 per cent of the area; and 57 million people (15 per cent) will live in the open spaces on the remaining 96 per cent of the country.[1] The high degree of population density produces stress, which is manifested in many ways.

To understand how the family is influenced by its surrounding community, let us examine more closely the community and its changing functions. In the following chapter, we will consider the resources that the community offers to your patient and the patient's family.

Defining Community and Culture

One definition of a community is, "A local area where individuals live together and influence each other. It is an area of distinct culture."

Culture refers to the total way in which a group of people organize their lives from the cradle to the grave. It includes social, emotional, and intellectual learnings. Culture differs from country to country and from North to South, from East to West within a country. Culture differs from family to family.

The cultural barriers are gradually being lowered today through television, movies, newspapers, improved transportation, more people traveling, and

[1] *U.S. News and World Report*, December 18, 1967, p. 47.

worldwide advertising. You can buy a "Coke and hot dog" in Paris, France; Tokyo, Japan; or Buenos Aires, Argentina. However, enough differences remain to be significant.

The metropolitan cities have always been noted for their unique communities, such as San Francisco's Chinatown and "Old Mexico" in Albuquerque. Montreal, Canada's bilingual city, has not only huge French- and English-speaking quarters, but large settlements of Jewish, Chinese, and Japanese people. Each ethnic community follows many of the customs of the native land and may speak its own language.

The word "ghetto" is now being used to describe the slum areas of big cities in the United States, areas that are often occupied by Negroes and Puerto Ricans. The original ghettos were walled-off areas of ancient cities, such as Rome, where Jews lived. The gates were closed at night, and Jews were officially forbidden to live outside the ghetto. Today's ghetto in an American city is not the walled prison that the name ghetto suggests, but it may house people who live there because they cannot find anywhere else to go. Usually, the reasons are economic.

The city you know best probably has its own unique communities, and possibly a ghetto. Perhaps everyone in your city speaks the same language, more or less, but differences in habits, values, and moral codes exist. A nurse needs to make allowances for cultural background in her approach to patients. She must be sensitive to local customs. You are trying to help the people to help themselves, but not by expecting them to give up everything dear to them.

Health in the Community

Economic factors are possibly the greatest influence on health in a community. People who live in crowded slums, without money to obtain the decent basics of life, have many health problems. The federal government's attack on poverty began with an attack on the health problems of the poor. Poverty-stricken rural areas have disclosed pockets of malnutrition and an alarming lack of medical care. People who are sick cannot solve other problems wisely. What appears to be a case of child neglect could be a case of a mother suffering from an undiagnosed illness.

Nurses have always had reasons to be interested in the community. The hospital is a community facility, designed to serve the health needs of the people in a certain area. Public health nurses must know how a community operates and its peculiarities in order to get a good health program adopted. Licensed practical nurses are employed as public health nurses in some areas and are making worthwhile contributions to their community. As a hospital or public health nurse, you need to understand how health is affected by community attitudes and community affluence (or lack of it).

The part of culture that deals with food and its preparation particularly influences health in the community. The nurse must be aware of the dietary customs of a community and not make the mistake of brushing them aside lightly.

Community Influences on the Family

An obvious influence of the community on the family is the manner of speaking. A true linguist could listen to someone talk, then fairly accurately describe his native state, or even the section of the state. Vocabulary, pronunciation, and colloquialisms are clues to our home communities.

Moral and ethical codes of behavior vary from one community to another. The family is influenced by, and tends to accept, the socially approved behavior of its community. Social status may be determined by ancestry in one community and by occupation or income in other communities. Certain less-privileged areas may have codes of living that differ greatly from middle-class values. In some moneyed circles, wealth is valued for itself alone, and austerity prized; in others, wealth is sought for the material possessions it buys. Money is spent freely.

Etiquette rules are observed more closely in some communities than in others. Generally speaking, in the United States the eastern section adheres the most to formality. The farther west one travels, the more informality one finds. If you are the nurse in a community new to you, you might well note carefully what is considered to be socially correct and what is not done. If you respect local customs, the citizens may more readily accept you and your nursing suggestions. Informal, casual dress may be acceptable in Los Angeles shopping centers, but perhaps not in more metropolitan San Francisco. Women in New York City and on the West Coast appear to adopt new fashions before they are worn by women in midwestern towns.

Religious beliefs and racial consciousness are shaped by community forces. Little children do not show racial prejudices. They acquire negative attitudes, as well as positive attitudes, from the adults they imitate.

The Urban Community

Upheaval and unrest in urban communities have created headline news. Whether you live in the city, town, or country, you are probably aware of the problems existing in the cities: overcrowding, breakdown of law and order, poor living conditions for many people, air pollution, traffic and transportation difficulties, strikes that paralyze a city, increased traffic in illegal drugs, more solid wastes to be disposed of, and urban renewal or highway construction dislodging hundreds of people from modest homes. Problems of such magnitude require solution by combined efforts of federal, state, and local governments, plus the cooperation of private industry and business.

Years ago the rural community was drastically different from the urban community. Today the difference between farm and city life is more theoretical than physical. Farm homes have electricity, furnaces, modern kitchens, bathrooms, and television sets. Automobiles and good roads give the rural people access to city shopping. Yet differences still exist.

The growth of cities is called urbanization. Urbanization is far more than mere shifting of people from country to city. Some cities are like large country towns, and some small communities have all the features of the city.

The urban society is highly interdependent, as contrasted with the independence of the rural family. Employment to produce money income takes on high value for fathers and mothers. Organizations in the city have grown and adapted to meet the needs of interdependence.

The urban community now assumes many of the tasks once performed by the family or kinfolk. In previous years the family, relatives, and neighbors were the guardians and sponsors of the young families or the families in distress. Today the newly married couples, the needy families, the junior executive and his family new in the city – all are very much on their own. They turn to community organizations for help. (In the next chapter we shall consider the organizations that offer help.) A community may be considered more urban as it increasingly emphasizes public solutions to problems, rather than individual and private attempts to cope with them.

The basic reason for existence of urban areas is the opportunity to earn a living. Increased technology, job specialization, and improved agricultural methods are among the factors causing the migration of rural people into the cities. In 1920 one American farmer produced enough food to feed 8 people. Today, he produces enough food for nearly 40 people.[2] People leave farms, bypass the small towns where job opportunities are dwindling, and head for the cities. They do not always realize the adjustments awaiting them.

The majority of people in the urban community are employed by business or industry, generally in a "service" occupation. The services include banks, beauty shops, hospitals, stores, entertainment, and public administration. Few people own their own business. They are not concerned with the price of wheat. The weather is important as it affects their flower gardens, getting back and forth to work, or the weekend camping trip. In a true city, we find an increasing number of people in nonservice occupations, and more libraries, symphonies, and adult education courses. Artists, musicians, and intellectuals are found at the core of great population centers.

The urban citizen has shown willingness to accept people who are different

---

[2] *U.S. News and World Report*, December 18, 1967, p. 47.

from himself at his place of work. He does not get unduly excited over cross-cultural marriages or interfaith groups. He is more prone to join freely with different kinds of people when studying in a classroom, listening to a symphony concert, or playing a game of baseball. He pursues activities with culturally different people as long as this does not threaten his identity.

The urban citizen is a "joiner." He seeks identification as a group member. He — or she — is a nurse, a teacher, a secretary, a Democrat, a Protestant, a Jew, a Negro, or a Greek. A modern urban citizen may belong to several organizations, some with conflicting interests. Sometimes his right hand does not know what his left hand is doing.

A nurse should realize that city life has always had the potential for complications. Many forces lead toward instability, confusion, despair, loneliness, and boredom. Your patient may be trapped in a way of life that he cannot control.

The Suburbs

The suburbs were planned and built for people who needed to live close to a city for employment, yet wanted to escape the problems of city life. It has been estimated that nearly one-third of the nation's population lives in the suburbs,[3] the area adjacent to a city and outside the city limits. At first the suburbs were only houses on private lots in somewhat open countryside, with schools built at appropriate intervals. In recent years many community services have moved into the suburbs. One finds shopping centers, high-rise apartments, and offices. Clinics, hospitals, and doctor's offices have been opened, although the big-city hospitals and medical centers continue to offer the greatest speciality treatments.

Once thought to represent the ideal way of life, some suburbs have developed many problems — crime, high taxes, even some racial troubles. The older suburbs have become more congested and less attractive. Many residents object to time-wasted commuting. Often businesses located in the suburbs have had trouble getting help. Some parents feels their children are deprived from being so far away from the center city and its cultural advantages.

As a result, many middle-income groups are returning to center city living. At the same time, poorer people in cities find that housing values in close-in suburbs are more attractive and are beginning to move outward. This trend continued may help to break up slums and ghettos, and to produce a better population mix.

People have always felt more comfortable with their own kind than with people who are different. Barriers are being lowered today, and this is no longer

[3] *U.S. News and World Report,* August 12, 1968, p. 32.

possible. Many communities, urban and suburban, are meeting the challenge. Some suburban communities have turned their backs on the problems and have isolated themselves, just as some urban communities find it difficult to face problems realistically. The typical human attitude is to resist change, to say: "Let change come later, after I retire or with the next generation." Some changes will not wait.

Stable and Unstable Communities

Most cities have both stable communities and disorganized, slum, or ghetto, areas. The stable community has immeasurable benefits for the family with school-age children. In a stable community, each family is known and each child is known. Reputations have to be maintained, and behavior is governed by neighbors and acquaintances as well as by members of the family. It is this extended reinforcement of standards that is lacking in a disorganized area[4]

TABLE 3/URBAN AND RURAL DWELLERS, HOUSING IN THE UNITED STATES, 1960–1970

Numbers of Urban Dwellers Increase

	1970	*change since 1960*
Americans in urban areas	149,300,000	up 19%
Americans in rural areas	53,900,000	down 0.3%

Nearly 3 out of 4 Americans now live in cities or suburbs. The western part of the U.S. is most urbanized: 83% of the people live in urban areas. Southern U.S. has the highest percentage of rural people: 35%.

Better Housing in America

	1960	*1970*
Decline in crowded homes		
Share housing units with more than one person per room	11.5%	8.2%
Better Sanitation		
Share housing units which lack complete plumbing facilities	16.8%	6.9%

From the 1970 Census Report, as reported in *U.S. News and World Report,* March 15, 1971, p. 25.

[4] R. W. White, *Abnormal Personality* (New York: Ronald Press, 1956), p. 385.

In disorganized areas people have difficulty improving their lot. The mother and children receive inadequate medical care; family breakdown is common. There are few opportunities for work, and welfare can become a way of life. Children grow up with an inadequate education and a clouded self-image. When they become adults, their children are likely to continue the same pattern of life.

In slum areas there is a high rate of crime, illegitimate births, drunkenness, suicide, prostitution, divorce, and desertion. All surveys report a high rate of juvenile delinquency and mental retardation in blighted areas.

United, community action is needed to improve these situations. Your patient from the slum area probably cannot solve his problems alone, but the situation is not hopeless.

Cities Are the New Frontiers

Human resources are concentrated in the cities, and the urban challenge presents great opportunities to adventuresome, imaginative people. New trends such as the rising level of education and the growing demands for services indicate that solutions to the urban problems are possible.

These factors may help: do more and better planning for new suburban areas; replace city slums with decent housing at lower density; improve mass transportation; make more money available to municipal governments or assign the responsibility for the city to a higher level of government that controls the revenues; and establish industry in midwestern rural areas to keep farm people there. Also, if migration of untrained Negroes from the rural South to central cities of the North slows down or ends, the big-city problems can be gradually brought under control.

Families with many problems, problems that have been handed down from one generation to the next, can be helped. Encouraging results came from a three-year experiment by the Family Service Association of Indianapolis.[5] Community residents had been shocked to learn that a few families were producing the majority of the juvenile delinquents. These so-called sick families were being contacted by various social agencies and branches of the law after tragedy had occurred. The Family Service Association selected 16 families with multiple problems, and in cooperation with various agencies, sought to improve their situations.

At the end of the three-year experiment, 11 of the 16 families had been helped. Lives of the parents, aged 30 to 40, had mostly stabilized, with improvements being painfully slow and only partial. But lives of the children had improved immensely. Of the 100 children involved in the 16 families, 72 had been influenced and directed toward a better life. Some of the changes were

[5] *A Three Year Demonstration in the Rehabilitation of Sixteen Families* (Indianapolis: Family Service Association of Indianapolis Feb. 22, 1961).

difficult to measure statistically. One malnourished infant had a better chance for life after the caseworker prevailed on the mother to prevent the older preschool children from quietly helping themselves to the contents of the baby's bottle. A slight change in parental behavior or a small improvement toward more tranquil family life brought a significantly important change in the schoolchild's life. He was less hostile toward brothers and sisters; his schoolwork improved; he participated more in church and recreational activities; his health improved and he cooperated better with his parents. Within a period of three years, one adolescent moved from commitment in a delinquency institution to enrollment in college extension courses on a scholarship. The social workers felt that the lives of these children were directed to more responsible adult life. When they married, they would be less likely to beget "sick families" and more likely to give their own children a good start in life.

Another project, "Operation Family," was initiated by the Family Service Agency of Southwestern, Illinois, serving East St. Louis.[6] Several thousand severely disadvantaged Negro families living in the area were unable to use counseling service effectively. The agency sought the help of volunteer families, matching one middle-class family with one disadvantaged family. The volunteer family was not expected to perform professional social service or to supply money, but to help by being themselves, to show personal interest in the family, and to use "middle-class know-how" to support them through ups and downs. For example, they made a special effort to add to the vocabulary of the children, thus reducing a severe problem of disadvantaged youngsters at school. At the end of one year the agency felt that the disadvantaged families had enhanced their own self-image; they had a feeling of being accepted and worthwhile. Several families previously troublesome to the police and courts improved their social behavior. The volunteer families had greater understanding of racial problems and changed attitudes.

These are only two examples of projects initiated to help people living in slums to improve their ways of living.

The Family Expects from the Community

People want to live in a stable community because of the substantial benefits they receive.

The family expects protection of property and civil rights; enforcement of public health measures such as providing safe water to drink and reducing air pollution; good, substantial housing; acceptable and creative schools for both children and adults; recreational facilities, such as parks, playgrounds, and golf

---

[6] Michael H. Dalton, "Operation Family," *Highlights* (April—May, 1968) p. 112.

courses; cultural advantages, such as libraries, museums, and concerts; transportation; and the church of their choice. They also seek shopping centers, and a conveniently located doctor, dentist, and hospital.

Where many people own their own homes, social relationships are more stable, and fewer people move from one house to another. A high rate of moving is one indication of a disorganized community.

Individuals often need personal references from someone in their community. No doubt when you applied for admission to your practical nursing school, you were asked for references from people in your community. This is another example of a community benefit.

Contributions of the Family to the Community

The family who has a sincere interest in "my town" willingly shares obligations to its community. It tries to be flexible in helping with community activities, to assist where needed.

Of course, we all pay taxes, or face penalties. However, we have other debts to our community. Everyone needs to abide by the community regulations. The 30-mile speed zone applies to all of us. The father who has a traffic ticket "fixed" should not be shocked if his son tries to change a grade on his school report card.

Every family should participate in community activities. We need to give our time as well as our money. Election day means voting day — but it also means work for someone. Voters have to be preregistered, voting lists must be checked, and votes have to be counted and tabulated. Somebody has to head the PTA, serve on the school board, help with the community fund drive, support the churches, and assist new residents to get acquainted.

We also make a contribution to our community when we maintain our property and the appearance of our home. Parents who regard the community as the larger family will convey to their children the idea that everyone has a responsibility to his community.

Questions for Discussion

1. What is the attitude in your community towards nurses participating in politics? (Some school boards have regulations against schoolteachers taking part in politics.)
2. Describe any unique communities within the city you know best.
3. Many of your class mates will have moved from one community to another. Describe differences in communities that have been observed. Did the newcomer ever feel she was an "outsider," hence unwelcome?

4. Has specific progress been made in your community toward improving slum areas? What organizations participate in attempts to improve life for the less fortunate people?

5. Contact either the Family Service Association or a health and welfare council in your city for published reports of important community projects. Note the roles that have been assumed by nurses.

6. What changes have occurred in your community during the past 20 years, or possibly the past 10 years?

Additional Readings

Hartley, Ruth E., and Robert M. Goldenson. *Complete Book of Children's Play*. 2nd ed., "Recreation in the Community," pp. 362–368. New York: Thomas Y. Crowell Company, 1963.

Hasler, Doris, and Norman B. Hasler. *Personal, Home, and Community Health*. Part IV, "Community Health and Hygiene." New York: The Macmillan Company, 1967.

Hayes, Wayland J., and Rena Gazaway. *Human Relations in Nursing*. 3rd ed., Chap. 5, "Society in a Changing World"; Chap. 12, "We Are at Home in Communities." Philadelphia: W. B. Saunders Company, 1964.

Mead, Margaret, and Ken Hayman. *Family*. New York: The Macmillan Company, 1965.

Sellew, Gladys. *Sociology and Its Use in Nursing Service*. 5th ed., Chap. 7, "Social Institutions: The Family." Philadelphia: W. B. Saunders Company, 1962.

Recommended Audiovisual Aids

FILMS

Children of Change (31 min., International Film Bureau, B&W)

The film shows how a good day-care center can be the answer for the lonely, unguided children who roam the streets while their mothers are working. It shows both the problems of the children and how a good day-care center should be operated.

The Neglected (35 min., International Film Bureau, B&W)

This excellent film shows how the problems of poverty, parental abuse, and neglect are passed on from generation to generation. Community children's service agencies can be effective in helping neglected children. Sometimes the threat of having their children taken away will shock parents and influence them to improve.

FILMSTRIP

Family Portrait (29 frames, Stanley-Bowmar Company, B&W; from series: Marriage and Family Living)
    This filmstrip stresses that strong family units make a strong, sound society. It illustrates the development in families of good and bad citizens, happy and unhappy persons, and how changes in society threaten family unity and strength. Preparation for marriage and family living is a necessity.

CHAPTER 20 / COMMUNITY RESOURCES:

LAWS AND AGENCIES

AFFECTING THE FAMILY

Laws and agencies — local, state, and national — are the tools by which the community shares with the family its problems and its responsibilities. The responsibility of the community to help the child to develop into a well-adjusted adult and citizen is generally accepted. For example, public school education began many years ago. It has taken people longer to realize that the community also has a responsibility toward the aged and the indigent family.

In cities, where most people live today, the family without money cannot work the soil or hunt game for food; they cannot sleep under a tree; nature's resources are no longer available for survival. Also in the cities the extended family — with aunts, uncles, and cousins — rarely exists today, to help when an emergency arises. The small, nuclear family — parents and children — turns to the community for help. The nurse needs a thorough knowledge of the agencies in her community so that she can guide the family in getting the best help available.

Laws have been passed that provide for agencies to work with families in many capacities. A variety of services are offered. For example, your practical nursing school may be partly supported by tax dollars.

In addition to tax-supported agencies, many volunteer or private agencies are supported by funds from individuals or organizations. Volunteer agencies vary from one community to another, although many are national, with state or local chapters.

Volunteer or government agencies seem especially necessary in the urban, industrial areas, where people are less likely to be friendly with their neighbors and less likely to know if the family in the next block needs help.

In many rural communities and among certain religious groups, people generously and unselfishly look after their own people. They help one another.

In the more complex urban areas — where most nurses are employed — such help is ordinarily given through agencies. Hence the nurse needs to be thoroughly acquainted with the laws, public agencies, and private agencies designed to work with families.

Laws

Society places a value on the child and considers his potential as an adult. Laws have been passed to protect and safeguard children. Some states have passed laws requiring adults to provide for aged parents.

State laws hold that parents are legally responsible for the welfare of their children. The laws define punishment for child neglect and child abuse.

Nurses have long been concerned about the battered children they see (as discussed in Chapter 7). All 50 states and the District of Columbia now have laws requiring physicians or other professional people to report cases of suspected child beating to welfare agencies, or to the police in some states. Such reporting is mandatory in 44 states, and in one-half the states, failure to report is a misdemeanor. The reporting physician, professional person, or hospital is granted immunity by law. The nurse should become familiar with the law in her state and the procedure recommended for reporting.

The child labor laws were passed to prevent many child abuses that were common practices years ago. History records how little children worked long hours in dark, poorly ventilated factories or from sunrise to sunset in the fields. These children had little chance to grow into healthy adults. Today, abuses of the child labor laws are not widespread, but need for the laws still exists. Nurses have noted exceptions to the law.

The compulsory school laws help to give each child educational opportunities. Great differences still exist in the quality of education that children receive, but extensive efforts are being made in almost every community to improve the education of its youth.

Social Security Act

Passed by the federal government in 1935 and since amended many times, the Social Security Act has many provisions related directly to the family. It provides that federal aid be given to the states for maternal and child health services; for services for crippled children; and for aid for dependent children. The Old Age, Survivors, Disability and Health Insurance is also part of the Social Security Act. The individual pays into the social security funds during his working years and receives benefits after he retires at the age of 62 or 65; or if he dies leaving small children, the wife and mother receives support payments until the children are 18 years old. Medicare and medicaid were also voted by Congress in amendments to the Social Security Act. Medicare and social security benefits are explained more fully in Chapter 26.

The Social Security Act provided for a Social Security Administration, which is now part of the U.S. Department of Health, Education, and Welfare.

DEPARTMENT OF HEALTH, EDUCATION AND WELFARE

Office of the Secretary
Office of the Undersecretary

Facilities Engineer & Construction Agency				Office of Civil Rights Office of Public Information		
Asst. Sec. Health & Scientific Affairs (Surgeon General)	Asst. Sec. Community & Field Service	Asst. Sec. Legislation	Asst. Sec. Planning & Evaluation	General Counsel	Assistant Secretary for Administration (Office of Child Development)	Asst. Sec. Comptroller	Asst. Sec. Education

PUBLIC HEALTH SERVICE	SOCIAL SECURITY ADMINISTRATION	SOCIAL AND REHABILITATION SERVICES	OFFICE OF EDUCATION
Environmental Health Services	*Staff Offices & 6 Bureaus:*	*Office of Administrator (Juvenile Delinquency & Youth Development)*	*Bureaus of:*
Sets antipollution standards, Gives grants to states to enforce them.	Data Processing & Accounts	Administration on Aging	Elementary & Secondary Education
Finances studies to combat pollution.	Disability Insurance District Office Operations	Assistance Payments Administration (welfare, AFDC)	Adult, Vocational and Technical Education
Health Services and Mental Health Administration	Health Insurance (Medicare)	Medical Services Administration (Medicaid)	Education for Handicapped
Maternal & Child Health Services	Hearings & Appeals	Rehabilitation Services Administration	Higher Education
Family Planning Services	Retirement and Survivors Insurance	Community Services Administration	Educational Personnel Development
National Communicable Disease Center (Atlanta)			Libraries and Educational Technology
National Institute of Mental Health			Other centers for research, development and planning in education
Community Health Services	*Food and Drug Administration*		
Health Facilities Planning & Construction Services	Bureaus of:		
Indian Health Services	Foods, Pesticides & Product Safety		
Federal hospitals	Drugs		
	Veterinary Medicine		
	National Institutes of Health		
	10 research institutes		
	Health manpower programs		
	Finances other medical research		
	National Library of Medicine		

Fig. 26. Organization of the U.S. Department of Health, Education and Welfare.

Community Resources

Established in 1953, the U.S. Department of Health, Education, and Welfare has grown into an agency that touches or affects nearly every American. Figure 26 shows its organization, with the various agencies and the wide scope of problems that they touch.

The *Social Security Administration* operates social security and Medicare programs. In late 1970 benefits were paid to more than 26 million people.

Social and Rehabilitation Services handles welfare and medicaid operations. In November 1970, 12 million individuals were receiving public assistance. Payments to welfare recipients totaled almost 13 billion dollars in the fiscal year that ended June 30, 1970.[1] The primary welfare assistance program is in aid to families with dependent children (AFDC). In 1970, 2 million families with 6 million children received $4 billion per year in money payments. The welfare rolls were comprised of 50.5 per cent white people, 47.5 per cent black people, and 2.1 per cent other races. The typical family remained on welfare for less than 24 months.[2]

Medicaid, or Title 19 of the 1965 Social Security Act, was designed as a federal-state-local operation to help the "medically indigent" people of all ages. This includes people who have enough money to meet everyday needs but cannot pay the costs of major illnesses or accidents. The individual states set their own standards for indigence, with the federal government paying at least 50 per cent of the cost. The original estimate was $238 million annually; today it costs almost $5 billion.[3]

The Social and Rehabilitation Services also runs vocational rehabilitation programs, with more than 12 million beneficiaries in 1970. It directs youth development and delinquency projects, and administers the crippled children's services. The Administration on Aging planned and directed the 1971 White House Conference on Aging. (Further description of the Administration on Aging is given in Chapter 27.)

The *Office of Child Development* was established in April 1969. Its director is also Chief of the Children's Bureau and has administrative responsibilities for Head Start Programs.

The Children's Bureau was founded in 1912 when child labor was the deep concern. The concern later broadened to the entire well-being of all children. The wide range of services were designed to help families protect children against danger to their health, safety, and economic well-being. Standards for care and protection of children, and research conducted on conditions affecting children, are reported to the public in the "best-seller" child-care booklets, such as *Infant Care* and *Your Child from One to Six*.

Child day-care services will likely be expanded in the years ahead. Nurses should be interested in following such new developments.

---

[1] *Journal of Home Economics*, December 1970, p. 712.
[2] *Welfare Review*, October 1970.
[3] *U.S. News and World Report*, December 7, 1970, p. 33

The Head Start Program was organized to help disadvantaged children overcome their lack of vocabulary and other basic learning skills. The ghetto child can be a potential dropout in the first grade. The goal of this direct service program became, however, the improved development of the whole child in the context of his family, relating to his health, nutrition, self-esteem, and experience.

The role of the Office of Child Development (OCD) functions more as a guide to the states than a controlling factor. An advocator and innovator, the OCD sets standards for quality services, provides technical assistance to the states, and drafts model legislature to aid state and federal legislature in areas affecting children.

Various functions of the *Public Health Service*, with its four divisions, will be studied frequently during your nursing career. The *Mental Health Services and Mental Health Administration* operates many programs of interest to nurses. Those particularly related to the family are family planning services for 1.1 million low-income people and child health programs for 2.9 million people.[4]

The *Office of Education* conducts research and makes loans and grants — for building construction and teaching materials — that help college students and grade and secondary school children. It also insures private loans to college students, provides special help to schools educating low-income children, is responsible for much vocational education, and finances the training of teachers in specialized fields.

Except for social security spending, the large bulk of the Department of Health, Education, and Welfare's work is in grants to states, localities (such as Model Cities programs), universities, school systems, hospitals, laboratories and foundations.

Other Federal Resources

The family-food-assistance program (food stamps) of the U.S. Department of Agriculture is another direct aid to needy families.

Several programs that began under the Economic Opportunity Act of 1964 continue to touch the lives of many American families. Among those are the Head Start preschool programs for needy children; Upward Bound, to help young people prepare for college; Community Action Against Poverty (CAAP), local agencies that guide antipoverty activities and include representatives of the poor; Volunteers in Service to America (VISTA), which sends volunteer teachers and workers into poverty areas; the Job Corps, to provide job training and basic education for ghetto youths in rural and urban centers; and Legal Services, to supply legal help for needy families.

---

[4] *U.S. News and World Report*, December 7, 1970, p. 34.

State Department of Public Welfare

Individual states have established departments of public welfare through acts passed by state legislatures, within limitations set by the Social Security Act. The state and local governments implement federal tax dollars with local and state tax money, as meant by the "grants-in-aid."

Through the program for *aid to families with dependent children* (AFDC), needy children can remain in the homes of the remaining parent or the home of near relatives instead of being placed in boarding homes or institutions. This program is based on the philosophy that the child did not ask to be born and that every child has a right to proper food, clothing, health service, education, and a share in the life of the neighborhood and the community. The funds may be used for vocational training of the mother, thus enabling her to provide for her children. Many fine practical nurses have had their training financed in this manner. AFDC is financed cooperatively, with the federal government bearing approximately 68 per cent of the cost, the state government approximately 19 per cent, and the county 13 per cent.

In *child welfare services,* emphasis is now on casework services that help parents to give their children better care and, if at all possible, permit the children to remain in their own home. Formerly, children were taken away from parents who neglected, abused, or exploited them. Now the caseworkers strive to safeguard and build strong parent-child relationships whenever possible. This is done for many children by providing social services to them in their own homes and to their parents; for some, through foster care; for others, through adoption.[5]

Social agencies cannot take children away from parents. Only the court has jurisdiction to remove children from their home when there is legal evidence that the parents are not willing or are unable to provide adequate protection and care.

Foster care is no longer regarded as the answer to all the difficulties surrounding children — lack of finances in the family, illness, death, desertion, neglect of parents, or behavior difficulty of the child. But when a child is deprived of the care of his own parents, or for various reasons should not remain in his own home and is not available for adoption, foster care may be the anwer. Foster care is not an end in itself but should be part of a long-range plan for the child to return to his own home, be adopted, or live permanently elsewhere. Foster parents are carefully chosen by the agency, and a specific home is selected that is best for the particular child and his parents. In a foster home, the child can receive warm, affectionate care on a continuing basis. Parents are not asked to give up their parental rights. The separation may be painful for the

---

[5] Children's Bureau Publication No. 359, *Child Welfare Services,* 1957, p. 8.

parents and for the child, but if everyone sees that this is the best way, foster placement can fulfill a purpose. The child needs to feel that his parents want this for him, and that they are not trying to get rid of him. Frequently children cling to parents who abuse and neglect them. It is as though the child needs to think well of his parents in order to feel adequate himself.

Services for crippled children are financed cooperatively by the country, state, and federal governments. If handicapped children receive medical care and treatment, they can become useful, independent adults. The program renders service for orthopedic disabilities; for congenital or acquired defects that will respond to plastic surgery; for rheumatic or other types of heart disease, including congenital heart disease that is amenable to surgery; for neurological disturbances, including cerebral palsy and epilsepsy; and for speech defects associated with organic defects.

Hospital care is followed by home visits of the nurse and doctor as needed, and social factors that may affect the child's recovery are worked out. If the crippled or sick child has some permanent handicap that will limit his employment, he may be referred to the rehabilitation division of the state department of education for vocational training.

The *blind assistance* program provides a monthly stipend and necessary medical care to needy persons whose eyesight is limited to a certain degree. Blind assistance is financed cooperatively, with the federal government paying approximately 55 per cent of the cost and the state approximately 45 per cent. In addition, the welfare departments of many states pay for any medical or surgical care given to the needy person for the purpose of restoring vision or preventing loss of vision. If the necessary medical attention is given to children when the eye diseases or handicaps are discovered, blindness in adulthood may be reduced and dependency decreased.

The *old-age assistance* program provides a monthly stipend and necessary medical care to needy persons who are 65 years of age and older. This program is financed cooperatively, with the federal government bearing approximately 65 per cent of the cost, the state 20 per cent, and the county 15 per cent.

Medical assistance may be handled in different ways, but most state welfare acts permit payment for medical care of persons receiving old-age assistance, blind assistance, or assistance to dependent children. Most of the states have medical programs which help the medically indigent.

Public Criticism

Welfare programs have met with criticism. Certainly any complex program shows weaknesses, can be misused, and needs continual revision. Real effectiveness is influenced by the interest and support of the people. The nurse has a responsibility to help the patient and his family receive deserving help. But she also has a responsibility to report abuses to the proper authorities.

Public Health Nursing

The Bureau of Public Health Nursing, under the Division of Public Health, offers many services to the family. Licensed practical nurses are hired in the field of public health; so consider carefully the type of services involved. You may choose public health nursing after graduation.

Public health nurses staff the well-child clinics sponsored for infants and preschool children whose parents cannot afford a private doctor. The well-child conferences may be held weekly or monthly at various community centers. Prenatal clinics and postpartum clinics are held at the county medical center. The number of such clinics may be surprising. At one state medical center, 45 adult and child outpatient clinics are scheduled.[6] At the county medical center a short distance away, 41 outpatient clinics are held.[7]

Public health nurses make home visits to show a new mother how to feed and bathe her newborn baby. They follow through on many referrals from the hospital, for many types of patients. Public health nurses are particularly needed to examine the home situations for possible early release of the hospital patient for home care. The public health nurse works with the schools and makes home visits to schoolchildren ill at home.

Schoolchildren receive brief examinations to detect vision, hearing, or dental defects. The nurse seeks to interview the parents of children who need medical help. She may refer them to the dental, eye, or health clinic. Cases of communicable diseases, such as tuberculosis, are brought to the attention of the public health nurse.

Visiting Nurse Association (VNA)

In some areas the visiting nurses and the public health nurses are united under one agency. In other areas, they are separate agencies.

For patients who do not require continuous nursing attendance throughout the day, services of the visiting nurse may allow them to remain at home rather than be hospitalized. The visiting nurse follows orders from the patient's doctor for injections, surgical dressings, or special treatments. Other services include bed baths, rehabilitation of handicapped persons, and health guidance for expectant and new mothers.

The visits are scheduled in advance, and the patient is charged a fee. If the patient cannot pay the fee, arrangements are made with the public health agency for the payment.

---

[6] Indiana University Medical Center, Indianapolis, Indiana.
[7] Marion County General Hospital, Indianapolis, Indiana.

The shortage of both nurses and hospital beds makes the services of the VNA a vital contribution to the health of the community.

Many VNA staffs include licensed practical nurses as well as registered, professional nurses.

Child Guidance Clinic

Children with extensive emotional and behavioral problems may be referred to a child guidance clinic for help. These may be parent-child relations or behavioral problems at home or at school.

Behavioral problems indicating emotional disturbances include destructive tendencies, excessive fears, and chronic naughtiness. Some children cannot progress in school, and the inability to read or lack of motivation may indicate an emotional block to learning. Children with extreme personality problems need help – the child who is excessively shy and withdrawn, who is extremely sensitive and distrustful, or who cannot get along with others. Children may have psychosomatic illnesses, just as adults. Sometimes the child's symptoms appear only at school. At home, he may be well-behaved because he is afraid to express himself.

The typical child guidance clinic uses the team approach. Usually, the social worker explains the facilities of the clinic to the person applying for the service. If it is agreed that the service may benefit the child, the social worker arranges the interviews for the child and his family. The psychologist sees the child for psychological testing; the psychiatrist observes the child in the playroom and may meet with the mother; the social worker interviews the mother and takes the family history. After sufficient information has been collected and reviewed, a case conference is arranged. The psychiatrist, the psychologist, and the social workers give their contributions toward the interpretation of the difficulties of the child and his family. Treatment is discussed and planned, with one of the three working actively with the child and the family.

Sometimes the child guidance clinic diagnoses only, referring the child to another agency for treatment. More frequently, the series of interviews results in working with the child, the mother, and the father toward improving the situation. Often helping a troubled child includes treatment of the parents. Frequently a parent expects too much from a child or from himself as a parent.

The child guidance clinics were first organized to combat juvenile delinquency by helping the delinquent to overcome his personal problems. The delinquent child is often an emotionally disturbed or maladjusted child. The scope of the clinics broadened as it became understood that the same methods might help the emotionally disturbed, nondelinquent child.

Child guidance clinics may be sponsored and supported in a variety of ways. Many large school corporations support a child guidance clinic; most large

Community Resources

schools employ a school psychologist. Usually a clinic is operated in connection with the state children's hospital. In some areas community mental health clinics have been successfully established. Fees may be charged based on the family's ability to pay, and services may often be arranged for those without the ability to pay.

Children are referred to a child guidance clinic from the schools, the juvenile court, the welfare department, private social agencies, or the medical doctor.

Dr. Gerald Alpern has encouraging words for the nurse. He says:

> The nurse cannot expect to be able to handle all the emotional problems of children. She can, however, serve the important role of a professional observer who is able to spot atypical, or irregular, behavior which may indicate emotional illness. At the point that the nurse becomes concerned or suspicious about a child's behavior, she should begin seeking a professional consultation. The hospital nurse should report to the ward physician, and this may lead to a psychiatric referral. Many psychiatric referrals emanating from hospital wards, schools, and homes begin with the careful observations of a ward nurse, a school nurse, or a visiting nurse.
>
> Good nursing notes always include behavioral observations, such as drastic mood swings, peer relationships, responses to frustrations, in addition to the usual physical data, such as fluid intake.
>
> However, whether the nurse's observations are written or not, they are an extremely valuable tool by which she can improve her skill as a nurse. The experienced pediatric nurse is able to judge whether a child's reactions are typical (normal fear of some medical procedure) or atypical (indicating emotional disturbance).[8]

If a child can overcome extreme behavioral problems, he is more likely to become a mentally healthy adult. This is one of many approaches toward prevention of mental illness, a problem of national concern.

Family Service Association

Since it is a nationwide agency and found in almost every community, the Family Service Association is one of the first and best sources of help to which to direct your patient with personal problems. Trained staff workers are available for private counseling on all matters that touch the family, such as marriage problems, adjustment to aging, behavioral problems with children, care of children, mental or physical illness, death in the family, personal problems, and problems of financial planning. Fees charged are based on the ability of the individual to pay. Often a homemaker service is available through the Family Service Association. If another agency in the community can give better and more appropriate service, the person is referred to the other agency.

[8] Written for this publication by Gerald Alpern, Ph.D., Director of Research, Child Psychiatry Services, Indiana University Medical Center, Indianapolis.

National Voluntary Health Agencies

Many voluntary health agencies work with families. They help to strengthen family life by improving health conditions. The national organizations usually have state or local branches. During your year of study as a student nurse, notice and learn as much as you can about the following:

American Cancer Society, American Heart Association, American National Red Cross, The Arthritis and Rheumatism Foundation, National Foundation supported by March of Dimes, National Multiple Sclerosis Society, Myasthenia Gravis Foundation, Inc., Muscular Dystrophy Association of America, Inc., and United Cerebral Palsy Association, Inc.

Other National Agencies

If you are an active citizen of your community, doubtlessly you have contacted some of the following national organizations, which help families in many ways: Boy Scouts of America, Camp Fire Girls, Girl Scouts, 4-H Clubs, and others.

Local Agencies in Most Communities

Every community has service organizations striving to make it a better place to live. Some of these are:

United fund, state association for mental health, community service council (sometimes called health and welfare council), sheltered workshops, day nursery association, speech and hearing centers, legal aid society, community settlement houses, and association for retarded children. Many religious denominations offer services, such as Jewish Social Service, Catholic Charities Bureau, Lutheran homes for girls, and a pastoral care and counseling center open to all denominations.

Rehabilitation Centers

Although rehabilitation centers are increasing in number, the need for these services still exceeds the availability. Sometimes the rehabilitation center is a separate agency in its own building; sometimes it is a department within a hospital. Most rehabilitation centers concentrate on restorative services for the physically handicapped. This is accomplished through physical therapy, occupational therapy, speech and hearing therapy, social services, and psychological evaluation. Some centers have more facilities to help mentally handicapped patients than other centers. The better-equipped and larger-staffed rehabilitation centers include social services, vocational evaluation, counseling, vocational training, and job placement. Sometimes a nursery school for handicapped children is operated. Generally, the patient must be referred by his physician. Rehabilitation services are so vital to the patient's complete recovery that the nurse should be well informed regarding the services available in her own community.

Home-Care Programs

Patients can be cared for in their own homes. In the days of spare rooms and large households, this was taken for granted. Recently, the benefits from organized medical services at home have received attention because of the rise in chronic illness, the increase in the older age population, the increased cost of institutional care, and the shortage of hospital beds.

Home care is the extension of hospital services to patients in their homes. Typical services to the patient include supervision from the physician as when he is hospitalized; nursing services from a registered, professional nurse or a licensed, practical nurse; social services; laboratory tests; drugs and medical supplies; sickroom supplies; X rays; oxygen; and supervision of diet by hospital dietary staff as needed.

These services are available in some, but not all, home-care programs: physical and occupational therapy, orthopedic appliances, speech therapy, and homemaker or domestic service.

Home-care programs require teamwork among the personnel giving service and among the different community health and welfare organizations. Not every patient can be cared for at home. A survey of one private hospital indicated that 15 per cent of the patients would be eligible for home care. The home of the patient must be suitable, with adequate space for the home sickroom. The patient must have relatives or close friends who are willing and able to assist in his care. The patient's need of hospital services must be limited enough to make it practical to provide them in his home.

A favorable report was issued by the Associated Hospital Service of New York on home care after hospitalization for the first 1000 patients to be cared for in the home under the expanded Blue Cross program.[9] The patients and their families liked home care because it shortened the hospital stay, reduced the costs of illness, and enabled the patient to be with his family. Hospital administrators felt that patient care was improved in two ways: continuity of service between hospital and home was improved, and early evaluation of patients for potential

---

[9] *Home Care Following Hospitalization,* annual report of Associated Hospital Service of New York, New York, June, 1962.

home-care fostered more individual care. From a community viewpoint, home care makes for more effective use of existing hospital beds and services.

Communities that have had the services of a visiting nurse seem to adopt the home-care program more readily than communities unacquainted with the services of a visiting nurse.

A growing number of insurance plans include coverage for home-care service. As this coverage increases, the potential of home-care programs may be more fully realized.

Homemaker Service

When the mother in a family becomes ill in a rural community, neighbors, relatives, or friends come to the aid of the family. Almost always someone volunteers to take over management of the home until the family can get organized.

In the urban community, the motherless family turns to a community agency for help. Homemaker services have been organized to help families in time of stress. The homemaker service provides qualified, mature women to substitute for the ill or absent mother, thus enabling the family to stay together as a unit. Many public welfare and voluntary health agencies employ specially trained women to serve as homemakers.[10] The families are expected to pay for her services if they are able to do so.

The homemaker service may be provided on a temporary basis, sponsored by a Family Service Association. The service enables the family members to stay together in their own home while they make long-range plans for the absence of the mother. It may allow the mother to convalesce without worrying about her family. It may enable the father to keep his job rather than taking time off to care for children, an elderly parent, or a sick relative. It sometimes enables motherless adolescent children to learn to manage the household.

Homemaker service on a more permanent basis may allow the elderly couple to maintain their own home. The disabled or chronically ill person may be able to remain in his home rather than be institutionalized.

The homemaker will prepare meals, do the marketing, and do the normal daily household tasks, such as straightening the house, making beds, and washing dishes. She is not expected to do heavy lifting or extensive laundry. If homemaker service is available for day care of children, a responsible adult must be in the house at night and on weekends. The homemaker will supervise small children, feed and bathe the baby, and get older children ready for school. The homemaker works under the supervision of the sponsoring agency.

Home-care programs for the sick person usually require housekeeping service if the home-care program is to succeed.

[10] Also called home aides, housekeepers, visiting homemakers, etc.

Community Resources

Since 1958, the amount of homemaker service has greatly increased. More agencies are providing service to the chronically ill. Part-time services have been extended. Many families can and do pay for the services of a homemaker for a few hours a day, a few days a week, although they could not afford to pay for a full 40-hour week. The part-time help also encourages the sick or aging person to recapture his strength.

In most communities, homemaker service is not yet available to everyone. There is widespread agreement that this service is needed by all age and economic groups. Many European countries consider homemaker service a necessity, not a luxury.

Meals-on-Wheels

Hot, attractive, well-balanced meals brought to his home daily can be a big boost to the person physically unable to prepare his own food. The meals-on-wheels program was particularly designed for the elderly person who lives alone and who may have difficulty buying and preparing food. Any convalescing or handicapped person confined to his home might benefit from the service. Loneliness and malnutrition often go hand in hand. There is not much incentive to cook a complete meal to be eaten alone. Sometimes cooking requires too much effort, especially for the man in front of a stove for the first time.

The nonprofit service may be sponsored by a civic organization or by a public or private health or welfare agency. Payment can be made by the recipient, friend, relative or spouse. The service may cost the shut-in as little as 25 cents per meal or as much as $3 a day. In some communities, volunteers act as cooks and chauffeurs. In other places, dietitians or chefs prepare the meals, and taxi drivers or automobile dealers deliver them. Special diets, such as diabetic or low-sodium, may be prepared at the direction of the recipient's physician.

Usually two meals a day, one hot and one cold, are delivered at noon. With the meals come a cheery greeting and a friendly contact with the outside world.

In the future, diet counseling and market services may be added.

A great need exists for more communities to operate the meals-on-wheels program and to reach more and more people.

Questions for Discussion

1. Relate specific contacts that you have had with one of the agencies described.
2. One member of the class should report on the mechanics of obtaining the services of a visiting nurse.

3. Find out the relationships (or differences) of the school nurse, public health nurse, and visiting nurse in your community. Are they united under one agency?
4. What are the child labor laws in your community?
5. Bring to class newspaper clippings describing parents arrested for child neglect. What penalties have been imposed?
6. What homemaker services are available in your community?
7. Where are the child guidance clinics in your area?

Additional Readings

Benz, Gladys. *Pediatric Nursing*. 5th ed. Unit VII, "The Child in the Community." St. Louis: C. V. Mosby Company, 1964.
Child Welfare Services. Washington, D.C.: U.S. Department of Health, Education, and Welfare, Children's Bureau Publication No. 359, 1957
Fuerst, Elinor V., and LuVerne Wolf. *Fundamentals of Nursing*. 4th ed. Chap. 3, "Health Agencies in Which Nurses Function." Philadelphia: J. B. Lippincott Company, 1964.
Hasler, Doris and Norman B. Hasler. *Personal, Home, and Community Health*. Chap. 22, "Voluntary Health Agencies." New York: The Macmillan Company, 1967.
Home Care Following Hospitalization. New York: Associated Hospital Service of New York, 1962.
Turner, C. E. *Personal and Community Health*. 13th ed. Chap. 27, "Your Government and Your Health." St. Louis: The C. V. Mosby Company, 1967.

CURRENT PUBLICATIONS

Homemaker Services Bulletin
Welfare Review.
Various bulletins from U.S. Department of Health, Education, and Welfare.

Recommended Audiovisual Aids

FILM

Angry Boy (33 min., International Film Bureau, B&W)
This film shows how a guidance clinic operates to discover the problems of an emotionally disturbed boy. The guidance counselor, psychiatrist, and clinical psychologist, working together, learn that the boy's problem is his mother. She gives him too much attention, the result of the lack of attention she received from her own mother.

PART V / The Family in the Later Years

CHAPTER 21/**NURSING AND THE AGING**

POPULATION

You have only to look among your family, your neighborhood, and your community to realize that, today, more people are living to an advanced age.

In previous years, a couple made news when they celebrated their golden wedding anniversary. Today, we may pay homage to a couple on their sixtieth wedding anniversary.

Personal observations are supported by statistics. People really are living longer today. Let us examine these statistics and then see how nursing is affected.

Life Expectancy

A white female baby born today has a life expectancy of slightly more than 74 years; a white male or a nonwhite female baby slightly less than 68 years.[1]

It is estimated that a baby born at the time of Christ had a life expectancy of 23 years. For 1900 years the life expectancy increased a little more than 20 years. In the next half century it increased almost as much, another 20 years (Fig. 27). Since 1956 the life expectancy has improved by less than a year.[2]

This has more personal meaning if you examine Table 4 and see how many more years of life the statisticians predict for you.

The longevity outlook of the nonwhite population is considerably less favorable than that of the white population. Among nonwhites, the expectation of life at birth in 1965 was 61.1 years for males and 67.4 years for females. The poorer record for nonwhites is even more noticeable when mortality rates are compared. The death rates for nonwhites is at least twice that for whites at ages 25 through 46 for men, and ages 23 to 67 for women.[3]

Proportion of Population Over 65 Increased

Currently, those aged 65 years and older make up about 9.5 per cent of the total population. In 1900 the older age group was 4.1 per cent of the total

---

[1] *Statistical Bulletin*, Metropolitan Life Insurance Company, August 1967, p. 8.
[2] Ibid.
[3] Ibid., p. 10.

TABLE 4./EXPECTATION OF LIFE AND MORTALITY RATE AT SINGLE YEARS OF AGE BY RACE AND SEX, UNITED STATES, 1965

	Expectation of Life in Years						Mortality Rate per 1,000					
		White		Nonwhite				White		Nonwhite		
Age	Total Persons	Male	Female	Male	Female		Total Persons	Male	Female	Male	Female	
0	70.2	67.6	74.7	61.1	67.4		24.5	24.2	18.3	44.2	36.0	
1	70.9	68.3	75.1	62.9	68.9		1.5	1.3	1.1	2.8	2.6	
2	70.0	67.4	74.2	62.1	68.0		.9	.9	.8	1.6	1.4	
3	69.1	66.5	73.2	61.2	67.1		.7	.7	.6	1.2	.9	
4	68.1	65.5	72.3	60.2	66.2		.6	.6	.5	1.0	.8	
5	67.2	64.5	71.3	59.3	65.3		.6	.7	.4	1.1	.7	
6	66.2	63.6	70.3	58.4	64.3		.5	.6	.4	.8	.6	
7	65.2	62.6	69.3	57.4	63.3		.4	.4	.3	.7	.5	
8	64.3	61.7	68.4	56.4	62.4		.4	.4	.3	.5	.5	
9	63.3	60.7	67.4	55.5	61.4		.3	.3	.3	.5	.4	
10	62.3	59.7	66.4	54.5	60.4		.3	.3	.3	.5	.4	
11	61.3	58.7	65.4	53.5	59.5		.3	.4	.3	.5	.4	
12	60.4	57.7	64.4	52.6	58.5		.4	.4	.3	.6	.4	
13	59.4	56.8	63.5	51.6	57.5		.5	.6	.3	.8	.4	
14	58.4	55.8	62.5	50.6	56.5		.6	.8	.4	1.0	.5	
15	57.4	54.8	61.5	49.7	55.5		.7	1.0	.4	1.2	.6	
16	56.5	53.9	60.5	48.7	54.6		.9	1.2	.5	1.4	.7	
17	55.5	52.9	59.5	47.8	53.6		1.0	1.4	.5	1.7	.8	
18	54.6	52.0	58.6	46.9	52.7		1.1	1.5	.6	1.9	.9	
19	53.6	51.1	57.6	46.0	51.7		1.1	1.6	.6	2.2	1.0	

20	52.7	50.2	56.6	45.1	50.8	1.2	1.7	.6	2.4	1.1
21	51.8	49.3	55.7	44.2	49.8	1.3	1.7	.6	2.7	1.1
22	50.8	48.3	54.7	43.3	48.9	1.3	1.8	.6	2.9	1.3
23	49.9	47.4	53.7	42.4	47.9	1.3	1.8	.7	3.1	1.4
24	49.0	46.5	52.8	41.6	47.0	1.3	1.7	.7	3.3	1.5
25	48.0	45.6	51.8	40.7	46.1	1.3	1.6	.7	3.6	1.6
26	47.1	44.7	50.9	39.8	45.1	1.3	1.6	.7	3.8	1.8
27	46.1	43.7	49.9	39.0	44.2	1.3	1.5	.7	4.0	1.9
28	45.2	42.8	48.9	38.1	43.3	1.4	1.5	.7	4.1	2.1
29	44.3	41.9	48.0	37.3	42.4	1.4	1.6	.8	4.2	2.3
30	43.3	40.9	47.0	36.4	41.5	1.5	1.6	.9	4.3	2.5
31	42.4	40.0	46.0	35.6	40.6	1.6	1.7	.9	4.5	2.8
32	41.5	39.1	45.1	34.8	39.7	1.7	1.8	1.0	4.7	3.0
33	40.5	38.1	44.1	33.9	38.8	1.8	1.9	1.1	5.0	3.3
34	39.6	37.2	43.2	33.1	37.9	1.9	2.0	1.2	5.5	3.5
35	38.7	36.3	42.2	32.3	37.1	2.1	2.2	1.3	5.9	3.8
36	37.7	35.3	41.3	31.5	36.2	2.2	2.3	1.4	6.4	4.1
37	36.8	34.4	40.3	30.7	35.4	2.4	2.6	1.5	6.9	4.4
38	35.9	33.5	39.4	29.9	34.5	2.6	2.8	1.6	7.3	4.8
39	35.0	32.6	38.4	29.1	33.7	2.8	3.0	1.8	7.8	5.1
40	34.1	31.7	37.5	28.3	32.8	3.1	3.3	1.9	8.2	5.5
41	33.2	30.8	36.6	27.5	32.0	3.4	3.7	2.1	8.7	6.0
42	32.3	29.9	35.7	26.8	31.2	3.7	4.1	2.3	9.3	6.4
43	31.4	29.0	34.7	26.0	30.4	4.0	4.5	2.6	9.9	6.8
44	30.6	28.2	33.8	25.3	29.6	4.4	5.0	2.8	10.6	7.1
45	29.7	27.3	32.9	24.5	28.8	4.8	5.5	3.1	11.4	7.5
46	28.8	26.5	32.0	23.8	28.0	5.2	6.1	3.4	12.2	8.0
47	28.0	25.6	31.1	23.1	27.3	5.7	6.7	3.7	13.0	8.5
48	27.1	24.8	30.3	22.4	26.5	6.3	7.5	4.0	14.0	9.1

TABLE 4. (Continued)

Expectation of Life in Years

Age	Total Persons	White Male	White Female	Nonwhite Male	Nonwhite Female
49	26.3	24.0	29.4	21.7	25.7
50	25.5	23.2	28.5	21.0	25.0
51	24.7	22.4	27.6	20.4	24.2
52	23.9	21.6	26.8	19.7	23.5
53	23.1	20.8	25.9	19.1	22.8
54	22.3	20.1	25.1	18.5	22.1
55	21.6	19.4	24.2	17.9	21.4
56	20.8	18.7	23.4	17.3	20.7
57	20.1	18.0	22.6	16.7	20.1
58	19.3	17.3	21.8	16.1	19.4
59	18.6	16.6	21.0	15.6	18.8
60	17.9	16.0	20.1	15.1	18.2
61	17.2	15.3	19.4	14.5	17.6
62	16.5	14.7	18.6	14.0	17.0
63	15.9	14.1	17.8	13.5	16.5
64	15.2	13.5	17.0	13.0	15.9
65	14.6	12.9	16.3	12.6	15.5
66	14.0	12.4	15.5	12.2	15.0
67	13.4	11.8	14.8	11.9	14.6

Mortality Rate per 1,000

Total Persons	White Male	White Female	Nonwhite Male	Nonwhite Female
6.9	8.3	4.4	15.1	9.8
7.6	9.3	4.8	16.2	10.6
8.3	10.3	5.1	17.4	11.4
9.1	11.3	5.6	18.7	12.3
10.0	12.5	6.0	20.1	13.2
10.7	13.7	6.5	21.5	14.2
11.7	15.0	7.0	23.1	15.2
12.7	16.5	7.6	24.9	16.4
13.7	17.9	8.2	26.5	17.7
14.9	19.5	8.9	28.1	19.2
16.0	21.1	9.6	29.6	20.8
17.3	22.8	10.3	30.8	22.5
18.6	24.6	11.2	32.3	24.2
20.2	26.6	12.2	34.9	26.4
22.0	29.0	13.5	38.9	29.2
24.2	31.6	15.0	44.1	32.6
26.5	34.5	16.7	50.5	36.4
28.9	37.5	18.6	56.8	40.2
31.4	40.6	20.5	62.0	43.1

Source: Division of Vital Statistics, National Center for Health Statistics. From Metropolitan Life Insurance Company, *Statistical Bulletin*, August, 1967.

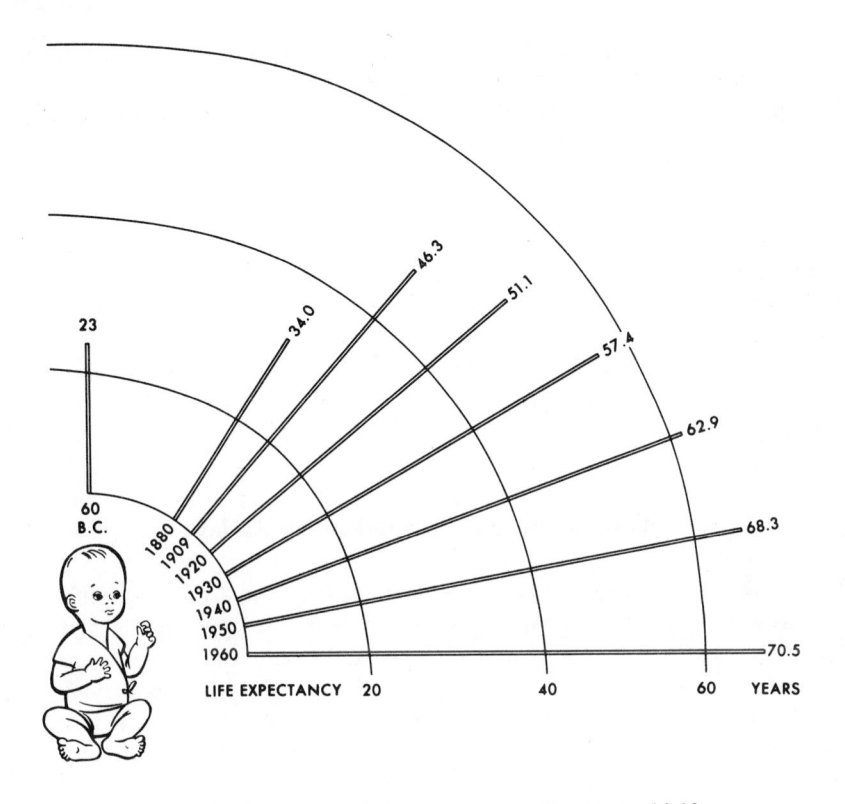

Figure 27. *Increase in life expectancy, 60* B.C. *to 1960.*

population; by 1950 they comprised 8.1 per cent. It is anticipated that by 1985 the elders will make up 10 per cent of our total population.[4]

While the total population of the country increased by 18.5 per cent from 1950 to 1960, the population aged 65 and older increased by 43.7 per cent. In the next few years, between 1967 and 1975, those 65–69 years of age will be the fastest growing segment of the country, increasing by almost 15 per cent. In the following decade, those persons aged 70–74 will experience the most rapid rate of growth, in excess of 20 per cent increase.[5]

Number of People Living to Age 65

Because of the increase in the total population of our country, the large number of elderly people may have more meaning to us than the proportionate

[4] *Statistical Bulletin*, Metropolitan Life Insurance Company, June 1968, p. 3.
[5] Ibid.

percentages. When we consider the number of elderly people needing medical care and hospital beds, we realize that new problems face our country.

In 1900 there were 3,100,000 people aged 65 or older in the United States. In 1967 there were 18.8 million people aged 65 or older, or six times as many. It is expected that by 1975 the number of aged will increase to more than 21 million and may reach 25 million by 1985.[6]

It is the number of people living past 75 or 80 that particularly concerns the younger generation and the nursing profession. Many people live independently and purposefully for 10 to 15 years beyond the age of 65. From 1950 to 1960 the number of persons from 75 to 84 years old increased by 41.1 per cent, and the number of persons 85 years of age or older increased by 60.8 per cent. There are now 6 million people aged 75 or older, and more than 10,000 beyond the age of 100.[7]

Why People Are Living Longer Today

Innumerable changes in our lives have made possible the longer life-span. People who longingly sigh for "the good old days" are only part remembering life as it used to be. Those reminiscing usually omit the unpleasantness of pioneer and earlier life, as do the glorified movie and television productions.

If you honestly think you might like to have lived 100 years ago, make a visit to a cemetery, preferably your own family cemetery. Note the birth and death dates inscribed on the tombstones. Also note how often you see a man's grave surrounded by the graves of more than one wife. His first wife died in childbirth; he married again, his second wife died in childbirth; and so it went.

You and I benefit immeasurably from the vast progress made in medical science. The new drugs effectively prevent and cure infections. Acute illnesses can be prevented and treated. We know the causes of communicable diseases and how to control them. New surgical methods produce almost miracles. Rehabilitation transforms the lives of handicapped people.

Health and hospital insurance plans place improved medical care within the reach of the working man. During the depression years of the 1930's, people often knew they were sick but could not afford to go to the doctor or the hospital for expensive treatment. Today, this is different. More people can afford to pay medical bills, and help is available for the medically indigent. Medicare is available for those 65 and older. Medicaid operates in most states.

Also, Americans are gradually being educated to heed symptoms of illness. One general practitioner was asked, "Doctor, do you receive many urgent calls

---

[6] Ibid.
[7] From Message from the President of the United States to House of Representatives, 88th Congress, relative to "The Elderly Citizens of our Nation," Document No. 72, Feb. 21, 1963.

Nursing and the Aging Population

for help in the middle of the night?" He answered, "Few, except for maternity cases. Most people seem to be seeking help with the first indication that something is wrong. They come to me before their condition is an emergency."

Safer Childbirth

More live babies are born and fewer mothers die during childbirth today, which has appreciably increased the average life expectancy. The number of babies who died at birth, the infant mortality rate, in 1968 was 21.7 deaths per 1000 live births. The current infant mortality rate is one-fifth below the rate of ten years ago and almost one-third below that of twenty years ago.[8]

In the general population of the United States, maternal mortality (death of mothers in childbirth) now is about 3.4 per 10,000 live births in 1964, as contrasted with 60 deaths per 10,000 live births in 1915.[9]

These figures are for the United States of America. A missionary couple told with justifiable pride that in 1962, in their hospital in Nigeria, Africa, 1248 live babies were born, and 721 babies were lost. Not all nations of the world benefit from scientific knowledge. Not all Americans benefit equally from scientific progress. Look again at Table 4 and note the difference in mortality rates for white and nonwhite women.

Doubtless during your first days of clinical experience, you will tour your hospital. As you see the tiny premature babies, ask yourself: Would these babies have lived 30 years ago?

Better Living Conditions

People live better today. They do not work as many long, exhausting hours to obtain food, shelter, and clothing. Work is less likely to be physically dangerous.

Improved sanitation means good water to drink and waste disposal in the cities. Organized fire fighting helps to prevent tragedies. You learn in your study of community health that we still have progress to make, but our country has made great improvements in living conditions.

Improved Nutrition

A variety of plentiful food is within the reach of more people today. Eating habits can be better, as discussed elsewhere in this book, and nutrition

---

[8] *Statistical Bulletin*, Metropolitan Life Insurance Company, February 1969, p. 5.
[9] Vital and Health Statistics, U.S. Public Health Service Publication No. 1000-Series 20-No. 1, U.S. Government Printing Office, 1965.

throughout life has improved. The pregnant woman is taught what to eat to help herself and her baby, and we know what to feed infants. Improved transportation makes it possible to have fresh fruits and vegetables the year around.

New Problems for Our Country

A larger population of elderly people brings new economic, social, and medical problems to our country.

Who supports the elderly people? Should a person be forced to retire at the age of 65? What kinds of part-time jobs are available to older people? Where do elderly people live?

What about recreational facilities for older people? What is to be done with forced leisure time? Does this increase the demand for television sets? How can elderly people be included in social activities? In a variety of ways, the aged represent a highly specialized market — a market for homes, for services, for special foods, and for travel programs.

As people get older, they have more health problems and need more medical services. What is the family to do when an elderly parent needs prolonged, expensive nursing care? With an increased elderly population, our country will need more doctors, more nurses, more hospitals, more convalescent homes, more medical schools, and more nursing schools.

Since the licensed practical nurse seems to be particularly suited to the care of the elderly person, everything seems to point to increased demands for trained practical nurses. Apparently you have chosen a field of work in which your services will be needed as long as you care to work.

Definition of Terms

Your study of elderly people will be easier if you are familiar with terms that are frequently used.

Aging is the normal, biological process of growing old. It begins at birth and continues through life. A baby is getting older, hence is aging.

Aged refers to those who show the results of aging. This can be at any period of life, but usually it is in the advanced years.

Senescence is the process or condition of growing old. It is normal, healthy old age. The spry, alert woman of 80 who does her own housework typifies senescence.

Senility is the state of bodily failure (physical and mental) due to old age. It is abnormal old age.

Defining the next few words requires explaining derivations:

Nursing and the Aging Population

Geron is the Greek work for "old man."
Geras is the Greek word for "old age."
ology at the end of a word means "study of."
iatrike means "medical treatment of."
iatricos means "medical care of."

Geriatrics is the medical care of the elderly person, including consideration of his physical, social, and emotional health. It is the care of the total person. Just as pediatrics includes care for the well child, so geriatrics includes concern for the well older person.

The *geriatrician* is a specialist in the medical care of elderly people. The pediatrician is a specialist in the care of children.

Gerontology is the scientific study of the aging process.

A *gerontologist* is the scientist who specializes in the study of the aging process.

Aging Is Relative

Just as there can be no fixed point at which adolescence ends and maturity begins, there can be no fixed point at which maturity ends and senescence, or old age, begins. You probably personally know one person who seems old at 45, while another seems young at 70. Aging is a continuous process.

Setting the age of 65 as the division between middle age and old age can be traced back to a historical accident. Back in the 1880's, Bismarck, a ruler in Germany, developed a program of social reward for his soldiers which would materialize when the soldier reached the age of 65. This age has been accepted since then and was codified in our own country when the Social Security Administration set the age of 65 for retirement in the middle 1930's. Now, tax laws, retirement programs, and many legal matters use the age of 65 to designate the older person.

As this term is used in the following pages, remember that it is a relative term.

Aims of Geriatrics

The statistics quoted earlier prove one fact: the aged are *here*, in increasing numbers. If people are going to live longer, those years should be worth living.

An old man neatly summarized the problem when he said: "I don't think people live longer today. It just seems longer."

Geriatrics should add more life to the years, as well as years to life. Geriatrics should strive to help the individual maintain physical and mental health, through maturity and senescence.

Geriatrics strives to minimize and control the diseases and disabilities of the advancing years. To prevent chronic illness, with no hope for recovery, is important. Everyone wants "to die with my boots on." Or, we prefer "to wear out, not rust out."

Both the geriatrician and the gerontologist agree that usually the elderly person should be kept in his own home as long as possible. That is, he shouid be kept out of the hospital and out of institutions when practical.

Almost a basic, instinctive desire of old people is to die in their own homes. The elderly person wants to be independent in mind and body as long as possible. Geriatrics helps the individual to maintain a feeling of personal worth and dignity. It has been said: "Geriatrics is the art of helping people to live better for a longer time."[10]

Questions for Discussion

1. What is the age of the oldest person you have ever known?
2. Compare your standard of living with that of your grandparents when they were young. What are the improvements?
3. What are some of the health hazards present in our urban, industrial society that were not a problem to your grandparents?
4. Describe someone you know personally who is young in spirit although advanced in years. Do you know a person who is young in years, but seems old in spirit?

Additional Readings

Aging with a Future. Reports and Guidelines from the White House Conference on Aging, Series No. 1. Washington, D.C.: U.S. Department of Health, Education, and Welfare, Special Staff on Aging, April 1, 1961.
Facts About Older Americans. U.S. Department of Health, Education, and Welfare, Administration on Aging Publication No. 410, May 1966.
Statistical Bulletin. Metropolitan Life Insurance Company. Monthly publication.

Recommended Audiovisual Aids

FILMS

Ready for Edna (23 min., U.S. Public Health Service, Produced by Center for Mass Communication of Columbia University. Available free from Department of Program Utilization, N.E.T., 10 Columbus Circle, New York, N.Y. 10019; B&W, 1965)
    This film depicts the history of the care of the aged in the United

---

[10] Pamphlet, *Medical Problems of Aging*, Indiana State Board of Health, p. 12.

Nursing and the Aging Population 235

States, and tells why life expectancy has increased. It might be used during any phase of geriatric study. It is the story of an elderly couple who move from their house to an apartment. The wife has a stroke. She comes home to the new apartment, where her husband, John, helps to rehabilitate her. John is killed instantly in an auto accident, and Edna is taken to a nursing home for her remaining years. The question is asked, "How many communities are ready for Edna, who will live 10 or 20 years after a stroke?" The film shows available services that might be useful, and how Edna herself can learn to help others, less fortunate, in the nursing home.

Don't Count the Candles (CBS television documentary, 1 hour, 1969)

Directed and filmed by Lord Snowdon, husband of Princess Margaret, the documentary is a moving and visually stunning essay on the joys and anguishes of growing old. It shows the faces of elderly English people — rich and famous, poor and obscure. Basic truths are illustrated: an elderly man who has attained distinction is treated with reverence; others less fortunate are not. Filmed for television, this beautiful documentary would be excellent for student nurses to see.

CHAPTER 22/SOCIAL AND EMOTIONAL

NEEDS OF OLDER PEOPLE;

USEFUL ACTIVITIES

This old adage appears appropriate: "Everyone needs somewhere to live, something to do, and someone to care." The needs of older people are really no different from those of people of all ages. Everyone wants to feel loved, wanted, useful, and important. We all need to have respect for ourselves and a feeling of personal worth.

Many signs indicate that the basic, deep needs of a large proportion of the 20 some million people in our society over 65 are not adequately met today. Are we being too smug, perhaps? Ours is an affluent society.

Why Life Is Unsatisfactory for Some

Many changes in our way of living affect older people, their status, and their ability to be useful. We live a fast pace today. The tempo is far beyond that of the old person who moves and thinks slowly.

In the predominantly rural society of former years, the aged person had a genuine place, but he does not fit well into today's urban, industrialized society. Household appliances have replaced the need for an extra pair of hands to help with repetitive tasks. Old people are no longer needed to teach the young people how to cook, weave, mend a fence, or shoe a horse. The store is operated by a chain of administrators. In some parts of the world the elders still teach the youngsters a trade. In Switzerland, the art of cheesemaking may have been in one family for centuries and is still taught to the new generation. This is rare in America. The adult of middle years finds it increasingly difficult to keep up with the technological advancement in his own field. It is said that the store of knowledge doubles about every 7 years. Also, a man's occupation may require that he move to another state, miles away from elderly parents.

Money is the resource most valued today. It takes money to buy food, clothing, and housing. Houses and apartments are too small for three- and four-generation living. There are fewer big houses today with room for the extra adult. In many ways, the family has lost something very precious. It was the extra adult in the household who had time and patience to spend a leisurely hour with a child discovering the joys of nature. The extra adult could often relieve the pressure between parents and children. (Of course, the extra adult could cause pressure, too.)

But of all the changes, perhaps the most significant is the changed attitude toward older people. Elderly people are often rejected. Even in Jewish communities, where the elders are traditionally held in special devotion and respect, social workers note less interest and respect given to elderly parents. Our society is both work-oriented (jobs give status) and youth-oriented, idolizing young people. Pick up any popular magazine or turn on a television set and note the advertisements offering to help you "to stay young and beautiful."

Possibly there is too much talk about the negative aspect of retirement, giving a grim, bleak picture of later years. We may frighten people into avoiding the appearance of age, not letting them see the rewards and advantages of chronological maturity.

We need a change in attitude to give the recognition to achievement, wisdom, and experience. Dr. Edward Bortz, a physician specializing in geriatrics, refused to write an article for a popular magazine on "How to Stay Young." His answer was, "I am not interested in arrested development."[1]

Dr. Bortz describes the retirement years as ". . . a gentle and pleasant period which might be designated as the Indian summer of life, when with mild waning of physical interests, there is increased clarity, expectancy, and efficiency in intellectual activities. There are fewer distractions from the tempests and passions of earlier years, lending a clearer sense of values and a philosophical calm and willingness to live the quiet life."[2]

When we universally accept the philosophy that maturing is growing and that age is growth, the elderly people will have their respected and deserving place in society.

Let us examine more closely how some of the basic needs of older people are met today.

Companionship

The elderly person needs someone to talk to every day and someone with whom to share experiences. We noted earlier that the 6-to-12-year-old and the adolescent need their peer groups, that is, people of their own age. The older person also needs satisfactory peer relationships. He likes to reminisce and to

---

[1] From a speech by Dr. Bortz at the Purdue University Conference on Aging, September 1962.
[2] Edward L. Bortz, *Creative Aging* (New York: Macmillan, 1963) p. 13.

talk over old times with his friends. The older person needs to talk with people of the opposite sex, too. One charming widow in her seventies remarked after her first visit to a senior citizens' day center, "How good it is just to sit and talk to a man." But constant contact only with other elderly people is not good. It is more wholesome, more normal for a person to be around people of all ages.

Yet many elderly people will not seek companionship. They hesitate to join senior citizen clubs. It is estimated that only 8 per cent of Chicago's elderly people belong to one of the many church-sponsored or park district clubs for the elderly. Another 5 per cent live in various kinds of institutions. Most of the elderly people avoid associating with other old people because this would be admitting to their own old age. The young avoid them because they are old. So the elderly spend their days alone.

Sometimes a person is so lonesome and so miserable living alone that he cannot eat or function as a human being. Living in a home with other older people furnishes companionship and may be the solution for many.

The elderly person wants someone to talk to him as a real person. He probably does not feel old, only when other people treat him so. The geriatric patient in a hospital benefits from a two-bed room. A single room can be very lonely, especially when the nurses are busy, work under pressure, and have little time to stop and talk.

Stimulating Experiences

Stimulating, happy experiences contribute to the well-being of an individual. The elderly person who lives a slower, more restricted life does not require an earth-shattering event to stimulate him. The author recalls spending an afternoon with a favorite aunt, sharing pictures taken on a trip through Europe. Three years later, the aunt still talked about the pictures.

Television can bring the outside world into the room of the elderly person. The view of the presidential inauguration or the White House reception for the astronauts may be better on the television screen than it is for the actual spectator. Watching the television scenes of the funeral, the tributes, and the homage given to Dwight David Eisenhower was important to many older people who had their own memories of world events during Ike's long career of public service. Yet, too, much television viewing can be harmful. An observant nurse noticed a group of elderly county home residents watching a blank screen, not even aware that the picture had disappeared.

Recognition

To be recognized for what he is — a special person whose survival marks him as worthy of respect — this is the need of older people. Many elderly people are happier remaining in their home community than they would be in moving into a new community. In her old community, the widow has status. People see her not only as she is now, but as she used to be. They may notice trembling hands and a cross reply, but remember the tasty cherry pies she used to bake, and the time she came to sit with them in their sorrow. Although a man's memory fails and he becomes confused, people still recall him as a clear-headed lawyer or professor, whom younger men admired and imitated.

One retired minister was asked, and agreed, to return to a community where he had been minister many years earlier. The couples now the bulwark of the church had been teenagers and young people at that time. He had guided, counseled, and married many of them. These people recognized the fine life of service of their retired pastor. He was not just another old man to them; he was a very special person.

Sense of Achievement

The sense of achievement for the elderly person may come from his past. The individual who has lived to serve others, to give of himself to others, has a store of rich memories to draw upon. Certainly the nurse who helps people through the years is building a storehouse of memories. Few types of employment give personal satisfaction equaling that of bedside nursing.

Yet living in the past alone is not good. Older people need to retain a feeling of self-worth and of self-respect. They need to feel important as individuals.

Love

To love and be loved is part of the feeling of personal worth. Love and affection are expressed in many ways. The elderly couple still in love are a precious part of our society to be preserved. We should help them to stay together. After the children have left the home, after retirement from active work, many elderly couples tend to disengage themselves from friends and other family members. They seem to need and to prefer only each other, as they did on their honeymoon and during early years of married life. They most nearly represent the Chinese interpretation of yin and yang — the one complements the other. Together they form a complete circle, a complete life. Separated they are incomplete.

With the loss of one partner, the other has truly lost part of himself. The shock can be traumatic. Children, friends, relatives, and familiar surroundings can be a source of comfort, but recovery is not immediate. Five years will be a short time after 45 years of happily married life.

Some single people have less difficulty filling the need for personal affection because they have developed substitutes through the years. Other single people may be bitter because they feel they have not lived a fulfilled life.

Freedom of Movement and Decision

Because the older person is often dependent, it is sometimes easy to push him around, control him, and tell him what to do. It takes patience and time to help him make his own decisions, but he should be encouraged to do so. Coddling an elderly person only encourages dependence.

However, probably the majority of elderly people resent others telling them what to do. Since they have made decisions all their lives, they believe that they know what to do and what is best for them. It requires wisdom on the part of a son or daughter to know when to intervene.

Economic Security

Economic security is a basic need so important to the older person that an entire chapter — Chapter 26 — will be devoted to it. Lack of finances causes much of the unhappiness and many of the troubles of older people.

A Feeling of Belonging

When older people gradually lose out on the activities that were formerly important to them, life can be meaningless. Organized clubs for older people represent one kind of effort to help them feel that they belong somewhere. Some people feel that these clubs are abnormal ways of getting older people together. Yet the clubs flourish, so the need must exist.

One minister discouraged the church's women's society from forming a "circle" for elderly women because he felt that they would benefit more from associating with younger women. But once started, the circle was immediately popular. The elderly women loved the special attention they received on this one day of the month. The younger women furnished them transportation to the church, and prepared and served a pleasant luncheon.

The family who has an aged relative living with them should share problems as well as triumphs with him. The natural impulse may be to shield the frail and ailing one from further worry, but he is likely to be aware that something is wrong. He will feel that he is still part of the family circle if he takes part in, or at least listens to, the discussions of problems.

Religious Faith

When the need for love is not met by human beings, many elderly people find peace with the assurance of God's love. Sometimes the older person feels that, through his church, he expresses his love for all humanity.

Death is a little closer to the elderly person than to the young person. A fatal accident can happen to anyone of any age but is more likely to occur to the older person. Many people need to believe in life after death.

The older person may not fear death. Many loved ones and dear friends have gone before him. He has seen his children established as adults. He has known his grandchildren and possibly his great-grandchildren. A young person probably cannot comprehend the feeling of having lived a fulfilled, completed life. Perhaps no one can know how the elderly person feels about approaching death until he is old himself.

Nor perhaps can you, the nurse, understand the tenacity to live that you will see in some elderly patients. The aging body may be completely deteriorating, and you view death as inevitable. Yet the person clings desperately to life, refusing to give up.

Experienced church and social workers do not attempt to change an elderly person's views or attitudes toward religion.

Mr. Robert White writes:

> We expect elderly people to continue the pattern of behavior and thought which they have followed and developed over the years. Old age is no automatic guarantee that a person will turn to religion. At such a time, religion will have about the same importance and the same significance it attained during the course of his life. Given time and encouragement, religious growth can continue to the end. The elderly person is most likely to continue all the patterns of his existence, relatively unchanged, up to the moment of death.
>
> A lingering death might effect religious changes. All of the person's response patterns are modified, and this includes religion.
>
> There is little reason to seek to transform the elderly person. No matter how clearly the person caring for him sees the value of change, the aged have grown accustomed to their life pattern. They depend upon it for security.[3]

If the elderly person wants to see a clergyman, the nurse should arrange for this. It does little good to pressure the aged.

---

[3] Former Minister of Education, Broadway United Methodist Church, Indianapolis, Indiana.

Interest in the Present

The older person who finds life barren, boring, and discouraging will tend to withdraw from the present and relive the past that was so much more satisfying. When the older person feels loved and secure and has something that he is eager to do, he is interested in today. He cares about the present. Family and friends can encourage the person and avoid mentioning the past but primarily he must do this for himself.

Some people can stay interested in a profession and follow its development. Others find satisfaction through hobbies, craftwork, and community service. Purposeful activity helps the person to live in the present. This is one of the big problems facing elderly people today.

Useful Activity

Someone said that "uselessness is the disease of old age." Most old people have one thing in common — an abundance of leisure time. It does not have to be, but it can be too much time for self-pity, for worrying about health and finances, to be bored, and worst of all, to blame others for one's dilemma. People need to be busy. The human body and the human mind are not built for idle existence. They are designed to be used.

Many older people grew up with the Puritan philosophy that it was not exactly nice or moral to enjoy oneself. Pleasure was regarded almost as a sin. Such an elderly person may feel guilty about having so much leisure time. She does not enjoy playing cards or sewing for herself. She may feel better about sewing for another person or helping in a service project.

Employment for Older People

If the person can and wishes to continue working, he has less of a problem of surplus leisure time. Not all elderly people want to continue working. Many elderly people held routine, uninteresting jobs in factories or offices, jobs they disliked at the time. They are relieved to have freedom from a nagging boss or the tyrannical alarm clock. The money is about all some retired people miss from their old jobs. Women who spent their lives as housewives and mothers do not want to start working for wages, even if work could be found. Age means narrowing of interests, and gradual withdrawal from society. An elderly man who wishes to eliminate some activities may welcome losing the social contacts associated with work.

But it is a fact that compulsory retirement at a set age prevents many talented, capable people from continuing to make a worthwhile contribution to society. Everyone loses thereby.

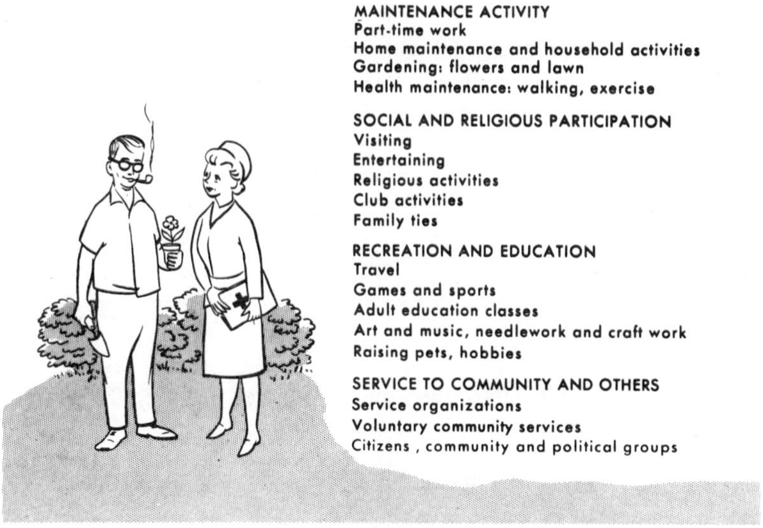

MAINTENANCE ACTIVITY
Part-time work
Home maintenance and household activities
Gardening: flowers and lawn
Health maintenance: walking, exercise

SOCIAL AND RELIGIOUS PARTICIPATION
Visiting
Entertaining
Religious activities
Club activities
Family ties

RECREATION AND EDUCATION
Travel
Games and sports
Adult education classes
Art and music, needlework and craft work
Raising pets, hobbies

SERVICE TO COMMUNITY AND OTHERS
Service organizations
Voluntary community services
Citizens, community and political groups

Figure 28. *The aging period offers a challenge to use wisely the increased leisure time. (Adapted from Chart 63, 1961 White House Conference on Aging,* Chart Book, *Federal Council on Aging.)*

Research comparing the elderly worker with the younger worker does not show that sudden changes occur in the worker's performance or capacity at the age of 65. The elderly worker's performance might be inferior if rated according to physical strength, speed, or agility. He is slower when learning new materials and new methods of work. But the older worker usually excels in terms of experience, judgment, responsibility, accuracy, stability, and other less easily measured traits. Skills perfected are usually retained. Absentee records and accident rates of older persons compare favorably with those of other workers.

But regardless of these arguments, facts indicate that government and industry rules are working toward earlier, not later, retirements. Industry generally requires workers to leave their jobs at age 65. Some key industries — autos, steel, and farm equipment — offer early retirement at 55. Reduced social security payments can be taken by men and women beginning at age 62. A widow can get social security retirement benefits at 60. To some people with good health, the idea of loafing away their remaining years has little appeal.

PART-TIME EMPLOYMENT

For those who wish to work, a partial answer lies with more part-time employment or a job that has shorter hours and fewer responsibilities and requires less physical energy.

Many self-employed people have successfully spread retirement over a period of years. They gradually give up responsibilities and shorten their working hours. Perhaps they continue in an advisory capacity. Many professional people serve as advisors to their own company or to others. Retired high school teachers occasionally serve as substitute teachers. A nurse nearing retirement age may find work as a companion to a handicapped person, in a doctor's office, or with private-duty cases. People in many fields of work, including nursing, have turned to writing.

The hobby followed during working years may lead to a vocation upon retirement. A man who has equipped his home with a workshop might spend many happy hours refinishing old furniture or making new furniture.

Some government projects offer jobs to retired people. Several states are cooperating with the federal government on "Operation Green Thumb," which puts retired farmers to work helping to beautify highways.

Community Service

At the White House Conference on Aging, in January 1961, community service was held to be the answer for useful activity for the elderly. The elderly were to be diverted with volunteer work in hospitals and institutions, or by helping the young or the handicapped. Just as some people find the answer by working full or part time, some undertake community service.

The elderly person who feels guilty about using forced leisure time for recreational purposes may appreciate the chance for community service. A typical remark is: "Oh, thank you for asking me to help."

Most elderly people are accustomed to giving, and they find it embarrassing to be receiving. They want to be useful. However, they are suspicious of "made work."

Many community projects need an extra pair of hands. There are always bandages to be cut and rolled, sewing for the sick or poor, envelopes to be stuffed for community drives, workers needed at the polls on election day, and people needed to serve as jurymen for court trials. Many professional organizations make an effort to include retired members in their activities. Most church leaders manage skillfully to fit the elderly people into the church activities.

Most community service projects are not a source of income, but a way of enabling a person to contribute to society. Jury duty is one community service that offers income. Another offering small pay is the government-sponsored "Foster Grandparent" program. Elderly people work with mentally retarded adults and children in state and church institutions. The small pay supplements a meager income – but the most important reward is the boost to the morale, the knowledge that the person is still useful and needed.

Retired Man's Problem

Retirement from active employment can be a terrific blow. It calls for reorganizing the routines in life, adjusting to reduced income, and possibly replacing business associates with other friends. Frequently women adjust more easily than men because women spend more time on their clothes, homemaking duties, and social activities such as card parties, club activities, and church functions.

Men believe in work, and their lives have been centered around work. Perhaps the elderly man feels useless because he is useless. We need to be patient, to help him find himself. In the over-65 population, women outnumber men 2 to 1; in the over-75 population, women outnumber men 4 to 1.

Successful leisure-time activities may be as unique as the individuals themselves. One elderly trio watched court trials as a hobby. The men relished the details of the robbery trials, the murder cases, and contested divorce suits. Sitting in the courtroom did not cost money, and they could find many more disagreeable places to be than the beautiful new city-county building with its ultramodern furnishings.

The elderly man with a little extra cash might purchase a few shares of stock and discover the excitement of following the stock market. One 74-year-old retired plumber, with an assured adequate income, felt that he could afford to invest an occasional $100 in stock. Each weekday morning, he walked to the brokerage office and spent a pleasant hour or two there. He attended stockholders' meetings and visited the factories of firms in which he owned stock. He had found a stimulating new interest in life.

The hobby that benefited a working man does not always suit his needs for a retirement vocation. A factory worker loves fishing because it takes him out into the open air, and he finds peace and quiet on the water. But he may find loneliness in retirement days and need something to bring him into contact with people.

Creative Hobbies and Craftwork

The wise person harbors interests that he secretly yearns to try. When retirement comes, he has the time for them. If people develop hobbies and varied interests during their working years, the hobby can become the focus of their life at retirement.

A schoolteacher bought a new sewing machine immediately before retiring. She said, "My granddaughters can hardly wait for me to retire so I can sew for them." From the twinkle in her eyes, it was obvious that this grandmother was anticipating eagerly the chance to make blouses for her granddaughters.

Many people find joy and satisfaction in creating a design. One does not have to produce a masterpiece to enjoy painting, sculpturing, photography, or music. Women are more likely than men to be interested in knitting, crocheting, tatting, needlepoint, or hooking. However, there is no reason why a man should not crochet if he is interested. Both men and women enjoy working with wood, metal, ceramics, leather, basketry, and cord knotting. Mosaics offer endless possibilities. Nurses should always be alert for potential projects for men patients. The man who likes detail may be fascinated with paint-by-number pictures, which require precise movements. This of course, requires good eyesight and muscle control or dexterity.

Collecting curios and antiques intrigues many people. The best collections are those requiring the person to study, classify, or arrange. When collecting stamps, one learns dates of historic events and names of famous people. An ordinary collection of matchfolders can be organized according to origin by states, cities, or countries.

Reading can be directed to one subject. The person may enjoy being an authority on a topic not related to his work. Many new stories have been published about Lincoln with a different interpretation of the Civil War or a refreshing picture of Mary Todd Lincoln.

Writing short stories or magazine articles is within the ability of many people. Almost every experienced professional person has at least one pet idea that could be developed into a magazine article.

Growing plants and vines can transfer a dreary room into a cheerful place. As the patient waits for the bud to flower, he looks forward to tomorrow. Such simple events can give a person reason to want to go on living. The list of creative activities is unlimited. A good hobby challenges the imagination and the skills of the person. Again, it is useless to try to hurry the older person. One elderly resident in a home for the aged took four years to decide that he wanted to learn to weave.

Creative hobbies are fine for those who have the talent and the interest. But we must remember that many aged adults lived when working hours were long, and they have had no experience with art hobbies. Thus it might be inappropriate — or even insulting — to suggest craftwork to them.

CONTINUING EDUCATION

More than three-quarters of a million people over 65 enroll yearly in formal education programs. They enroll in adult education courses in the public schools and the university extension centers. They expand personal horizons through educational programs of churches; personnel departments of business, industry, and government; fraternal and service organizations; and clubs and voluntary agencies. The public libraries often organize weekly reading and discussion groups for "senior citizens."

Today, less than one-half of the retired people have a high school education. It is estimated that by 1980, more than half of the elderly citizens will be high school graduates. A higher educational level of the retirees will mean that more of them will enjoy reading and studying. Continuous education may prove to be the key to satisfying later years.

Motivating the Elderly Person

Many elderly people are able to develop skills and interests on their own; others need outside help and stimulus. A well-organized activity center in the community has many values.

Nursing homes and homes for the aged should offer some kind of diversional activities for their people. One director of a home for the aged explained that the success of an activity program depends on the staff — the registered professional nurse, the licensed practical nurse, and the aides. If the nurses and the aides believe the activity is important, they usually succeed in getting the patients to participate. If the nurses and the aides think it is unimportant, the program usually fails.

When the patient shows absolutely no interest in doing anything, getting him started is not easy. The nurse may have to attempt more than one approach.

Making a gift for someone else may appeal to the elderly person. The woman with a loved great-grandchild may spend hours clipping pictures to paste in a scrapbook for the child.

Show the person a finished project, and he may be intrigued with the thought of making a similar item. Ordinary gingham yardgoods and floss may not appeal to a woman, but she may be fascinated by a pretty pillow top made of smocked gingham. "That looks easy. I could do that," she may say.

Get the patient to talk about himself. Often a man will volunteer information regarding a previous activity. Most women have crocheted or knitted at one time. If the nurse knows enough of the basic stitches to encourage the person to start again, she will find it comes back to her.

Occasionally, a patient can be "needled" into attempting a project. A family member might use this approach more safely than the nurse. One woman of 89 finally started an advanced knitting project after her daughter unwittingly said exactly the right thing, "Mother, I don't think you can." The mother snapped a reply, "Well, I'll have you know I *can* knit these slippers." And she did.

The nurse must be realistic when suggesting activities. For example, many elderly people are not interested in community service. A person who was self-centered before 65 will not turn into an altruistic person, concerned for his fellow men. A woman who finished the tenth grade in 1918, and never went to school again, will not be interested in adult education classes. The man who never read anything more challenging than the sports page in the daily newspaper will not suddenly enjoy a great books discussion group merely because he is now 65 years old.

We cannot help elderly people if we expect them to become very different people from what they have been all their lives. The aged cannot change.

Senior Citizens' Charter

From the report of the White House Conference on Aging, held January, 1961, came this statement of the rights and obligations of senior citizens:[4]

RIGHTS OF SENIOR CITIZENS

Each of our senior citizens, regardless of race, color, or creed, is entitled to:
1. The right to be useful.
2. The right to obtain employment, based on merit.
3. The right to freedom from want in old age.
4. The right to a fair share of the community's recreational, educational, and medical resources.
5. The right to obtain decent housing suited to needs of later years.
6. The right to the moral and financial support of one's family so far as is consistent with the best interests of the family.
7. The right to live independently, as one chooses.
8. The right to live and die with dignity.
9. The right of access to all knowledge as available on how to improve the later years of life.

OBLIGATIONS OF THE AGING

The aging, by availing themselves of educational opportunities, should endeavor to assume the following obligations to the best of their ability:
1. The obligation of each citizen to prepare himself to become and resolve to remain active, alert, capable, self-supporting, and useful so long as health and circumstances permit and to plan for ultimate retirement.
2. The obligation to learn and apply sound principles of physical and mental health.
3. The obligation to seek and develop potential avenues of service in the years after retirement.
4. The obligation to make available the benefits of his experience and knowledge.
5. The obligation to endeavor to make himself adaptable to the changes added years will bring.

---

[4] *The Nation and Its Older People*, Report of the White House Conference on Aging, Jan. 9–12, 1961 (Washington, D.C.: U.S. Department of Health, Education, and Welfare, Special Staff on Aging, April 1961), p. 118.

Questions for Discussion

1. Describe occupations of persons over 65 whom you know who are working.
2. What are the arguments given in favor of, and against, compulsory retirement?
3. What part-time employment is available in your community for people over 65?
4. Describe unique hobbies of people past the age of 65.
5. What community service projects in your area can use retirees?

Additional Readings

Arthur, Julietta. *Retire to Action*. Nashville, Tenn.: Abingdon Press, 1969.

Donahue, Wilma, ed. *Free Time, A Challenge to Later Maturity*. Ann Arbor: University of Michigan Press, 1958.

Donahue, Wilma, and Clark Tibbits, eds. *Planning the Later Years*. Westport, Conn.: Greenwood Press, Inc., 1968. Michigan University Conference on Aging.

Free Time Activities, Recreation, Voluntary Services, Citizen Participation. Reports and Guidelines from the White House Conference on Aging, Series 6. Washington, D.C.: U.S. Department of Health, Education, and Welfare, 1961.

Havighurst, Robert J. "The Natures and Values of Meaningful Free-Time Activity," in Robert W. Kleemeir, ed., *Aging and Leisure*. New York: Oxford University Press, 1961.

Westberg, Granger. *Nurse, Pastor, and Patient*. Rock Island, Ill.: Augustana Press, 1955.

Recommended Audiovisual Aids

FILMS

Adventure in Maturity (22 min., International Film Bureau, University of Oklahoma production, Color)

Not a modern setting, but the film conveys an important message. An elderly woman — rejected, and living in the past — is convinced by a friend to accept suitable work. With new clothes and fashionable coiffure, she acquires confidence and a new life for herself. The film advises people to be useful, to like what they are doing, and to grow with the years.

The Steps of Age (25 min., International Film Bureau, presented by Dept. of Mental Health, South Carolina, B&W)

The dress shown is slightly old-fashioned, but the main theme is appropriate today. Elderly people should try to adjust to old age and to living with a younger family. It depicts an elderly couple who had made no plans for their retirement years. The husband had no interests outside his job. He finally attempted to go back to the iron works, but could not handle his tools. He threw his tools into the river, and died soon afterward. His wife moved in with her daughter and family, where she felt, and actually was, unwanted. Finally, she decided to make an effort to fit in with the younger family, to make herself useful to others — and she succeeded.

CHAPTER 23/**PHYSICAL CHANGES WITH AGE**

One geriatric specialist[1] believes that today's 70-year life-span will reach 100 years within the next generation. He says the human body is built to last much longer than most people think. Different organs and systems have different life-spans. The eyes have a life expectancy of 120 to 130 years. The skin may be even longer-lived. Some cell reservoirs (such as the bone marrow) apparently never age. Women age more slowly than men, have a longer life expectancy, but require more medical repair work.

Some facts of the aging process are generally accepted, even though we do not yet know the complete answer to "what is aging?"

The outward, physical appearance of a man of 80 differs from that of a man of 30. Look carefully at the next elderly person you see.

Outward Physical Changes with Aging

Old people look different. Many old people have lost both weight and height. They seem to shrink. However, many obese people survive to old age despite insurance statistics showing that overweight is a detriment to long life.

The elderly person is weak physically. He has lost vitality and vigor. He moves slowly. He lacks coordination and a sense of balance. He can often push down, when he cannot pull himself up. He becomes short of breath on exertion. The body sags, the shoulders droop, and the spine curves or becomes bowed with kyphosis. The joints are stiff and the muscles flabby.

The hair turns gray, grows thin on top, and may fall out. The skin becomes thin, dry, wrinkled, and withered-looking. Elasticity diminishes, and sometimes the skin resembles crepe paper. Eyesight changes, and the eyes appear faded and blurry. The elderly person's eyeballs seem recessed, and the eyelids droop. Hearing losses are almost universal with aging. Often the teeth become loose and are eventually lost. The sense of taste, touch, and smell decrease, as do sensations of heat, cold, and pain.

These physical infirmities of later life are evidences of chemical changes within the body. Let us examine further these changes to understand more fully the struggle for good health that your elderly patient faces.

---

[1] Dr. Edward L. Bortz, "Take a New Look at Your Elderly Patients," *RN* (April 1962), p. 53.

Age and the Body Cells

In your study of body structure, you learn that the human body is composed of many types of specialized cells, such as muscle cells, gland cells, and nerve cells. These specialized cells join together to form "tissues" of the body, such as muscle tissues, connective tissue, and glandular tissue. Different kinds of tissue are grouped together as "organs." Organs grouped together to do certain work in the body are called "systems."

Let us see how aging affects cells and then what is known about the effect of aging on the body systems.

The cellular units are constantly being replaced. When cells are replaced at the same rate as cells die, the tissues show no apparent change with the passing of time. When the cell division occurs faster than cells die, the total number of cells increases and the growth of youth results. When the regeneration rate is slower than the rate at which cells are worn out or injured, atrophy occurs. Also during senescence, the cells become smaller and function at a lower, less efficient level.

The normal rate of cellular replacement varies with the tissues. For instance, epithelial tissues show a greater rate of cell division than do the cells making up the supporting tissues of the body, such as muscle, bone, and fibrous connective tissue.

The tissues of the brain and nervous system are the exception to this general pattern. Nerve cells do not multiply after growth of the individual is complete. These cells, therefore, are nearly as old as the body itself. Once the body of a nerve cell is destroyed, it is never replaced. If the nerve cell is injured, it may slowly repair itself, or it may not. Parts of the brain may cease to function without causing death. These cells are apparently not necessary for the continuance of life, but essential if life is to be consciously enjoyed.

One of the goals of the medical field, one of the goals of geriatrics, is to bolster the renewal powers and to slow down destruction of the cells, that is, to postpone aging.

Changes in Body Functions

Changes in the organ systems due to aging lead to changes in function. At rest, bodily functions of the aged person are normal.

Response of the aging body to stress and strain is limited. That is, homeostasis is lost. Homeostasis is the power of the body to regulate itself and to maintain a constant internal environment. Hence the aged person does not tolerate excessive cold or heat. He cannot adapt to extreme environments. His heart functions well when little demand is made on it, but it cannot respond to extreme demands.

Physical Changes with Age

The aged person cannot react quickly to change in body position. When a person rises after lying flat on his back, the nervous system normally increases the heart rate and constricts the smaller arteries and veins so rapidly and efficiently that he is not aware that the blood pressure falls for a few seconds. In older people, the effect of gravity is not compensated as quickly, and the fall in blood pressure on standing may cause dizziness, faintness, dangerous falls, or inability to walk.

Because of decreased homeostatic ability (plus arteriosclerosis), the aged are drastically and immediately affected by dehydration, starvation, sudden loss of blood, oxygen deprivation (anemia, surgical shock), and damage from certain irritants.

When bodily reserves are used, the aged body cannot respond as well. A young person can abuse his body and overtax his strength with little effect. For the aged, this leads to disaster.

Old people complain of being cold more often than young people. The older body apparently produces less heat and cannot prevent heat losses as well as the younger body. An interesting study in England[2] concluded that the oral temperatures of a group of apparently healthy older people ranged from 95.2° to 100.2°F. Hence in an older person, a temperature of 98.4 F might be equivalent to two or three degrees of fever.

Resistance to Disease

Not only does the elderly person recover slowly after body injury, he is also more susceptible to infection than the younger person. A gradual change occurs in the body's natural resistance to infection. This is partly due to atrophy of structures concerned with immunity, such as glands of internal secretion, spleen, phagocyte cells, bone marrow, and lymphatic tissue.

Pathological changes in various organs cause lowered resistance to infection. For example, poor circulation in extremities often leads to serious infection and gangrene.

Nutritional deficiencies common in old age, usually inadequate vitamin and calcium intake, also lower resistance to infection.

Skeletal System

The bones of elderly people are more brittle, predisposing them to fractures that are slow to heal. Elderly people are subject to osteoporosis (bone thinning and weakness) and arthritis, possibly due to insufficient calcium utilization and

---

[2] Ernest W. Burgess, *Aging in Western Societies* (Chicago: University of Chicago Press, 1960), p. 159.

endocrine imbalance. These conditions are less likely to develop when people remain physically active, eat well, and take glandular supplements (if prescribed).

That the bones become more firm and lack elasticity affects other parts of the body, such as the spinal column and the rib cage. The cartilages contract, harden, and may finally ossify. People lose about one-half inch in hieght for every 20 years of adult life. The stooped posture so often seen in elderly people means that the upper thoracic vertebrae are bowed. The ribs fall downward and forward, decreasing the chest capacity and leading to respiratory difficulties.

Muscular System

In senescence, the muscles themselves shrink from the gradual drying-out that occurs in all the body's tissues. The muscles become less elastic, lose tone, and undergo some atrophy. Some muscle strands are replaced by fibrous tissues. Body tissues change in composition to relatively more fat and less muscular tissue.

Lack of hormones affects muscular strength. The strength of the arm biceps at the age of 60 is about 50 per cent of that at the age of 25 to 30. The trunk muscles decline in power somewhat more slowly. Because the muscular structure is weakened, hernias occur. Reflexes are less sharp; the whole body slows down. Gradual deterioration is unavoidable, but the rate can be slowed and atrophy postponed by maintaining good physical fitness programs throughout life. Muscles must be used at all ages to keep in good tone.

Circulatory System

The failure of the circulatory system is often the direct reason that man does not live his normal life-span. The heart degenerates somewhat with aging, as do other muscles. Because it has to work harder, the size and weight of the heart actually increase, lessening its efficiency. The greater trouble, however, is with the blood vessels and the two diseases, hardening of the arteries (arteriosclerosis) and high blood pressure (hypertension), which tend to increase with age.

In arteriosclerosis, the arteries and veins become less elastic, more rigid, and more elongated. The walls thicken, the inside diameter of the blood vessel narrows and the blood flow is diminished or restricted.

Atherosclerosis is a typer of arteriosclerosis characterized by fatty degeneration or thickening of walls of the larger arteries. Atherosclerosis affects the coronary arteries.

The resistance of the entire vascular system is decreased by arteriosclerosis. The heart has to pump harder to force the blood through the constricted blood vessels. When the pressure in the arteries remains high, the condition is hypertension. In hypertension, the heart muscle becomes thicker and the heart enlarges. The heart may have to work so hard to force blood through the narrowed vessels that it destroys itself in the process. Not enough blood gets through the lesser vessels to nourish tissues and remove waste products. Many people with arteriosclerosis also have hypertension, but some do not. Some people have hypertension, but very little arteriosclerosis.

The calcified, thickened, and less elastic blood vessels are inclined to clog or rupture. When this happens in the brain, a "stroke" results. Little "strokes" involving little blood vessels are quite common in old people, and they cause impaired memory and many other mental and physical infirmities. Large "strokes" cause paralysis or death. Even without the major closures or breaks, the condition causes a chain reaction of damage throughout the body. Arteriosclerosis is probably the cause of more physical and mental damage in the aging than any other factor.

Loss of elasticity in the arteries begins earlier in some people than in others. The real cause is not known, but observations indicate that heredity, diet, and metabolism are involved. Women often develop high blood pressure in their forties; it occurs more frequently in men after 50.

Because the aged person makes fewer demands on the circulatory system, he may not realize that his heart is weaker and his system is less efficient until he is faced with an emergency. Then he finds that he cannot respond to the stresses of a physically active life. People who maintain an active life help to keep all cell tissue healthy.

Unfortunately, some degree of anemia is often found among the elderly. Anemia is more serious for the elderly person than for the young person. Content and quality of the blood assume a critical role in cardiac diseases, cerebral arteriosclerosis, and any circulatory insufficiency. Anemia may be caused by poor eating habits or other factors than can be remedied.

The nurse should remember that the elderly person is likely to have poor circulation in the extremities. Because he has difficulty adjusting to temperature changes, he needs an even room temperature and warm clothing to prevent heat loss.

Respiratory System

Changes in the nose and throat due to aging are few and result largely from simple atrophies of the mucosa, the glands, and the muscles similar to those found elsewhere in the body. The changes are more likely to cause annoyances and discomforts rather than real disabilities. Atrophy of the muscles of the pharynx and the larynx may render the voice flat, hard, and even shrill. Vocal changes are even more pronounced when accompanied by hearing losses. When one is deaf, his voice sounds weak and far away to him, so he compensates by forcing it.

The elasticity of the lung tissues decreases, as does the lung expansion, making the elderly patient a likely candidate for pneumonia. When lying flat, secretions may fill the lower portion of the lungs and increase the danger of infection.

Atrophy and fatigue of the respiratory muscles cause poor respiratory action, as does the poor tone of the abdominal musculature, which interferes with the action of the diaphragm. Arteriosclerotic changes in the blood vessels make circulation through the lungs less efficient.

If the lungs do not function properly, an extra burden is placed on the heart. Heavy bed covers may mechanically impede respiration.

Digestive System

Various changes in the digestive system cause elderly people to lose interest in food, but malnutrition does not have to be the result. The nurse who understands how digestion is affected will give more help to her geriatric patient.

Basal metabolism (the rate at which oxygen burns food in the body) tends to slow down with age and the rate of excretion usually decreases. Again the slow-down is delayed if the individual keeps active physically and involved with life.

Changes in the mouth make coarse, dry food less acceptable. The quantity of saliva decreases, the quality changes, and swallowing may be difficult. The tongue and the cheeks also change, and some taste buds disappear.

The stomach loses muscular strength and takes longer to empty. The digestive fluids decrease in volume and efficiency. From 23 to 65 per cent of persons aged 65 and over lack free hydrochloric acid.[3] A reduction in acidity interferes with digestion and with absorption of calcium and iron. Fats are poorly tolerated because they retard gastric evacuation and because the pancreas secretes less lipase to break down fats. The loss of muscular tone in the small intestine, colon, and stomach increase the likelihood of constipation and abdominal distention from certain foods.[4]

The liver decreases in size and weight, and detoxifies drugs less efficiently. Liver diseases are common in the aged. The incidence of gallstones increases with age, but the gall bladder, free from disease, apparently empties normally even in very old people.[5]

The blood cholesterol is usually elevated as age increases. Research on the

---

[3] Kathleen Newton, *Geriatric Nursing*, 4th ed. (St. Louis: Mosby, 1966), p. 70.
[4] Corinne Robinson, *Proudfit-Robinson's Normal and Therapeutic Nutrition*, 13th ed. (New York: Macmillan, 1967), pp. 382–383.
[5] Edward J. Stieglitz, *Geriatric Medicine* (Philadelphia: Lippincott, 1954), p. 69.

role of cholesterol in cardiovascular disease is still inconclusive, but it appears important to maintain normal weight throughout life.[6]

The sugar level of the blood may be the same for both young and old people, but after it has been raised, the rate of dropping to normal increases with age. This is another illustration that the older body does not perform as well under stress.

However, one study revealed that a group of older persons were able to utilize 86 per cent of protein intake, and 92 per cent of caloric intake.[7] This implies that other factors are involved in malnutrition.

Not all old people are constipated. Constipation or indigestion may be due to poor teeth, poor eating habits, lack of exercise, or pathological conditions. Drinking sufficient amounts of water stimulates the flow of digestive juices and helps the bowel and kidney functions in removing body wastes.

Urinary System

Because the functioning of the circulatory and the digestive system affects all other systems, it is difficult to get a clear-cut picture of the changes in the urinary system.

The kidneys decrease in size with age. Some of the extracting units of the kidney atrophy, and kidney circulation deteriorates. The senile kidney has less ability to concentrate urine. The occurrence of nocturia may lead to drinking less fluids, making waste elimination more difficult.[8]

Because drugs are not as efficiently detoxified in the liver and excreted by the kidney, medications such as bromides and barbiturates are not tolerated well. Daily use of drugs may have an accumulative effect, as some of the drug may be retained each day.

General arteriosclerosis means a reduced blood supply to the kidneys and lowered efficiency. However, each kidney needs only 25 per cent of its healthy tissue to function normally.[9] In the absence of specific renal disease, the kidneys can function adequately when the individual is 100 years old.

Older people may have trouble voiding, but it is one of the fallacies regarding old age to believe that nothing can be done about it. Frequently in elderly men, the prostate gland enlarges and obstructs the emptying of the bladder. Corrective surgery is usually favorable, even on men who are in their nineties. Damage to the kidney and bladder will be prevented if the condition is detected soon enough.

---

[6] Corinne Robinson, op. cit., p. 383.
[7] Kathleen Newton, op. cit., p. 70.
[8] Corinne Robinson, op. cit., p. 383.
[9] Bertram B. Moss, *Caring for the Aged* (Garden City, N.Y.: DoubleDay, 1966), p. 12.

Endocrine Glands

The endocrine glands have a much shorter life than the total organism, and unlike other organs, the individual glands may atrophy partly or completely. In middle years or in old age, a gland may function inadequately but still not fail completely and cause death.

The complex glands of the endocrine system are extremely important in maintaining life. The subtle interactions of the secretions are not yet well understood.

Thyroid function is the endocrine activity that declines first in senescence, especially in the male. The basal metabolism rate begins to fall in the forties. The thyroid gland shows shrinkage and atrophy in old age. Since decreased thyroid function is associated with degenerative disease, the physician attempts to control the effect of the thyroid on the body. It is held that thyroid function controls occurrence of the menopause, with a decrease in estrogenic hormones. Signs of estrogenic deficiency are largely those of disturbances of the nervous system: hot flushes, sweats, and emotional instability. Thyroid deficiency commonly produces fatigue, weakness, and vascular degeneration. The elderly person may not complain about these feelings because he expects to be less energetic.

Often people approaching the age of 70 have many changes representing senility: extreme fatigue, lack of strength, symptoms of menopause or male climacteric, atrophied skin, bent posture, and energy loss until the person is bedridden. This results from failure of the reproductive organs (the gonads), the adrenal cortex, and sometimes the thyroid. Physicians do not accept this as normal aging when the vital organs are still capable of functioning. Supplemental therapy with the deficient hormones may help to restore the health of these patients.

At the time the gonads decline and cease to function (menopause or climacteric), the adrenal cortex normally compensates for reduced secretion. When the anterior pituitary decreases stimulation, the adrenal cortex is not capable of compensation and the results of aging begin to show.

The pancreas tends to slow insulin production, and diabetes is likely to increase in incidence with age, at least up to the age of 50 or 60. This may be caused by generalized arteriosclerosis, which reduces the blood supply to the pancreas, making the pancreas less effective in secreting insulin; or it may be caused by decrease in male or female hormones, which contributes to the atrophy of specialized organs. Again, there is less diminishing of hormones with physically active and physically strong people.[10]

---

[10] Edward L. Bortz, *Creative Aging* (New York: Macmillan, 1963), p. 68.

The individual glands, however, have remarkable durability and reserve powers, and as a system, should be able to last for 100 years or more.

Reproductive System

The gonads are organs that attain their special functions in late childhood and lose their functions in middle life, roughly a span of 30 years.

The rate of decline of the female ovaries at the normal menopause may be as rapid as a few months or prolonged for several years. When ovarian atrophy appears much earlier than 34 or 35, usually one finds a specific disease contributing, although heredity is not completely eliminated as a factor. The life-span of the testes is longer, and the decline more gradual.

The older woman is affected both by atrophic changes in the genital system and by lack of hormonal influence. The rate of change varies greatly with the individual. The genitals lose tone and gradually become smaller. Pubic hair becomes scanty. Because muscles lose supporting power and tone, good support for the abdominal muscles is sometimes lacking.

The menopause and the climacteric, with the slow atrophy of structures, do not mean that sexual activity ceases. For many persons, participation in sexual activity continues after 65 years of age.

Nervous System

Evidence suggests that some degeneration and atrophy of the nervous system occur with age. How much impairment is caused by normal aging and how much is caused by pathological conditions are difficult to know. We do know that the nerve cells do not replace themselves once destroyed.

Different areas of the brain control different functions. Certain cells of the cerebellum have been known to atrophy, a factor in muscular weakness of old people. Part of the cortex of the frontal lobe concerned with memory and general integration of the human personality may deteriorate or be damaged, a factor in the general mental deterioration associated with age. If the hypothalamus in the base of the brain can no longer stimulate the pituitary gland, a chain of deterioration begins. The anterior pituitary no longer stimulates the adrenal cortex; hence it cannot compensate for lack of male or female hormones. Evidence supports the suggestion that the condition of the central nervous system, especially the hypothalamus in the diencephalon, determines sensecent changes throughout the body.[11] General atrophy has been found in the cerebrum and in the spinal cord.

It has been estimated[12] that the human brain has lost 20 per cent of the

---

[11] Edward L. Bortz, op. cit., p. 78.
[12] Howard J. Curtis, *Biological Mechanisms of Aging* (Springfield, Ill.: Charles C Thomas, 1966), p. 70.

cells by the seventh decade of life. Fortunately the brain has tremendous reserve capacity and may continue to function well. Particularly, the people within the upper 5 per cent of intellectual ability show very little change in advanced years.[13]

Specific senescent changes may be nueromuscular weakness, slowed reaction time, slower speed of learning, loss of memory for recent events, and less mental endurance. An elderly person may not be able to learn as quickly as he once did, but this does not mean he is incapable of learning.

An older person can have the advantage over the younger person in correlating and evaluating new experiences, greater accuracy, greater motivation, and more past experiences with which to judge and to compare. In other words, he retains the capacity to learn.

Eyes and Ears

As age advances, the individual relies more on sight to perform tasks previously accomplished through touch alone or by habit. Yet vision fails with age.

Most people over 60 years of age need eyeglasses, the result of accumulated damage to the eyes, degeneration of fibers within the optic nerves, and the onset of cataracts and glaucoma.

Color perception is reduced, and the eyes have less ability to adjust to different levels of light and dark.

The so-called "second sight" of people past 60 is caused by the following: (1) The lens continues to grow at the periphery (vertex) and approaches the cornea. (2) Material at the center of the lens becomes more dense. (3) The lens swell from increased water.[14]

In old age, the network holding the vitreous humor may degenerate, giving rise to floating opacities, called "spots before the eyes." The condition is not serious, and there is no special treatment for it. In very old people, senile degeneration of the retina may cause blindness.

Abnormal recession of the eyeballs into the sockets, enophthalmos, results from less orbital fat. Drooping eyelids are caused by loss of tone in muscles and skin. Cataracts, a clouding of the lens, commonly occur in older people.

The ability to hear high-pitched tones is usually lost by age 65, but this need not interfere with hearing normal conversations. There is gradual atrophy of the nerve cells in the basal coil of the cochlea. Other factors causing hearing losses are anemia, nephritis, and diabetes. Older people may be affected by the same ear diseases that affect younger people.

---

[13] Manuel Rodstein, "The Aging Process and Disease," *Nursing Outlook* (November 1964), p. 43.
[14] Edward J. Stieglitz, op. cit., p. 72.

HEARING AND SIGHT LOSSES PER 1,000 POPULATION

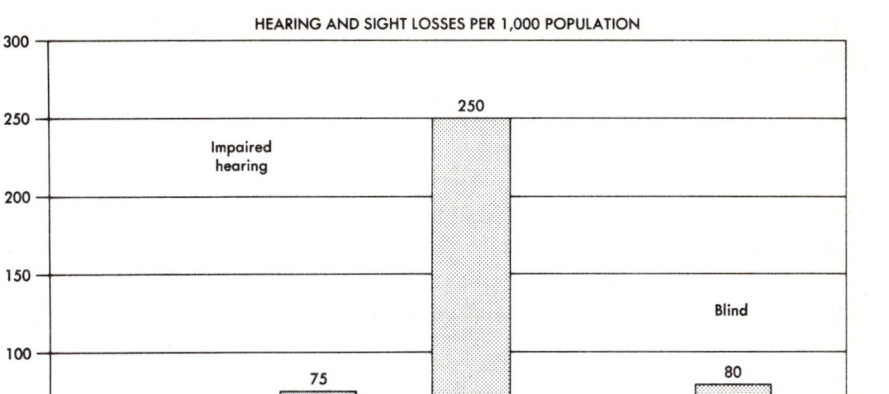

Age	Impaired hearing / Blind	Number
Age 20	Impaired hearing	10
Age 60	Impaired hearing	75
Age 80	Impaired hearing	250
Age 80	Blind	80

Figure 29. *Loss of hearing increases greatly between ages 60 and 80; one out of four of the very aged has significant loss of hearing. (From* Working with Older People, *Vol. II*, Biological, Psychological and Sociological Aspects of Aging. *U.S. Department of Health, Education and Welfare, Public Health Publication No. 1459, April 1970, P. 26.)*

Skin, Hair, and Nails

Skin changes with age are obvious, but the reasons are not as well understood. The derma gradually thins, and the tissues become less elastic. Much of the subcutaneous fat is lost. Because elasticity is lost, the skin springs back less readily. You can demonstrate this by pulling up a fold of skin on the back of the hand of an aged person. Note that the fold stays up for a while, then returns slowly and irregularly to the resting position in contrast to the marked resistance and quick return to normal of a younger person's skin. The elderly person's skin sags, and creases or folds resulting from habitual expressions become fixed as wrinkles. Exposed areas tend to develop pigmented spots.

The sebaceous (oil) glands gradually decrease their secretions, and this gives the skin a dull and dry appearance. Because the sweat glands gradually atrophy, there is less perspiration, and the skin is prone to be dry. Aging of the skin is influenced by nutrition, heredity, hormone balance, amount of exposure to the sun, and other environmental factors.

After middle age, fingernails and toenails become increasingly tough, thick and sometimes brittle. Because advanced senility is usually accompanied by circulation impairments, extreme caution is needed to cut carefully through the hard, tough toenails.

The hair grows thinner, especially on top, as the hair and sweat follicles atrophy. The scalp becomes dry. Diminished activity of the blood vessels also affects the hair. Causes of baldness and graying of hair are little understood. Heredity is involved, as are general health and nutrition.

Curiously, as the hair of the head and pubic and axillary areas tends to thin, other hair shows increased growth. Hairs in the nose and in the external ear become thicker, and the eyebrows become coarse and bristly. Hairs on the face of women are often one of the irritating aspects of aging.

Teeth

The majority of older people have lost most or all of their teeth, a loss not due to aging alone. Some people in their eighties and nineties still have their own teeth. Almost all dental decay is caused by poor food habits, neglect in oral hygiene, infection, and mechanical injury.

After the age of 34 years for men and 39 years for women, periodontal disease is the first cause of loss of teeth.[15] Malocclusion and defective bite result in absorption of bone surrounding the roots of teeth and lead to their loosening and being lost. If teeth remain, deposits form on the teeth and if not removed, they may progress under the gum margins and destroy the delicate fibers holding the tooth to the inner socket. This loosens teeth and may be the cause of losing teeth that are without cavities. Dental treatment in early childhood can help to correct malocclusion and defective bite.

In one respect, a person is fortunate who requires dentures in middle life. He is usually willing to learn to use dentures successfully. An aged person may not be willing to go through this prolonged and painful process. Also, the alveolar ridge is more narrow and more shallow with age; hence good fitting and proper use of dentures are progressively more difficult.

With improved, modern dentistry, loss of teeth is not necessarily a major tragedy, but in some people, it is a temporarily traumatic experience. Twice-yearly dental examinations and proper follow-up care will do much toward maintaining the teeth.

Questions for Discussion

1. Describe, in your own words, the physical characteristics of an elderly person whom you know.

2. Why might an anemic condition easily be overlooked in an elderly person?

[15] Kathleen Newton, op. cit., p. 59.

Physical Changes with Age

3. Of what significance is it to the nurse if her elderly patient's normal temperature is slightly above or below 98.6° F?

4. Of what value are the numerous beauty treatments toward maintaining a youthful-appearing skin?

5. Why do some people no longer agree, "You can't teach an old dog new tricks," and say instead, "You have to know more than the old dog"?

Additional Readings

Bortz, Edward L. *Creative Aging*, Chap. 4, "The Human Power Plant"; Chap. 5, "What Is Aging?" New York: The Macmillan Company, 1963.

Bortz, Edward L. "Take a New Look at Your Elderly Patients," *RN*, April 1962.

Moss, Bertram B. *Caring for the Aged*. Chap. 2, "Physical Aspects of Aging." Garden City, N.Y. Doubleday & Company, Inc., 1966.

Newton, Kathleen. *Geriatric Nursing*, 4th ed. St. Louis: The C. V. Mosby Company, 1966.

Positive Health of Older People. Chap. 2, "Investigation and Discovery in Physical Aging." New York: National Health Council, 1960.

Research in Gerontology: Biological and Medical. Reports and Guidelines from the White House Conference on Aging, Series No. 10. Washington, D.C.: U.S. Department of Health, Education, and Welfare, Special Staff on Aging, August 1961.

Rodstein, Manuel. "The Aging Process and Disease," *Nursing Outlook* (November 1964), pp. 43–47.

Steiglitz, Edward J. *The Second Forty Years*. Chap. 4, "Hazards of Senescence"; Chap. 8, "Sex and Age." Philadelphia: J. B. Lippincott Company, 1946.

Steiglitz, Edward J. "Personal Challenge of Aging: Biological Changes and Maintenance of Health," in Clark Tibbitts, and Wilma Donahue, eds. *Aging in Today's Society*. Englewood Cliffs, N.J.: Prentice-Hall Inc., 1960, pp. 44–53.

Recommended Audiovisual Aids

FILM

The Proud Years (28 min., Charles Pfizer & Company, B&W, 1956)

This film emphasizes that handicapped elderly people should be trained to care for their own needs and wants insofar as possible. With rehabilitation, they are happier and require less attention from others. Physical conditions of elderly people may be noted.

CHAPTER 24/MENTAL AND PERSONALITY

CHANGES WITH AGE

Nurses are justifiably concerned with the mental and personality characteristics of elderly people. Physical changes, studied in the previous chapter, directly influence the functioning of the person. Yet not all personality changes result entirely from physical reasons. The nurse needs to understand the many factors involved.

Adjustment to Aging

Every period of life requires adjustment from the individual. We said earlier that the period of adolescence was mainly a time of adjusting to adult life, with its increased freedom and greater responsibilities. Perhaps every individual has to accept and adjust to old age when it comes.

The person has to live with the fact that he has less strength, poor vision, limited hearing, and less taste for food. He may find it difficult to give up his beloved game of golf or to admit that he cannot shave as quickly as formerly. The elderly lady has to ask for help with her spring housecleaning. It may hurt her to admit that she cannot make as active a contribution to her church or her club work.

She may have to give up her own home and go to live with a younger family. Retiring from active employment is traumatic for many people. The person who has been making his own decisions all his life will find it exceedingly difficult to be dependent on others, financially as well as physically. Yes, old age requires many adjustments from the person at a time when making adjustments is extremely difficult.

Yet some people adjust very well. We all know mentally healthy people, psychologically strong with great inner resources. To these people, aging is another challenge and a new experience. In their added maturity and deepening values, they continue to love living and people. The nurse who cares for such a patient often finds that her inner life is strengthened and that she is the one who benefits. Although all old people are individuals, certain personality traits are noted among those who continue to enjoy life in old age. (See Table 5.)

But because the nurse wants to give the most help possible to the difficult patient, let us study and try to understand the somewhat negative character traits and behavior associated with old age.

TABLE 5./ADJUSTING TO OLD AGE

Less Successful	More Successful
Self-Hater Constantly criticizes self Blames self for limitations Unhappy	*Mature Type* Constructive approach to life Accepts facts of aging Adjusts well to losses Realistic about past and present Faces death with relative calmness
Angry Type Often hostile Blames others for limitations Sometimes gets along fairly well	*Rocking Chair Type* Tends to lean on others Accepts passivity Sits and rocks without guilt Number increasing as society has more leisure
Denies Existence Denies old age Refuses to alter style of living Imitates youth	*"Armored" Type* Well-developed defenses Clings to middle-age routines Keeps busy Manages to get along very well

From *Working with Older People*, Vol. II, Biological, Sociological and Psychological Aspects of Aging, U.S. Department of Health, Education, and Welfare, Public Health Service Publication No. 1459, April 1970, pp. 6, 33.

Personality Traits Associated with Age

Rigidity is commonly noticed in elderly people. The person has found a satisfactory way of doing certain things and sees no need to change. He dislikes change, for it represents the unknown, the fearful, or the awkward way. The elderly woman wants her living room furniture arranged the same way. The elderly man who has always drunk a bottle of beer before retiring intends to continue doing so.

The old person frequently *forgets* what happened yesterday, although he can remember clearly events of 20 or 40 years ago. Perhaps what happened yesterday was really not very important to him. A woman distinctly remembers her wedding day or her daughter's wedding day because she was a central figure then. Yesterday's event probably did not really involve her. People have less tendency to forget when they are vitally interested in the present and genuinely care what is happening. We can help by not mentioning the past; the old person will do so often enough.

Wakefulness can be annoying to the elderly person and to his family but is actually less harmful than it seems to be. When the person awakens at 2 A.M., the minutes tick by all too slowly. Yet if he gets up and moves about, he may disturb family members who need their rest for the coming working day. Sleep patterns of elderly people change, as will be considered later in Chapter 25. If it was understood that not everyone has to sleep eight successive hours, fewer sedatives would be needed.

Frugality may present a difficult problem. Many elderly people in comfortable circumstances begrudge spending money for bare necessities. They will not buy things that could make life more enjoyable — conveniences and comforts of which they are most deserving. Perhaps, however, the old person realizes that his working days are ended. He fears he will outlive his supply of money. Also, many people who lived through the depression years had to be frugal, and habits rarely change. Of course, the reverse may happen, and the old person may go on a spending spree. This indicates a genuine need for help. Sometimes the family ignores the situation until the elderly person has disposed of huge sums of money. It is a delicate decision to know when to take legal action.

Irritability may be a reaction to fatigue or to poor health. The elderly person may not be willing to admit that he needs more frequent rest periods. He resents restriction of his activities. A sympathetic family or nurse strives to help the person to accept his limitations gracefully.

Depression is usually due to lack of interests. Interests tend to narrow with age. The person who thinks only of himself — young or old — can easily become depressed.

Many undesirable traits of old age are caused by the person's desire to continue to be important. He resents his dependency.

Personality Traits Accented

In many respects, age does not actually change people. They seem to become more of what they have always been. The kind, generous, and thoughtful person becomes more kind, more generous, and more thoughtful. One observing student practical nurse summarized this well when she said: "Take the queer old people that you know. Most of them have been a little bit queer all their lives."

Perhaps when the person reaches this age, he no longer sees the need to pretend. He feels that he can act and behave as he wishes. If he disagrees with you, he will voice his opinion. If he approves, he will say so. Character and personality are not hidden. He seems to be saying: "Why bother to try to impress other people? I am not seeking a raise in salary or an advanced position. I have no ax to grind. I am just what I am, and I will do as I please."

Happiness or Unhappiness

The difference between the happy and the unhappy elderly person seems to lie in the memories each has. Those elderly persons who have a history of outgoing acts, of doing good for others or for worthwhile causes, are the happy ones. They are also the ones who are still active and interested, who meet new experiences willingly and adequately. The elderly person who has focused his life on himself, who has demanded that the world come to him — he is the unhappy one. Interestingly enough, the unhappy people apparently have great blanks in their chronological memory recall — as though many of the experiences they had while making personal demands resulted in unpleasantness, and the mind has sought to erase these results. It is a recognized psychological fact that the mind can erase memories of unpleasant experiences.[1]

Temporary Mental Disturbances

Extreme fatigue or an emotional shock cannot be tolerated well by an older person. Mental abnormalities may result, such as confusion, restlessness, or the sensation of hearing uncontrollable noise.

Fever or infection may cause an elderly person to become delirious. The confusion may persist for some time after the fever subsides. Confusion can also result from the body's retention of toxic products, such as occurs with disorders of the urinary tract or kidney disease. Inadequate nutrition and anemia both may be contributing factors. The nurse should always be alert for symptoms of anemia and malnutrition.

Certain drugs, for example, the sulfonamides, the barbiturates, and the bromides, are likely to have a cumulative effect on older people and may cause restlessness, confusion, and even maniacal states.

Sleep medication may be useful to ease the way through a difficult, traumatic experience. But to rely on such medication for ordinary sleep is unwise, particularly for the aged. Some sleeping drugs are habit-forming. Their effect diminishes and increased dosages are required. The latter may lead to mental confusion.

Organic Changes Affecting Brain Functioning

With cerebral arteriosclerosis, the brain cells receive a diminished supply of blood. This causes some of the characteristics of old age, such as dizziness or fatigue.

[1] By Robert G. White, written for this publication.

One kind of cerebral accident, "the little stroke" or hemorrhage, may cause sudden digestive or personality changes. The person may lose his appetite, or become mentally confused. An astute businessman may make unusual or unwise decisions, but his family may not be aware of what has happened. Sometimes the changes are temporary and the person recovers; sometimes he does not. The brain cells do not regenerate if damaged by an interruption of the blood supply for more than a few minutes.

It is generally believed that the brain degenerates with aging, reducing in size and weight, and causes behavior changes. Nerve cells disintegrate and various waste products of metabolism accumulate in the tissues.

Symptoms of Senility

"Senility" or "chronic brain syndrome" or "senile dementia" are not synonymous, but to distinguish them correctly would require more technology than is necessary. To understand their general meaning will help you, the nurse, to care for the patient at this stage.

Symptoms of decline include reminiscence, forgetfulness, disorientation for time, place, and person, and a return to early forms of coping with reality. In the later aspects of breakdown, it includes incontinence, undressing, a return to simple, softer food, and if the person lives long enough, a resemblance of neonatal and fetal stages.[2]

The person is more confused at night than during the day. He is frightened easily, often by things not bothering other people. He may become more crude, less refined in dress and actions.

Forgetting the day and the year, or one's age, may indicate a return to living in the past. It is not always possible to prevent further regression, but if the nurse emphasizes the present and helps the old person to enjoy living today, decline may be halted temporarily. One nursing-home operator placed a large calendar in the living room to remind her guests of the current date.

Anxiety may be expressed in many ways. Often the elderly person wanders away, sometimes covering an amazing distance by foot. Perhaps he is seeking the past that was so much more pleasant than the realities of today.

His emotions may resemble those of the child, in that he becomes angry or weeps easily, shouts and calls people names. But he is not a child and should never be treated as a child. An incident may appear trifling to another person, but to the aged person, the little things are his life.

Perhaps the aged adult is compared to a child because both are dependent. Reactions of the dependent adult may be similar to those of the dependent child. When the young child's parents take him to the hospital and leave him

[2] Morton Leeds, *The Aged, the Social Worker and the Community* (Cleveland: H. Allen, 1961), pp. 70–71.

there, he feels they have deserted him. Likewise, the dependent aged adult may feel his family has taken him to the hospital and deserted him. Nurses have observed this to happen.

Help the Family

The geriatric nurse faces many problems with the senile patient — among them, how to help the family as well as the aged relative. The family may be tragically aware of what is happening and have a sense of guilt. They may be consoled to realize that the aged person is not aware of his regression. It is as though nature is kind to those who live that long; they do not realize the difference.

One family had cared for the elderly grandmother as long as possible, and finally knew that hospitalization was necessary. When told, the "grand dame" said, "That is all right. I have been needing medication for some time." Later she was transferred to a good nursing home, and during a period of elucidation she said, "Am I not fortunate to be here in this nice place?"

You will find many ways to give support to the family.

Use of Tranquilizers

Certain drugs, commonly called tranquilizers, cause the person to relax and be less anxious without dulling the senses completely. Many lay people justifiably question the use of these drugs for the purpose of subduing a person. One doctor writes:

> Perhaps tranquilizers have been used too freely with some older people because the aged are not considered an important group in our culture. . . .
> It is now possible to separate organic brain syndrome, and functional reactions resulting from age, and those resulting from social pressures. . . .
> In a physically diseased individual, tranquilizers can be helpful. Older people are particularly vulnerable to stress. Worry over serious physical disease must be controlled, if treatment is to be effective. Both in the preoperative medication of elderly patients, and in postoperative control, tranquilizers can be helptul.[3]

But often, tranquilizers are prescribed to be given as necessary. A nurse must never be tempted to give the drugs when other measures will suffice. Perhaps the patient's fears and anxieties will be allayed by discussing personal problems with him, and close attention to physical comfort may make the drugs unnecessary.

[3] Thomas T. Tourlentes, *Positive Health of Older People* (New York: National Health Council, 1960), pp. 24–25.

For this reason, the diagnosis of brain damage is approached with caution. This implies irreversible change, usually followed only with supportive treatment, not therapeutic efforts. Frequently an elderly person is confused and irrational during the first week in a nursing home, then the symptoms disappear. Even partial recovery would not be possible if brain damage has occurred. Efforts are made today to distinguish between reversible and irreversible changes.

To Maintain Usefulness

Not all old people become senile. History records the lives of numerous people who were active, contributing members of society in their seventies, eighties, and even nineties.

Benjamin Franklin was active until he was 82; Michelangelo painted the ceiling of the Sistine Chapel when he was almost 90; Titian produced his masterpiece at the age of 85, and lived to be 99; John Wesley preached every day at the age of 88; and Oliver Wendell Holmes was 82 when he wrote *Over the Teacups*.

More recently, Sir Winston Churchill, Carl Sandburg, and Albert Schweitzer were active past 80. Pope John XXIII was 80 when he summoned the Ecumenical Council to Rome.

These people might be considered mental giants. Yet among our own friends, we know people who are living useful, purposeful lives past the age of 65. The secret of maintaining mental vigor is still a mystery, but certain factors may help.

The mind is like any other part of the body. When used and kept agile, it serves us better. People can always learn new things. The individual is more likely to remain useful to society to the end of his life if:

His mind has always served him well.
He has a wholesome personality.
He has a keen interest in the present.
He keeps in touch with progress of business or a profession.
He has formed the habit of looking forward.
He associates with young people, especially intellectually.
He maintains a sense of humor.
He maintains good physical health.

Questions for Discussion

1. Which personality characteristics have you personally observed in elderly people (such as rigidity, wakefulness)?
2. Describe incidents that indicate senile breakdown.

3. What should the nurse tell the family when the elderly patient has days of confusion, followed by days of mental clearness?

4. Describe an elderly person among your friends or relatives who is happy. Contrast him (her) with an unhappy elderly person. Can you explain the difference?

5. Interpret this old saying: "The face you have at 20 is the face God gave you; the face you have at 60 is the face you gave yourself."

6. Suggest ways that the nurse can help the family of a senile patient.

Additional Readings

Busse, Ewald W. "Mental Health in Advanced Maturity," in Wilma Donahue and Clark Tibbits, eds., *New Frontiers of Aging*. Ann Arbor: University of Michigan Press, 1957, pp. 143–152.

Havighurst, Robert J. "Personal and Social Adjustments in Old Age," in Wilma Donahue and Clark Tibbits, eds., *New Frontiers of Aging*. Ann Arbor: University of Michigan Press, 1957, pp. 172–179.

Leeds, Morton. *The Aged; the Social Worker, and the Community*. "The Mental Aspects of Aging," pp. 27–41. Cleveland: Howard Allen, Inc., 1961.

Mental Disorders of the Aging. Washington, D.C.: U.S. Department of Health, Education, and Welfare, Public Health Service Publication No. 993, 1963.

Moss, Bertram B. *Caring for the Aged*. Garden City, N.Y.: Doubleday Company, Inc., 1966.

Current Publications on Aging

Aging. Published every second month by the Social and Rehabilitation Services, Administration on Aging, U.S. Department of Health, Education, and Welfare. U.S. Government Printing Office, Division of Public Documents, Washington, D.C. 20402.

Geriatrics. Monthly. Lancet Publications, Inc., 4015 West 65th Street, Minneapolis, Minn. 55435.

Harvest Years. Monthly. Harvest Years Publishing Company, 104 East 40th Street, New York, N.Y. 10016.

Journal of the American Geriatrics Society. Monthly. The Society, 10 Columbus Circle, New York, N.Y. 10019.

Journal of Gerontology. Quarterly. Gerontological Society, 660 South Euclid Avenue, St. Louis, Missouri, 63110.

Quarterly Bulletin. National Old People's Welfare Council and National Council of Social Service, 26 Bedford Square, London, W.C.1, England. 8d.

Social Security Bulletin. Monthly. Social Security Administration, U.S. Government Printing Office, Division of Public Documents, Washington, D.C. 20402.

Recommended Audiovisual Aids

FILM

Life with Grandpa (20 min., March of Time, B&W)
    The problems of old age are depicted in this film, such as generative diseases, economic insecurity, and a feeling of loneliness and uselessness. Various solutions are presented.

CHAPTER 25/**GOOD HYGIENE FOR ELDERLY**

PEOPLE

Looking after one's personal needs is part of independent living. The person who continues to care for himself is helping to preserve his independence. Elderly people are easily treated as dependents because they are frail physically and have reduced incomes. These factors may cause humiliation, which in itself creates problems.

Good hygiene for an elderly person begins with his assuming the responsibility for himself as long as possible. When this is impossible, the nurse assumes the responsibility for the physical needs of the geriatric patient. The nurse encourages every patient to do as much for himself as his condition permits. She always strives for the cooperation of the patient, and this is doubly important with the elderly.

Effectively treating the ills of old age requires the active cooperation of the patient, so much so that he must be considered a respected partner rather than someone on whom treatment is imposed. As a matter of fact, he will probably not follow any treatment imposed on him. He will rebel and do as he sees fit unless the responsibility of his care is shared with him.[1]

The Health Consultation

The wise middle-aged person establishes the routine of regular physical checkups, as described in Chapter 18. The elderly person who has not done this, can still profit by having a thorough physical examination, and then returning at regular intervals. The aging person needs medical supervision more than he did in younger years, and he needs to realize how important it is to follow the doctor's advice. One ninety-year-old living alone in her own home took seriously her doctor's advice: "He said for me to drink more milk, so I drink milk. I also keep ice cream in my refrigerator."

One doctor recommends that an individual maintain his weight of age 26, and have tests twice yearly of blood count, blood sugar, blood cholesterol, and urine.[2] When changes are found in weight, blood pressure, or cholesterol, the

---

[1] Paul V. Lemkau, *Mental Hygiene in Public Health* (New York: McGraw-Hill, 1949), p. 309, adapted.
[2] Edward L. Bortz, *Creative Aging* (New York: Macmillan, 1963), p. 142.

physician can evaluate the deviation. He may recommend changes in the quality or quantity of food eaten.

Regular visits to the dentist may reveal an early dental cavity or a gum condition that can be corrected.

The doctor should also watch for any condition of stress in the person's life which could lead to trouble if prolonged.

It is a great comfort to a person over 60 years of age to be examined and found in good health.

Good Nutrition

Sensible eating habits are vitally important to the health and mental attitudes of elderly people. A diet of tea and toast is no more adequate for the elderly person than for the adolescent. They both need a well-balanced diet but not the same number of calories. Older people should have fewer calories. Nutritious, carefully planned meals can help the older person to maintain vigor, withstand disease, and retard senescence.

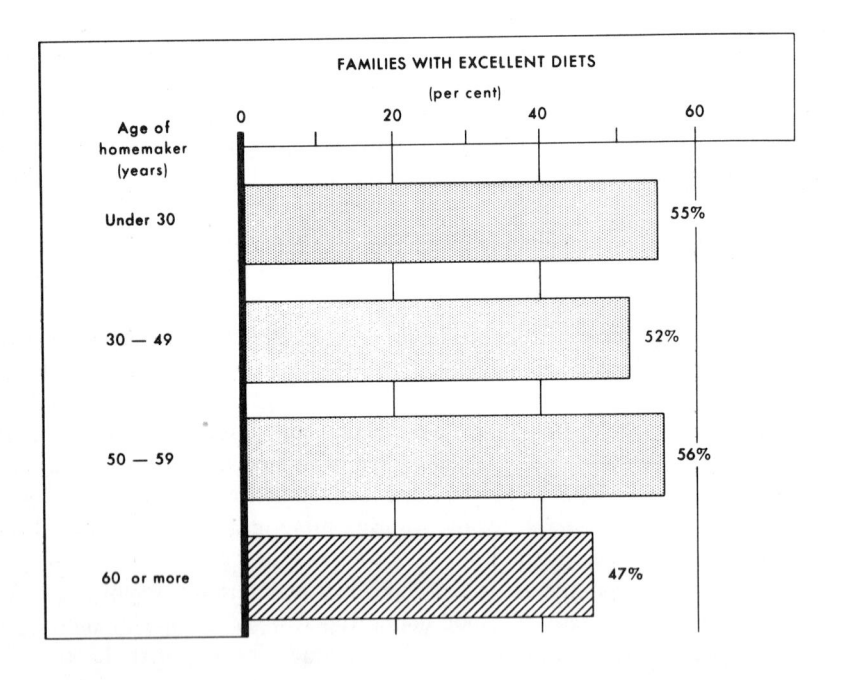

FAMILIES WITH EXCELLENT DIETS (per cent)

Age of homemaker (years)	
Under 30	55%
30 — 49	52%
50 — 59	56%
60 or more	47%

Figure 30. *Older persons are more in need of dietary improvements. (1961 White House Conference on Aging,* Chart Book, *Chart 49, Federal Council on Aging.)*

Good Hygiene for Elderly People

Poor eating habits can cause the elderly person to tire more easily, to gain extra weight, to be depressed and gloomy, to show needless anxiety, to lose sleep, or to have weakened skin, so that bedsores develop more easily. His complaints of acid mouth and sour stomach may stem from poor eating habits.

Reasons for malnutrition include emotional strain, physical changes, illness, loss of teeth, lack of money, and lifelong habits of poor eating.

Worry, anxiety, loneliness, and lack of activity can deaden the appetite. When a person has no interest in food, he does not eat well. Then he feels worse and has even less interest in food. The person living alone may have little incentive to prepare a complete meal because no one will be there to share the meal. A feeling of uselessness or insecurity can cause apathy toward food. This vicious cycle needs to be interrupted. Sometimes a person eats excessively because he is lonely, and he can think of nothing else that he wants to do.

Apathy toward food may be partly caused by physical changes, such as less saliva formed, which makes foods hard to chew; fewer taste buds, which decreases the enjoyment of food flavors; and less keen smell, which fails to stimulate the appetite. Ill-fitting dentures may also be a factor.

Edentia, the loss of natural teeth, prevents many people from chewing well. Older people often refuse to wear false teeth or will not try to adjust to wearing them. Cleaning the teeth carelessly can interfere with enjoyment of the food. An unclean mouth and unclean dentures can cause odor, destroy the appetite, and deaden the flavor of foods.

A low income may mean the elderly person has a diet composed of the cheaper carbohydrate foods, instead of the badly needed protein foods that are usually more expensive. The elderly person living alone finds that buying food for one person is not economical. He may find it difficult to get to the large supermarket, where foods are cheaper. Perhaps he cannot afford to have his groceries delivered. His cooking facilities may consist of a one-burner hot plate and a shared refrigerator (or none at all).

The individual with a lifetime of poor eating habits is not likely to change his whole pattern of eating. Many older people have not been exposed to nutrition education, which today begins in the elementary schools. Perhaps they do not know what a well-balanced diet is. They may insist on following food fads that are harmful, or they may have peculiar associations with certain foods. You learn in your nutrition class that cracked-wheat or whole-wheat bread is more nutritious than refined, white bread. But to some older people, white bread denotes a higher standard of living, for years ago, only the poor people ate brown bread. Nevertheless, even the person with poor food habits in a poor state of nutrition can benefit greatly if he can be coaxed into changing his eating in a few small, but important ways.

Food needs of older people are similar to those of persons of any age except that when calories are balanced to energy requirements, fewer calories are needed. Older people are less active physically; they are not growing. Their basal metabolism rate is reduced, and food is absorbed more slowly. Thus if the elderly person continues to eat the same quantity of food, he gains weight.

The woman who needed 2000 calories daily at age of 30 should have 1600 calories at the age of 65.[3] The man requiring 2800 calories at 30 years of age will get along better if he has 2300 calories at age 65. Past the age of 75, a further slight reduction is good. The overweight person who consistently overeats may not realize that losing weight would help to reduce his blood pressure, relieve dizziness and arthritis, and enable him to move about easier. Reducing is difficult at any age, but especially in old age.

Elderly people need a diet that is liberal in proteins, calcium, iron, and all the vitamins. Many of the disorders associated with old age are allied with inadequate protein intake. Evidence now suggests that the need for certain amino acids increases substantially with age.[4] Yet most people eat fewer protein foods as they get older. The meats easiest to chew are often too expensive for limited budgets. It is possible to cook the less tender and the less expensive cuts of meat so that they are easy to eat, but many older people do not know how to do this. As people age, they tend to drink less milk.

Diets of elderly people are commonly deficient in calcium, iron, and ascorbic acid. Because of the tendency of the aged to develop anemia, the diet should be adequate in iron. Good sources of iron are liver, lean meat, eggs, legumes, whole wheat, raisins, apricots, and other foods. Disturbances of calcium and protein metabolism leads to osteoporosis. A high proportion of women with this bone disease have been poor milk drinkers all throughout life.[5] Cheese is a fairly good substitute for milk in providing calcium. Generous amounts of vitamins are supplied in fruits and vegetables, especially those served raw.

It might seem that vitamin pills would be a simple remedy for dietary deficiencies. In a survey of food habits of elderly people conducted in Syracuse, New York, it was found that one-third of the householders used some kind of vitamin supplements.[6] However, only a small number effectively improved their diets with missing nutrients. This is an area of nutrition education needing more attention.

Older people need soft bulk, but not roughage, in the diet. Soft, indigestible bulk helps to give mass to the stool, to encourage peristalsis and prevent constipation. Rough, scratchy fibers and tough hulls may irritate the sensitive lining of the intestinal canal and are best omitted from the diet of the aged. Roughage is food that cannot be strained through a colander, such as corn on the cob, celery, and vegetables and fruits with hard seeds. Soft bulk is food that

[3] Foods and Nutrition Board, National Academy of Sciences — National Research Council, *Recommended Daily Dietary Allowance*, Rev. 1968.
[4] *Nutrition Abstract and Review*, Vol. 37, No. 1 (Jan. 1967), p. 207.
[5] Corrinne Robinson, *Proudfitt-Robinson's Normal and Therapeutic Nutrition*, 13th ed. (New York: Macmillan, 1967), p. 383.
[6] C. LeBovit, "The Food of Older Persons Living at Home," *Journal of American Dietetics Association,* 46:285 (1965).

Good Hygiene for Elderly People

can be strained — beets, turnips, carrots, parsnips, and leafy vegetables, such as spinach and lettuce. This does not mean that elderly people should eat only pureed food, but that they should eat only foods that can be pureed.

Extra fluids in diets of elderly people help the kidneys to function better. Dehydration frequently complicates the illnesses of the aged;[7] hence it is important to push fluids. The recommended daily intake of 2 quarts of liquids might include tea, coffee, milk, soups, and carbonated beverages.

To stimulate the appetite and aid digestion:

>   Encourage light exercise, such as walking in fresh air.
>   Create more interest in life.
>   Make mealtime sociable.
>   Have meals at the table whenever possible.
>   If not, serve food on attractive tray in pretty dishes.
>   Have meals at regular times.
>   Five light meals a day are preferable to three heavier meals.
>   Avoid excessively heavy meals.
>   Serve the heartiest meal at noon, with a lighter meal in the evening.
>   One hot food at each meal is desirable.
>   Serve meals in a pleasant, quiet, unhurried atmosphere.
>   Avoid saying, "This is good for you."

The food itself:

>   Prepare as the person wants it prepared. Humor him when possible.
>   If foods must be easy to chew, change the preparation, but not the food itself.
>   Meats should be chopped, ground, or minced with a sharp knife. Skillful use of a blender will add variety to meals.
>   Pay more attention to flavor and seasonings. Possibly "pep up" foods with onion, chives, parsley, mint, or chopped celery leaves.
>   Serve a food of distinctive flavor in the same meal with a mild-flavored food.
>   Serve something crisp to contrast with softer-textured foods.
>   Offer bright-colored foods for eye appeal.
>   Serve in small amounts.
>   Older people like moist food, not coarse, dry food.
>   Be generous with liquids — soups, eggnogs, blended foods, milkshakes.
>   Warm beverages between meals may be welcome — tea or broth.
>   Serve frequently: honey, applesauce, prunes, eggs, cottage cheese.

Offer fruit juices between meals.

Vegetable oils and fats (particularly polyunsaturated fats) are preferable to meat and butter fats.

---

[7] Bertram B. Moss, *Caring for the Aged* (Garden City, N.Y.: Doubleday, 1966) p. 143.

Avoid these foods if they cause distress:

> Rich salad dressings, gravies, and sauces.
> Fried eggs and other fried foods.
> Cabbage and beans, especially when cooked with salt pork.
> Excess sweets.
> Tea and coffee if they cause sleeplessness.
> Cucumbers, radishes, watermelon, onions, turnips (when not tolerated).

Oral Hygiene

Good oral hygiene helps the elderly person to retain interest in food and to maintain a healthy appetite. Many elderly people have ill-fitting dentures or decayed, broken, and missing teeth. When chewing is difficult, they often refuse certain foods, and a faulty diet can be the result.

Getting used to new dentures is a harder task for the elderly person than for the young person. Artificial dentures, at their best, are an imperfect substitute for one's natural teeth. The loss of teeth will affect the chewing of food, cause structural changes in the jaws, alter speech, especially the consonant sounds, modify emotional and facial expressions, and change the appearance.

Cleaning the teeth daily is important for every person, but particularly the person with dentures. One woman's entire hospital experience was unhappy because one time, her mouth was not cleaned. Food lodged under her dentures, her mouth became sore, and she was uncomfortable for days.

The nurse should make mouth care easy for the elderly patient. He must have a regular denture cup in which to place his dentures at night. The dentures should be covered with water. Dentures should be rinsed with cool water after each meal, especially if the person eats berry foods or drinks milk. Lost or broken dentures are expensive to replace; so they should be handled with great caution. In addition to the expense, the process of having new teeth made may be impossible for the infirm or chronically ill person to manage. Dental care is seldom included in the health services to the homebound.

Rest and Sleep

Older people tire easily. They need more rest and relaxation than people of middle age, but they are likely to have fewer hours of deep sleep at night.

It was once thought that older people could manage well with less sleep than when they were younger. It now appears that many complaints of the aged may result from too little sleep. A study[8] of a group of mentally alert and

---

[8] By Dr. Robert M. Teller, Jr., of Louisiana State University School of Medicine.

Good Hygiene for Elderly People

physically active older people showed that those who slept eight hours or more every night displayed less tension, fatigue, dizziness, gastrointestinal and muscle pain, and headaches than those who slept seven hours or less. When the sleep span of the "seven hour" group was increased, symptoms decreased and general comfort improved.

Older people will become fatigued more quickly than young people, and should rest when they are tired. An elderly person cannot go without sleep or continue working (or being active) when fatigued as a young person can. Frequent rest periods help to conserve the energy of the elderly person. However, daytime naps should be discouraged if they interfere with a good night's sleep. Sleep's restorative value appears to be greatest when it is deepest. The older people who supplement their nightly rest with daytime naps may not get enough real rest, even though they sleep a total of eight hours daily.

The elderly person often awakens in the early hours of the morning and then worries because he cannot sleep again. There are several reasons for this. He may be awakened by the need to void, then cannot go back to sleep. But probably the greatest reason is that the elderly person often dozes during the day.

Hospital patients who disturb the ward at night are often the ones who sleep during the day. They lie in bed with nothing much to do but sleep. Interesting activities may help to prevent this.

Also many elderly people have formed the habit of retiring early in the evening. In their younger days, no one had television or good lighting for reading. They had no reason to stay up after dark.

One nursing-home operator told how she tried to interest her guests in staying up later at night: "I even bought the second and third television sets, thinking a choice of programs might interest them. But no, they insist on going to bed immediately after the evening meal." Estimate this for yourself. If you went to bed at seven o'clock in the evening, and slept eight hours, at what time would you awaken?

Insomnia is common among old people and not easily remedied. Taking to bed one's worries and anxiety will prevent sleep at any age. Talking out problems may help. Those who have trouble sleeping should avoid drinking tea and coffee or excess liquids in the evening (drink extra liquids earlier in the day). They should establish a routine of slowing down before bedtime, avoid excitement, and possibly take a relaxing bath. Comfortable, warm bedclothes may help. If the elderly person understands he is resting, even if not asleep, he may worry less.

Although old people need more rest and relaxation than younger people, too much rest can be dangerous. The individual who does nothing but rest is escaping from the realities of living. He can easily regress. Excessive bed rest has other dangers, too.

Dangers of Too Much Bed Rest

Nurses should understand why bed rest is no longer considered "the cure-all" in the treatment of diseases or in convalescence, particularly for the elderly patient. Studies show that normally healthy young men suffer from being in body casts from six to seven weeks.[9] Almost every part of the body is affected, with greater hazards to the elderly.[10]

The respiratory system of the elderly patient is particularly affected by bed rest. When the body is maintained in one position, bronchial secretions collect in the bases of the lungs, and pneumonia may develop easily. Also, lack of exercise and deep breathing prevents reexpansion of a collapsed or diseased lung.

Extensive bed rest decreaesses the efficiency of the circulatory system. The veins clot more readily. The skin becomes tender, and bedsores may occur. Some muscles contract with bed rest, and other muscles stretch. Joints become "rusty," as shown by the hobbling, painful gait of the convalescent. When bones are not used, such as for weight-bearing, the calcium drains from them. Fractures take longer to heal. Both kidney and bladder stones may be due in part to bed rest. Urine retention may occur, especially in the man who finds that using a urinal is clumsy and embarrassing. Minor as these problems may seem, the elderly patient may eventually become incontinent, that is, lack bladder control. Getting an incontinent patient out of bed may turn him into a clean patient. Bed rest may also lead to constipation, especially harmful to the aged.

The influence of bed rest on the mental attitude is particularly noted in elderly people. At first, the patient may be irritable and fussy. Then he sinks into a lethargic, "I-don't-care" attitude, which may eventually cause him to lead a vegetablelike existence.

Exercise and Activity

Because of these many hazards from continued bed rest, elderly people should be encouraged to get out of bed every day and to continue being as active as their physical condition permits. Many managers of homes for the aged insist that their residents be up and about.

The bed patient needs to sit up every day and to change his position. He is getting some exercise when he turns himself, feeds himself, or helps with his bath. Many patients have prescribed exercises to be repeated every few hours during the day. The patient who cannot have active exercise may benefit from passive exercise as prescribed by the doctor and carried out by the nurse and the

---

[9] Bertha Harmer and Virginia Henderson, *Textbook of the Principles and Practice of Nursing*, 5th ed. (New York: Macmillan, 1955), p. 504.
[10] *British M. J.* Dec. 13, 1947, p. 967.

Good Hygiene for Elderly People

family. You will learn more about breathing exercises and passive exercise in your class on rehabilitation. Exercise for the geriatric patient is a significant part of his rehabilitation.

The healthy elderly person is wise to continue as much activity as feasible. Actually, every individual at every age needs exercise and activity. The sedentary life of most city people makes for insufficient exercise. People of middle years can become so engrossed with earning a living, looking after their families, and various required tasks that they neglect physical activities. Possibly the extremely strenuous sports, such as tennis and basketball, should be avoided after the peak of maturity. Golf, bowling, and archery are less competitive and more reasonable. The wisest choice is those sports that have no competition: fishing, gardening, horseback riding, swimming, and walking. The amount of exertion can vary each day: one can walk briskly or amble slowly. The benefits from walking are easily overlooked. Since the strength of an individual may vary from day to day, the elderly person should realize, when choosing activities, that his strength may vary from day to day.

Slower Pace

The older person needs a slower pace and a more tranquil, peaceful life than the person of early or middle years. The hustle and bustle of three-generation living can be too much for the grandparent, or, more appropriately, four-generation living can be too much for the elderly great-grandparent. A noisy, busy hospital can make life miserable for the elderly patient.

Elimination

Elderly people often suffer from constipation and many nursing home patients are incontinent.

Attention to good basic hygiene helps to prevent constipation. The patient should not smother or ignore his natural impulses. Eating the tender fibers of fruits, vegetables, and whole-grain cereals encourages normal peristalsis. Constipation may result from improper chewing of food, which, in turn is caused by poor teeth or ill-fitting dentures. Proper exercise will help. Walking is adequate exercise for many elderly people.

The elderly person should drink plenty of liquids. Water stimulates peristalsis and helps to combat constipation. The kidneys can more easily secrete a large volume of dilute urine than a small volume of concentrated urine. The concentrated urine is more odiferous and more likely to cause a bedsore if the patient wets the bed. When nocturia is a problem, encourage the individual to take as much water as possible early in the day.

The incontinent patient presents many problems to the nurse. Special precautions are needed to keep the skin in good condition. Dry-bed panties may be less offensive to the person who still understands what is going on than a type of diaper that is available.

The use of room deodorizers may help to improve the morale of both patient and nurse.

Cleanliness

Elderly people do not need a daily bath. They are less active physically, they perspire less, and their skin is not as oily. Cleanliness needs emphasis, of course, as some older people grow careless and neglect themselves. But cleanliness is maintained differently — with more frequent sponge or partial baths but fewer tub baths.

A tub bath is weakening to the extremely old person. Getting in and out of the tub is dangerous. Therefore, showers are preferred. Combination chair-showers are installed in many nursing homes.

The fragile and dry senile skin should be washed carefully with a gentle soap. Avoid harsh soaps, too much rubbing with towels, or incomplete drying of the skin. Do not use extremely hot or extremely cold water for the bath. The use of vegetable oil, cocoa butter, or lanolin will counteract the dry skin, especially areas such as heels, toes, and elbows. Because alcoholic lotions are drying, they are not good for the aging skin.

Similarly, hair shampoos are needed less frequently as people get older. The scalp becomes more dry and less oily with age. Nursing-home patients are often satisfied with a shampoo every three or four weeks. Use an extremely mild shampoo. The hair can be kept clean by brushing frequently with a soft brush. A damp washcloth run through the hair and gently rubbed on the scalp may help.

Nail Care

Fingernails should be trimmed with great care. The older skin is less resistant to infection, and any slight scratch or crack may be a source of infection. There is less danger from ingrown toenails if the nails are cut straight across, instead of rounding off the corners. Oiling the fingernails and toenails is good, as they tend to get brittle. Soaking the feet or applying pads soaked with warm oil will soften the nails. When neglected, the hard, tough toenails of elderly people are difficult to cut. Pedicures must be given with meticulous care and cleanliness. This caution is especially essential for elderly diabetic patients. A large percentage of cases of diabetic gangrene of the toes is caused by infection introduced when nails are carelessly trimmed. The senile person with

Good Hygiene for Elderly People

unsteady hands, faulty vision, and difficulty in bending should not attempt to cut his own toenails. Many good nursing homes schedule a weekly visit from a podiatrist for this purpose.

Foot Care

The feet should be washed daily. Warm socks are needed in cool weather. Discourage wool socks, unless the patient insists. Broad, comfortable shoes will help to avoid pressure sores and calluses. The elderly person's feet need support, especially arch support, but too heavy a shoe is cumbersome. Treat dry skin by rubbing with cold cream, lanolin, a commercial massage preparation, or cocoa butter after bathing. The geriatric patient may sleep better with extra warmth on his feet at night. If bed socks suffice, there is no danger from burning. Either a warm brick covered, or a hot-water bottle no warmer than 105°F will furnish warmth and will not get hotter. Do not use an electric heating pad.

Clothing

Elderly people want comfortable clothing, but attractive clothes will also encourage pride in personal appearance. Frequently elderly women stay away from social functions because they do not have the proper clothes to wear.

Socially active elderly women prefer one-piece dresses, long sleeves, hats, laced shoes with medium-height heels, and the color navy.[11] Garments should be loose for comfort; front openings are convenient. Clothes should be easy to dry-clean or wash. Elderly people also like sweaters.

The nursing-home patient may insist on having layers and layers of garments. He does need warm clothing, but watch the type of fabric used. Clothing in contact with the dry, fragile, senile skin should be soft and not irritating, or chafing of the skin will result. Wool is scratchy.

However, the geriatric patient may insist on wearing his familiar flannel pajamas. Such situations require wise decisions from the geriatric nurse. Who will be harmed if the elderly man wears his woolen underwear? He may be uncomfortable, but no one else suffers. Contrast this with the feeble man who persists in smoking in bed. When he endangers the safety of others, we cannot humor him.

Often the geriatric patient does not get out of bed in the hospital because the hospital robe is uncomfortable, cold, or out of his reach. He may be more active if a comfortable robe and substantial slippers are kept within easy reach.

[11] Suzanne Shipley and Mary Lou Rosencranz, "Older Women's Clothing Preferences," *J. Home Economics* (Dec. 1962), p. 854.

Good Grooming

A touch of glamor does wonders for the morale of people at all ages. Encourage the elderly woman to use her favorite cologne or her dusting powder with its delightful fragrance. Place colorful bows or pretty combs in her hair. The services of a beautician may be well worth the fee charged. An elderly woman can have an attractive personal appearance. Encouragement and compliments from those around her may be all that she needs to maintain pride in her appearance.

Everybody needs an occasional excuse to "dress up." Men should have a reason to be clean-shaven and to wear the Christmas tie. Women love to wear their earrings and jewelry. In some homes for the aged, dressing for dinner is the custom. The little things help to make life more enjoyable and more worth living. Happy people tend to be healthier people.

Safety

A minor accident can be a major catastrophe to an elderly person. Older people take longer to recuperate and longer to overcome effects of immobility. An accident can strain limited resources, both physical reserves and bank accounts.

Home accidents occur easily to elderly people. The many infirmities of age create extra hazards. The person may be unsteady on his feet, shaky, or dizzy, or he may lose his balance. Both eyesight and hearing are less keen; hence the person may not see or hear danger. His sense of smell is less acute; hence he may not detect smoke or the odor of escaping gas. For these reasons, we encourage elderly people to practice safety habits and to make their surroundings as safe as possible.

The elderly person should try not to hurry. It will take the woman longer to wash her breakfast dishes and the elderly man longer to shave. They should watch for fatigue and rest when they are tired. The older person should not move rapidly from one position to another, such as from lying down to standing up. He should hold on to something and move slowly. He should get help with household tasks that require bending, climbing, or carrying heavy loads. Such simple things as keeping clothing in good repair will help. A loose hem, torn sleeve, or broken heel can cause a fall.

Good housekeeping is a safety measure for everyone. The following help to prevent accidents: clean floors, rugs in good condition and firmly attached to the floor, nonslippery floors, stairs and halls free of clutter, traffic lanes clear, and equipment put away when not in use. Good lighting is essential, such as a light that can be turned on at the foot and head of the stairway, a night light in

Good Hygiene for Elderly People   285

the bathroom or hallway, illuminated switches, and a light that can be reached from the bed.

These extra measures add to the safety of living quarters of elderly people: handrails on halls and stairways, grab bars in the bathroom next to the tub and toilet, waist-high storage for dishes and personal belongings used daily, plenty of space instead of rooms crowded with furniture, and, if possible, no steps or door sills.

Elderly people will be more safety-conscious when they are convinced that someone really cares about their welfare. They might be careful just to please you.

Questions for Discussion

1. What chronic illnesses that often begin in middle age may be prevented, or arrested, by regular health consultation?
2. Describe unusual eating habits of elderly people that are not necessarily harmful. What food fads are harmful for elderly people?
3. What favorite foods of an elderly person might be made edible in a food blender? A class demonstration on the use of the blender might be arranged by contacting the home service department of your local electrical utility company.
4. Do you know how a confined or elderly person might have dental work done?
5. A geriatric nurse should be acquainted with name brands of satisfactory soaps, hair shampoos, dental powders, lotions, etc. Notice the supplies used in your hospital.
6. What special safety measures are observed in the geriatric hospital ward? If your class has an opportunity to visit a nursing home or home for the aged, look for the safety features.
7. Should an elderly couple select a small or large refrigerator if buying a new one? (Appliance salesmen often push the small refrigerator.)

Additional Readings

BOOKS

Bortz, Edward L. *Creative Aging*, pp. 56-80. New York: The Macmillan Company, 1963.
Mowry, Lillian. *Basic Nutrition and Diet Therapy for Nurses*. 4th ed. St. Louis: The C. V. Mosby Company, 1969.
Newton, Kathleen, *Geriatric Nursing*. 4th ed. Chap. 6, "General Hygiene"; Chap. 7, "Nutrition." St. Louis: The C. V. Mosby Company, 1966.
Peyton, Alice B. *Practical Nutrition*. 2nd ed. Chap. 15, "Food Needs of the Older Age Group." Philadelphia: J. B. Lippincott Company, 1962.
Robinson, Corinne H. *Basic Nutrition and Diet Therapy*. New York: The Macmillan Company, 1965.
Scott, Lou. *Clinical and Community Nursing*. Chap. 12, "Geriatric Nursing." New York: The Macmillan Company, 1968.

Shackelton, Alberta Dent. *Practical Nurse Education.* "Nutrition and Geriatrics," pp. 101–106. Philadelphia: W. B. Saunders Company, 1961.

Stevens, Marion K. *Geriatric Nursing for Practical Nurses.* Philadelphia: W. B. Saunders Company, 1965.

PAMPHLETS

Are You Planning on Living the Rest of Your Life? U.S. Department of Health, Education and Welfare, Administration on Aging, Washington D.C. 20201. AoA Publication No. 803, 1964.

The Fitness Challenge in the Later Years. U.S. Department of Health, Education, and Welfare, Social and Rehabilitation Service, Administration on Aging, Washington, D.C. 20201. AoA Publication No. 802, May 1968. An exercise program for older Americans.

Food Guide for Older Folks. U.S. Department of Agriculture, Home and Garden Bulletin No. 17, 1963.

Handle Yourself with Care. U.S. Department of Health, Education, and Welfare, Administration on Aging, Washington, D.C. 20201. AoA Publication No. 805, May 1969. Accident prevention for older Americans.

Recommended Audiovisual Aids

FILM

More Than Food (23 min., U.S. Public Health Service, produced by Colorado State Dept. of Health, Color)

This film stresses the importance of good food in a nursing home and how to encourage the patient to eat well. It would be good for food service personnel in a nursing home and also help the practical nurse to learn about geriatric food needs, including the mechanics of feeding.

CHAPTER 26/**FINANCES OF OLDER PEOPLE**

As people get older, financial security becomes more important. An assured income for food, rent, and medical expenses gives peace of mind. An older person can be so worried about money that he cannot eat and enjoy the food that he does buy with his limited income.

A little money above that needed for the essentials can make the difference between happiness and boredom, loneliness, and unhappiness in old age. It takes money to eat dinner in a nice restaurant, for bus fare to the senior citizens' center, for theater and movie tickets, for flower seeds, and for materials to make gifts.

You may be one of the countless student practical nurses living frugally now but looking forward to the status and the income of a licensed, practical nurse. You are reasonably thinking, "tomorrow will be better." A young married couple can live happily on a meager income because they have hopes and plans for a better future. But the elderly person has no hopes and plans for a better future. He cannot reason, "I will work harder. Tomorrow will be better." He cannot work harder. His earning days are probably ended, and he knows that.

Hence a lack of money can be a steady, gnawing pain that does not subside; it increases.

Incomes of the Elderly

Inadequate income is still the major problem facing most older Americans despite the benefits of social security, medicare, and medicaid. The U.S. Senate Special Committee on Aging released a study in 1969[1] disclosing that one-third of elderly people lived in poverty. A grave shortage existed in housing, nursing homes, and other forms of shelter. About five in ten families with an aged head of household had less than $4000 income in 1967; about one in five was below $2000. Of older people living alone or with nonrelatives in 1967, half had yearly incomes below $1480 and one-fourth had $1000 or less.

Most elderly people, especially those who had been retired for several years, could not afford the level of living set by the Bureau of Labor Statistics in its "Retired Couple's Budget."[2] This budget would require an annual income of $3869 for a moderate standard of living, for a retired, self-supporting couple in

---

[1] U.S. Senate Special Committee on Aging, headed by Senator Harrison A. Willims, working paper, "Economics of Aging," March 1969.
[2] *Retired Couple's Budget for a Moderate Living Standard*, U.S. Dept. of Labor, Bureau of Labor Statistics, Bulletin No. 1570—4, Autumn 1966.

urban areas in the autumn of 1966. It was estimated that an elderly person living alone in a city would need about $2130 annual income.

The Senate report showed that many elderly Americans of the minority groups lived in poverty, especially Negroes in ghetto areas and Mexican-Americans in southwestern United States.

Widows and other aged women living alone were often desperately poor.[3] In 1966 six out of ten had incomes below the poverty line.[4] The number of women living alone had increased since a previous survey in 1959, indicating the increasing number who live independently even at the price of poverty.

The difference in income between working families and retired families is widening. (See Figure 31.) Many older people living in poverty were not poor until they were old. Of the 7.1 million families with an aged head of household in 1967, almost 10 per cent had incomes under $1500 as compared with 3 per cent of younger families. Almost 37 per cent of older families had incomes of less than $3000 annually as compared with 8 per cent of younger families.

The largest single source of the total income for people 65 and older remains employment, even though fewer than one in five are in the labor force.

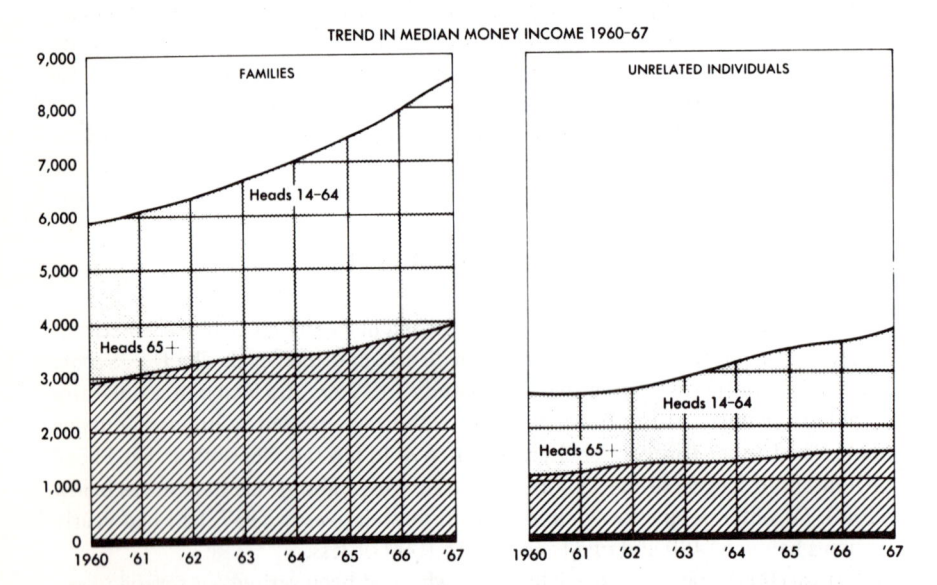

Figure 31. *The income difference between older and younger people is widening.* (From Economics of Aging: Toward a Full Share in Abundance. *Working paper for Special Committee On Aging, United States Senate, March 1969. p. xvi.)*

---

[3] U.S. Senate Special Committee on Aging, op. cit., p. 14.
[4] The poor (or poverty line) was defined in 1966 as having an annual income of less than $1975 for an elderly couple not on a farm, and less than $1565 for an aged person living alone.

(In 1965 it was 17 per cent, or more than 3 million working.[5]) The median annual income of $3928 for couples aged 65 and older includes those still working. As the person advances in age, he can no longer work. Concern exists because more and more Americans are living more and more years in retirement.

However, some older Americans are well off. Older families with incomes of $10,000 or more numbered 13.5 per cent of the older group, as contrasted to 38 per cent of younger families.[6] Among older couples, about one-third had assets (other than their home) of $10,000 or more. A little less than a third of the nonmarried had assets of $5000 or more.[7]

Personal Assets

Since older people have had a lifetime to accumulate savings, it might seem that they will have done so. But people now old were hampered in their efforts to save for the future by two world wars, a major depression, and generally low lifetime earnings. The facts available show that those who have low incomes also have little or no savings. The 1963 Social Security Survey revealed that 37 per cent of retired couples and more than half of the unmarried men and women had financial assets amounting to less than $1000.[8] Retired persons also had more financial assets and less debt than the population generally.

The major asset of older people is the owned home, an asset not readily convertible to cash for daily living. Selling the house to meet current living expenses would mean the need for another house or living quarters, perhaps at greater cost. More than half of the owned homes are modest houses, valued at less than $10,000.

Assets are reduced, in some cases exhausted, as people live several years on retirement incomes. Home ownership becomes difficult to maintain with advanced age, mounting taxes, and rising costs in general.

Social Security

Social security benefits are the major source of income for most older persons. At the end of 1968 about 16½ million people 65 or older were drawing social security benefits. Persons who received benefits (or were eligible) comprised 92 per cent of the total population of 65 or older.[9]

Congress passed the Social Security Act in 1935 to provide financial

---

[5] *Facts About Older Americans*, U.S. Dept. of Health, Education, and Welfare, Administration on Aging, AoA Publication No. 410, May 1966.

[6] U.S. Senate Special Committee on Aging, op. cit., p. 6.

[7] From the Social Security Administration 1963 Survey of the Aged.

[8] U.S. Senate Special Committee on Aging, op. cit., p. 11.

[9] U.S. Senate Special Committee on Aging, op. cit., pp. 7–8.

security in old age. The worker and his employer both contribute regularly to the system in proportion to the worker's earnings. The self-employed person also contributes a percentage of his earnings. When he stops work at the age of 65, the individual receives a monthly income based on previous earnings. Both workers and wives may receive reduced benefits beginning at age 62 (some at age 60). Recipients under the age of 72 who earn more than certain annual or monthly amounts will forfeit part of their benefits. Details concerning the earning limitations or "retirement test" are worthy of further study. After the age of 72, a person can earn any amount of money and receive social security benefits.

For the person between the ages of 65 and 72, careful distinction is made between income from working and income from investments. Income from investments, pensions, securities, and the like never affect the size of a person's social security benefits, or his rights to receive them.

In his message to Congress on January 14, 1954, former President Eisenhower explained the purpose of OASI, Old Age and Survivors Insurance (later OASDHI, Old Age, Survivors, Disability and Health Insurance): "The system is not intended as a substitute for private savings, pension plans, and insurance protection. It is, rather, intended as the foundation upon which these other forms of protection can be soundly built ... the system both encourages thrift and self-reliance and helps to prevent destitution in our national life."

For many people, however, the social security benefits are their only source of income, a situation likely to continue. Pension experts say that only one in five has a private pension to supplement social security.[10] The "1965 Report to the President on Private Employment Retirement Plans" projected that 21 per cent of persons aged 65 and over would be receiving private pensions in 1970; by 1975, 25 per cent; and by 1980, 28 per cent. Again, the coverage is concentrated among higher paid workers.

Another simulation project estimated that more than two-thirds of retired couples are expected to receive $3000 or less in social security benefits in 1980.[11]

Social security benefits paid at the end of 1968 averaged $98.50 monthly ($1182 annually) for the retired aged worker; $51.20 monthly ($614.40 annually) for the spouse; and $86.50 monthly ($1038 annually) for the aged widow.[12]

Medicare and Health Needs

The Medicare law became effective July 1966, and the extended care coverage effective January 1, 1967. With low incomes and almost no savings,

[10] *U.S. News and World Report*, August 5, 1968, p. 76.
[11] U.S. Senate Special Committee on Aging, op. cit., p. 41.
[12] U.S. Senate Special Committee on Aging, op. cit., p. 8.

Finances of Older People

older people have far greater medical expenses than younger people. One major medical expense is enough to wipe out savings and independence for an elderly couple. It is impossible to measure the value of medicare in freeing older people from fear of the heaviest costs of illness and in relieving younger people from the need to finance these costs for elderly parents. And of course, some elderly people went without. Despite imperfections in the law, results have made a great difference in many lives.

As a nurse, you need to know how Medicare operates and to keep informed of revisions. The 1965 Amendment to the Social Security Act established two complementary health insurance programs for persons aged 65 and over. One program provides for basic costs — for inpatient hospital services, outpatient hospital diagnostic services, posthospital extended care facilities services, and posthospital home health care services. It is financed under the social security program, through a separate payroll and tax fund. The patient pays some costs, such as the first $40 inpatient hospital expense.

The second part of the 1965 act established a voluntary supplementary plan providing for doctors' services and a few other specified medical expenses. This is financed through a monthly premium paid by the participant (initially 3 dollars monthly, since raised) and a matching amount from the federal

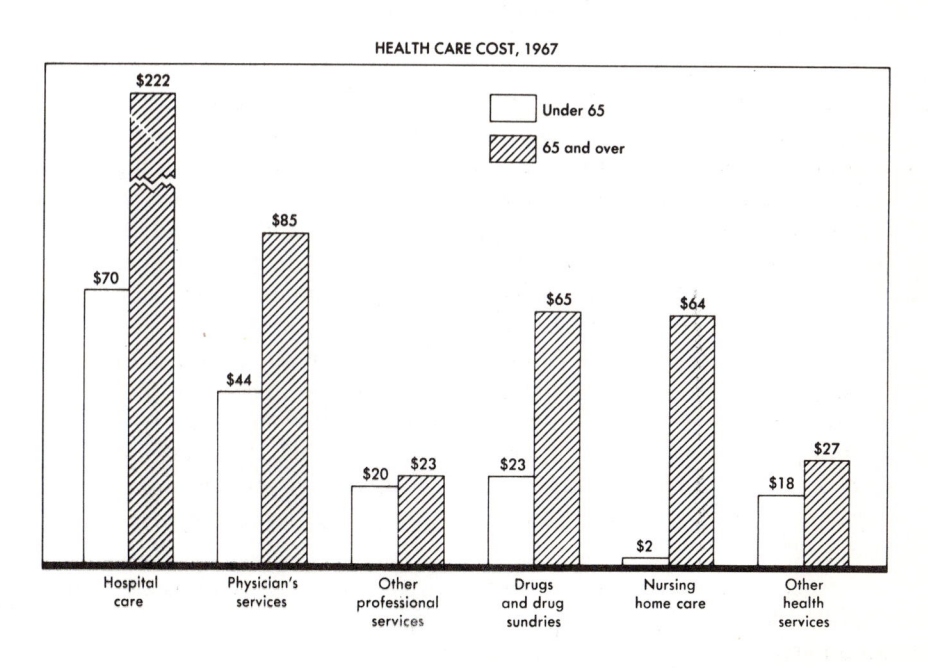

Figure 32. *Cost of health care per person by type of expenditure and age, 1967.* (Social Security Bulletin, *August 1968.*)

government. It covers approximately 80 per cent of the expenses in a year. (For example, the patient pays the first $50.)

Social workers for the aged point to two disadvantages in the Medicare program: the noninclusion of prescription drugs, and the patient must be hospitalized before being eligible for long-term care. More than 50 per cent of nursing home patients are age 80 or over.

After three years of Medicare, the Commissioner of Social Security reported that older people were getting 20 per cent more hospital care than before Medicare. This was needed care given in a dignified way to maintain personal self-respect. The participating hospitals and nursing homes must meet standards of quality.

Medicare was not meant to pay for all health care expenditures of the elderly. Medical expenses continue to take a significant portion of the retiree's budget. The "Retired Couple's Budget"[13] allotted $148 annually for out-of-pocket Medicare costs, and $136 for other medical care, totaling $284 annually. In the first full year of Medicare, fiscal 1967, private funds accounted for 41 per cent ($200.29 per person) of the medical bill of the aged. Public funds accounted for 59 per cent, or $285.62 per person.[14]

Old Age Assistance

The Old Age Assistance program (OAA) provides a monthly cash stipend to persons who are in need and can show that they have no means of support. In 1968 slightly more than 2 million people received old-age assistance, over half as supplement to Social Security benefits.[15] The program is operated by the state, usually the state department of public welfare. Funds come from taxes, with the federal government paying about 65 per cent of the cost, the state 20 per cent, and the county 15 per cent. Levels of assistance vary markedly from state to state. The person must be over 65 years of age and must meet the requirements for residency of the state. The state may require the person to agree to reimburse the state and county if it is ever possible. This agreement constitutes a lien on any property owned by the applicant, but the lien is not enforced during the lifetime of the person or during the lifetime of a surviving spouse.

For persons getting both payments in February 1967, the average monthly social security benefit was $52.95, and the average OAA payment was $56.75. For those receiving only an OAA payment, the average amount was $80.30.[16]

[13] *Retired Couple's Budget for a Moderate Living Standard,* op. cit.
[14] U.S. Senate Special Committee on Aging, working paper, "Health Aspects of the Economics of Aging," July 1969, p. 13.
[15] U.S. Senate Special Committee on Aging, working paper, "Economics of Aging," March 1969, p. 40.
[16] Social Security Bulletin, April 1968.

Income Needs

It has been recommended that incomes in retirement should be at least 50 per cent of preretirement incomes. The overwhelming majority of people retiring today receive total pension incomes ranging from 20 to 40 per cent of average earnings in the year prior to retirement.[17]

Some expenses are reduced, but needs of elderly people do not suddenly evaporate. The fact that older people spend less than younger people is not proof that they need less.

However, people often find that retirement income stretches further than they had anticipated. Once he gets used to the idea, the retiree may realize that many former necessities are really luxuries. A new car every other year does not seem as important as it once did. Activities of retirement years are less expensive than those of youth or middle age. Fishing, making ceramics, and flower raising tend to be less costly than raising a family, buying a house, or going to the theater.

For those retired, work-related expenses are eliminated, such as social security payments, retirement savings, union fees, and meals away from home. No more white uniforms or white nurse's shoes are needed.

The retirement income is partly tax-free. Social security payments are not taxable. Some states offer double income tax exemptions to those 65 and older, and also there are certain federal tax benefits.

Older people are more likely than younger people to own their homes, free and clear of mortgage payments.

However, medical expenses (despite Medicare) are considerably higher than for young people. Older people can do less for themselves as physical ability decreases, and they may incur higher expenses for maintaining their homes or for institutional living.

Expenditures of older people follow a pattern similar to that of low-income groups in general. The older families spend proportionately more on food, housing, household operation, and medical care than do younger families.

Smaller expenditures by older people frequently reflect low incomes rather than no need for goods or services. When younger and older households at the same income level are compared, few differences exist with regard to ownership of automobiles and major kitchen appliances.[18]

---

[17] U.S. Senate Special Committee on Aging, working paper, "Economics of Aging," March 1969, p. viii.
[18] U.S. Senate Special Committee on Aging, working paper, "Economics of Aging," March 1969, p. 13.

Savings

The retired people who have an adequate income probably planned and worked for it. Very few people inherit money or accidentally strike oil.

For most workers during most of their working lifetime, extra income over expenditures leaves little margin for savings. Self-employed, professional, and skilled workers are more likely to be able to save than clerical, semiskilled, or unskilled workers. To do without today's pleasures in order to save for old age has little appeal, especially with the prospects of continued prosperity. It requires discipline, but some people can do it.

A cash fund is an asset to a retired couple, a bulwark against emergencies, medical expenses, or a change in living quarters.

A small amount put aside monthly through the years will build up. If a man 35 years old begins purchasing a $25 U.S. savings bond monthly, investing $225 yearly, and if the bonds are reinvested as they mature, he will have an amount in excess of $10,000 when he is 65 years old.

A new car and new household appliances bought just before retirement are a form of savings that help to stretch the retirement income.

Annuities and Endowments

These may be purchased from life insurance companies as a source of income for old age. Endowment life insurance furnishes insurance protection and at the age of 65 pays the policy holder a lump sum of the face value of the policy. This might be the source of the $10,000 entrance fee required by some beautiful homes for the aged.

An annuity guarantees a certain monthly income to the person as long as he lives. An annuity can be purchased through yearly premiums or in one sum. Annuities are stable and permanent and eliminate the possibility of outliving one's capital.

Investments and Inflation

The retiree's purchasing power is reduced because part-time job opportunities disappear as he gets older, health services go up, property taxes are higher, and inflation increases the cost of living.

Inflation presents the biggest problem to the person with a fixed retirement income. An annual rise of only 2 per cent will reduce the purchasing power after one decade by 18 per cent, and after two decades, by 33 per cent. For this

Finances of Older People

reason, people hesitate to save dollars for retirement when the dollar will probably be worth less when they are ready to spend it.

Equities that pay good returns are also subject to risks that many unsophisticated savers with small amounts may not wish to assume. Of course, more fortunate people with generous incomes can turn to authorities in estate planning for guidance in buying stocks, bonds, and mutual funds.

Investments in real estate tend to fluctuate with the dollar. In long-term planning, people should consider two types of investments: (1) those that would furnish a money income, such as a pension, and (2) those that would rise in price if the value of the dollar were to rise, such as a farm or real estate. Many families of ordinary means have purchased a "double" house, with living quarters for two families. When retirement comes, rent from the other half of the house can help the retired person to maintain his half. His rent is free. This of course, implies that the house is located in a stable community. Even so, some return on the investment should be realized.

Home ownership is one kind of investment. If the house no longer meets the needs of the couple or individual, it can be rented or traded for other housing. The amount received if the house is sold may not be the original value, but remember, the person lived there for many years. His sale value will be more than empty rent receipts.

Unfortunately, some people are tempted to invest life savings in a small business at retirement time, a business that is new and strange to them. People should investigate carefully any such projects.

Live Only to Retire?

Some people believe that too much stress is given to "save money for retirement." A personnel man with a large company told about interviewing four young men, recent college graduates with advanced degrees. Three of the four asked first, "What is your company's retirement policy?" They hired the fourth young man who wanted to know about the future of the company, what he could offer to the company, and what type of work was involved.

Questions for Discussion

1. Define the term "median income." What does this mean regarding the numbers of elderly people who have an income less than that recommended for a moderate standard of living?

2. Plan a sample budget for an elderly couple or single person based on maximum social security pension. Would this provide comfortable living in your area?

3. How much of the preceding budget would be available for medicines, doctor bills, or health services?

4. What are the costs per week, per patient, in the skilled nursing homes in your area? What are the costs in a retirement home?

5. Describe an elderly person you know who is independent financially. In what way did he save or invest during his working years?

Additional Readings

Developments in Aging, 1968. A Report of the Special Committee on Aging, United States Senate. Report No. 91–119 to Senate, 91st Congress. U.S. Government Printing Office, Washington, D.C., 1969.

Economics of Aging: Toward a Full Share in Abundance. Working paper. Special Committee on Aging. U.S. Senate, March 1969.

Employment Aspects of the Economics of Aging. Working paper. Special Committee on Aging. U.S. Senate, December 1969.

Health Aspects of the Economics of Aging. Working paper. Special Committee on Aging. U.S. Senate, July 1969.

Retired Couple's Budget for a Moderate Living Standard. U.S. Department of Labor, Bureau of Labor Statistics, Washington, D.C. 20212. Bulletin No. 1570–4, Autumn, 1966.

You, the Law and Retirement. U.S. Department of Health, Education, and Welfare, Social and Rehabilitation Service, Administration on Aging, Washington, D.C. 20201. AoA Publication No. 900. Rev. 1966.

Recommended Audiovisual Aids

FILM

Retire to Life (20 min., International Film Bureau, B&W)

This film tells the story of the retired machinist who had looked forward to "loafing." His plans for fishing and for living with his son and family did not prove satisfactory. Retirement is more difficult for him than for his wife. The machinist finally locates a part-time job, and he and his wife move to their own home. This film depicts several activities and hobbies for retired people. It emphasizes that elderly people should plan for some work or activity after they retire from a regular job.

CHAPTER 27 / COMMUNITY

RESPONSIBILITY AND RESOURCES

FOR THE AGED

The major problems facing elderly people today are those that require united community action. Note how many of the rights of elderly people, as expressed in the Senior Citizens' Charter, depend on the community. For example: "The right to a fair share of the community's recreational, educational, and medical resources."

Examine the liberal provisions for youth that are found in almost every community: the schools, parks, YWCA and YMCA, 4-H Clubs, maternal and child health services, and others. Of course, the future of a nation lies in its youth, and children are the rightful responsibility of everyone. But also look at the community facilities directed to the working adult: civic theater groups, employment, housing, golf courses, adult education classes, and others.

Elderly people have been described as a "minority group" within the community. As a minority, they have a tendency to emphasize certain traits and to suppress others, in order to be accepted by the "dominant majority" of younger people. Elderly people should not be a neglected minority. Nor should community planning be centered on the needs of this group. However, a minority group may well have a proportionately larger number of problems than the general public. If their problems can be handled in the planning stage, both the community and the private citizen will benefit.

Community action is necessary if older people are to have suitable housing, health services, employment for those willing and able to work, decent nursing homes and homes for the aged, recreation and counseling, and participation in the activities of the community.

Both the elderly person and his family need the help of the community. Since more elderly people are living into their eighties and nineties, more families are confronted with the care of the dependent and the senile adult. The extended family and large houses are practically nonexistent; so the small family (the nuclear family) turns to the community for help.

With new problems facing our country, new solutions must be found.

Housing for Elderly People

Suitable, adequate housing for elderly people should offer a variety of choices: rental apartments, small homes, resident hotels, retirement villages, homes for the aged, group residential facilities, and nursing homes.

Fewer and fewer elderly people can look to their children for homes. With the shift from rural to city life that has taken place since 1900, three-generation living is less common. Smaller, more compact city housing simply does not allow space for the elderly parent. Household appliances have decreased the burden and number of household tasks, as well as decreased the usefulness of the elderly adult. Figure 33 shows that only 8.6 per cent of elderly men and only 17.8 per cent of elderly women live with relatives. Forty per cent of the elderly people live in non-metropolitan areas (Figure 34).

When elderly people express preferences, they usually indicate the desire to live alone in their own households rather than to live with their children. They want privacy and independence, but not segregation and isolation. Most of them want to continue to live in the community in which they spent their working life. For this reason, their housing becomes a community problem.

Good housing for the aged has the same basic principles of good housing for people of all ages, with these special features: living space on one floor without stairways or raised door sills, automatic heat, adequate storage space, equipment and shelving at proper height to eliminate bending and overreaching, nonslip

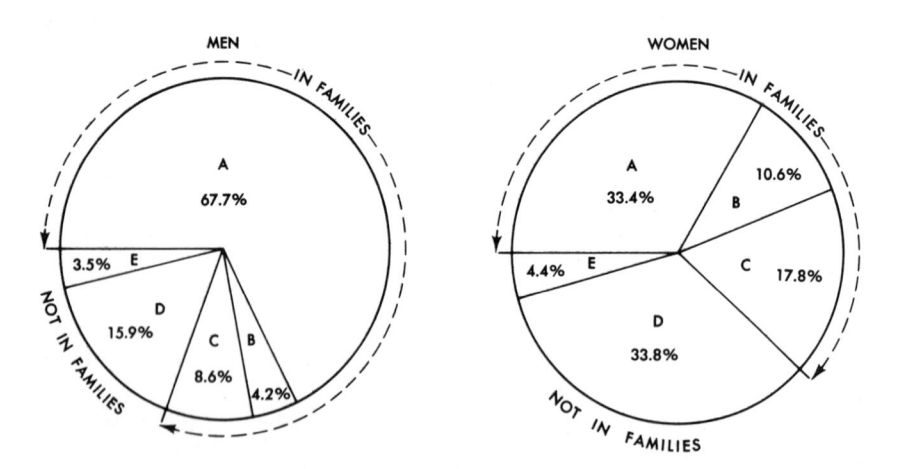

Figure 33. *How older people live, year 1967. A. In husband-wife families; B. family head, no spouse present; C. family member related to head, as elderly person living with son and his family; D. living alone or with nonrelatives; E. living in an institution. (Statistics from U.S. Senate Report,* Developments in Aging 1968, *p. 221.)*

Community Responsibility and Resources for the Aged 299

floors, good lighting, handrails for bathtubs, hallways, and entranceways, and probably a large kitchen with eating space instead of a separate dining room. All safety features are important.

Good, small homes and light, airy apartments are usually more satisfactory when located in the general community. People like to be "in the stream of life." For example, elderly people might offer services such as baby-sitting. The elderly person also needs contact with nature — to be able to see the green grass, the snow, or autumn leaves.

In the city, elderly people tend to live in the near downtown area in small apartments and rooming houses. Shopping is convenient and rent is low, but often the dwellings are dreary and substandard. There is a second fringe area in

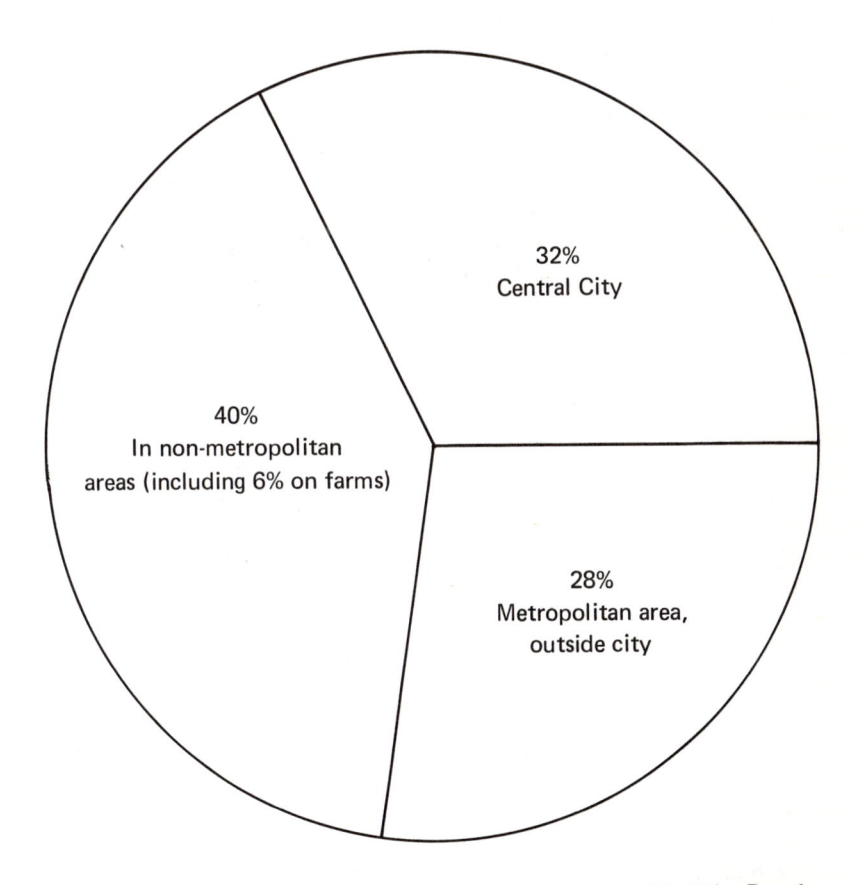

Figure 34. *Where older people live. (From* Working with Older People, *Vol. III,* The aging Person: Needs and Services, *U.S. Department of Health, Education and Welfare, Public Health Service Publication No. 1459, April 1970, p. 25.)*

which elderly couples often live in private homes, usually larger than they need.[1] Managing the large house may not be difficult until the couple reach the eighties, but after that, accidents can easily happen, and the work of the house is difficult.

In the more comfortable income groups, it is possible to have s small apartment within the larger home. Many houses built today have a second bathroom and a family room. After the teenagers leave home, the second living room may not be important. A small kitchenette could be added, making a truly small home within the larger home. The aged parent could have privacy and still be within convenient "checking range" of the younger family.

Retirement communities have both advantages and disadvantages. Older people require more medical services, and when large groups of elderly people are congregated in special communities, the medical facilities of the area are strained. Real estate developers frequently fail to make adequate plans for medical services.

Despite the arguments that retired people should not move away from lifelong friends, retirement-vacation communities are flourishing. People are buying property in an area where they enjoy vacations. They make friends, get acquainted with the community, and learn about the weather. When retirement comes, they sell their present home (probably mortgage-free) and build a compact, easy-to-care-for house. One Chicago-area couple frankly stated that their retirement income would not support their active social life. They moved to a vacation-retirement community in Florida and were happy living where their income was adequate. A visit from the grandchildren was an exciting event for everyone. Social life in these communities is usually organized to include everyone, and the physical design is often well planned.

Increasing numbers of homes for the aged are sponsored by church groups, fraternal organizations, professional groups, and labor unions. Many have extensive recreational programs and facilities for hobby and craftwork. Medical services are planned, often on an ambulatory basis, with arrangements for hospital or nursing care when necessary. Again, the lovely homes are not inexpensive, often requiring a substantial entrance fee.

Government housing is available in some areas for elderly people. Under programs administered by the Housing and Home Financing Agency, low-rent housing units have been and are being built that are specifically designed for aged persons.

Congregations of only elderly people have been regarded as depressing and undesirable, but Dr. Wilma Donahue of the University of Michigan, one of the founders of American gerontology, expresses another view. "The large housing projects built to rent at prices old people can afford have been noted to be effective in helping these people remain mentally well adjusted. With the support

---

[1] Morton Leeds, *The Aged, The Social Worker, and the Community* (Cleveland: H. Allen, 1961), p. 88.

of fellow residents, many of the mentally deviant are able to cope and go undetected by management, which views them generally only as complainers." Dr. Donahue points out that letting older people keep this independence amid familiar surroundings improves their chances of staying well.

Nursing Homes

Medicare is one of many factors helping to brighten the picture of nursing home care. A nursing home must meet standards to be eligible for medicare patients. Individual states have had requirements for licensure, requirements which have been raised. Also, commercial insurance companies are increasing payments for nursing-home care as well as hospital care.

People who dread to think of an elderly parent as a nursing home patient probably retain the old image of a dreary converted residence that did not meet health and sanitation requirements, let alone provide nursing care. Many of these were actually "living morgues" where the aged lived a vegetablelike existence.

One visit to a new, modern home may be necessary for people to appreciate the improvements possible. Today's nursing homes may be beautiful, modern structures with picture windows, resembling motels or trim apartment buildings. Inside, the rooms are airy, light, and colorful. Competent, trained staffs encourage each guest to do as much for himself as he can do. The emphasis today is on rehabilitation and restorative services.

Trained, practical nurses are desperately needed to staff nursing homes. If you are considering this type of nursing service, you will want to learn a great deal about nursing homes and the services they can offer.

The term "health facility" may be used to designate a home giving only custodial care. The health facility must meet the state sanitation requirements to be licensed, but does not necessarily qualify for medicare patients. Custodial care is for those with minor physical or emotional disabilities who have no one to take care of their needs. The nursing homes giving skilled nursing care usually qualify for medicare patients. Fees are related to the type of home and amount of service required. The more services, the higher the cost.

The large nursing home, offering skilled nursing care, may be almost hospital-size, yet differences exist. You will not see as many registered nurses per patient, and probably no interns. The nursing home will have no surgical facilities nor an emergency room. However, the nursing home must be equipped to handle emergencies required by the aged and chronically ill, such as oxygen and intravenous fluids.

Many nursing homes have working arrangements with nearby hospitals for handling major medical emergencies. Particularly if the home is located within a few blocks of the hospital, the affiliation encourages progressive patient care. The physician can supervise his patients in the hospital, then in the nursing home, and finally in the patient's home. The diagnostic services of the hospital might also be available.

The number of aged persons who require nursing care is difficult to estimate. Some say considerably less than 10 per cent of the aged need or want care in a nursing home, home for the aged, or other institution. When more varied living arrangements are available, better use will be made of existing nursing homes. Many an elderly person has gone to a nursing home because he had no other place to live.

Community Interest in Nursing Homes

When people in a community become interested in the fate of elderly people, improvements result. A minister's statement typifies the concern of the lay people: "In too many nursing homes, old people are given tranquilizers and put to bed. The situation is sad."

The wrong attitude is encouraged when the welfare department pays the nursing-home operator more daily for a bed patient than for an ambulatory patient. The margin of profit for a nursing home is slim, and such a policy encourages an unscrupulous operator to keep his patients in bed.

A state board of health nurse said: "We receive many calls from people asking us to name a good nursing home for an aged relative. These people never ask me about rehabilitation services."

Community Involvement in Nursing Homes

Not only community interest, but community involvement is needed to improve nursing home care. The operators of nursing homes need the cooperation of the entire health team — physicians, social welfare directors, health department personnel, and volunteer groups.

Most nursing homes are not subsidized by city grants, united fund monies, or tax-deductible gifts from wealthy citizens. They are managed by private citizens who must make a profit or go out of business.

The medicare program provides for many welfare patients, but not all. Social workers should strive to see that nursing-home operators are paid adequately for welfare patients. The local health department can offer help and guidance when inspecting nursing homes.

Nursing-home patients need visitors, entertainment, and religious services. Different church groups and neighborhood auxiliaries might help the nursing-home manager to provide social life and religious services for the patients. Outside contacts would help to improve the morale of the patients and employees, as well as the general appearance of the home.

In many communities, the Jewish people have been leaders in establishing good homes for the aged and good nursing homes for their people. At the Borinstein Home for the Jewish Aged, Indianapolis, Indiana, members of the Jewish Council of Women entertain the residents each Wednesday. Religious services are provided every week. These elderly people are considered an important part of the Jewish community.

The nursing-home manager might encourage family members to help with the social life of the patients. Two sisters, both schoolteachers, reluctantly admitted they could no longer care for their mother. They virtually "adopted" the nursing home to which they took her. They prepared the Thanksgiving turkey, decorated the Christmas tree, and took an interest in every guest in the home. Many people have guilty feelings because they can no longer look after an aged parent. Helping in such a way gives reassurance that this is the best course of action. Through active participation, the citizens of a community will become more aware of the needs of the patients and of the nursing homes.

Occupational and Physical Therapists

The expense of hiring an occupational therapist and a physical therapist is beyond the modest budget of most nursing homes.

One suggestion is for a group of nursing-home operators to hire jointly a physical therapist and an occupational therapist. These specialists could teach the nursing-home personnel the basic principles of physical and occupational therapy.

Another suggestion is for the consultant occupational therapist to combine occupational-therapy duties with other duties. If she can perform another service, she has a better opportunity to get acquainted with the home and the patients and to adapt a program to their needs. It is difficult for a stranger to make recommendations on the basis of one visit a week. A person in the home for a longer period of time might see that a woman could learn to use a dishholder and thus feed herself. The therapist might observe and suggest it, but the nurse would need to encourage her persistently to use the dishholder.

Of course, the nursing-home operator should not expect someone to combine another full-time job with part-time occupational therapy. The therapist needs time and energy for the work.

The hospital without an occupational therapy department and the nursing home probably have no budget allowances for craft materials. The cost of yarn for knitting may be prohibitive to the patient or the nursing home.

Frequently manufacturers will donate remnants if contacted by the therapist or nurse. She should explain to the company officials that the scrap materials will not be used to make a product of commercial value or to offer competition. They may be glad to contribute to the happiness and rehabilitation of nursing-home patients (this is community involvement again). A lumber company may have small pieces of hardwood lumber that are checked or cracked. An upholstery company may have leather or fabric in pieces too small for their use. A garment factory or woolen mill may have scraps of fabrics to give away. And weaving, for instance, can be done with scrap materials.

Recreation and Counseling Centers

Senior citizen centers originated to furnish social contacts and recreational activities for older people. The hours when working people are at business can be a lonely time for the retired person. He needs a place to go where he can relax over a cup of coffee or tea, and to chat with old friends or to meet new friends. He will continue attending if the center offers a variety of pursuits designed to afford meaningful use of free time and opportunity for social participation.

After several day centers were established, it became obvious that this was the logical place for counseling services and sources of information. Older people have difficulty getting around; hence it is practical and economical to provide many services within one setting. This was the start of the multipurpose or multiservice center.

Skilled social workers can offer counseling on employment, living arrangements, recreation, financial matters, family and social problems, and referral to other community services.

Medical and financial information of interest to older people may be featured in programs. Special-interest programs arranged at one center including a lip-reading class, hearing tests, discussion by a tax expert on tax exemptions for senior citizens, demonstration by state-board-of-health nutritionists on preparing food for one person, and visits to the eye clinic at the public hospital for members.

It is important that the center first be established in a central location, near public transportation. Later, the center may be moved farther from the center of the city.

Cheerful, colorful surroundings help to create a friendly atmosphere. Convenience, a place to hang coats at the entrance, one-floor design, safety features, plenty of space — all of these features attract and reassure the elderly person.

But the most essential requirement is for a friendly, trained staff capable of organizing a program of activities catering to the needs of members. A typical day center has at least one professionally trained social worker, preferably with experience in social group work with the aged.

At first, the elderly people who come may be the socially active people who are getting along fairly well anyway. But eventually, the isolated, lonely elderly person may be reached. More women than men flock in at first. Men are attracted by equipment, games, and things to do. Women are more likely to congregate to socialize. A center is not production-centered, hence the greater hesitancy of men.

At a truly successful day center, the members eventually plan the progress and make the decisions. They feel that "this is my club." Sometimes an elected council with regularly scheduled meetings will encourage members to become active and enthusiastic.

If the multipurpose center for elderly people is to prove worthwhile, it needs the active support of many different groups, such as church groups, state and local government bodies, service organizations, fraternities and sororities, trade unions, medical groups, business organizations, and social service people.

As a student nurse and as a graduate practical nurse, you will contact many elderly people. Not every elderly person needs a day center. But the ones who do need it are usually reluctant to go. If you understand the good results that can come from participation in a recreation and counseling center, you will be more likely to guide to it the elderly person who will benefit.

Federal Government Helps the Elderly

Help for elderly people is extended on all government levels – local, state and national. The first White House Conference on Aging, held January 1961, created national publicity concerning needs of our growing elderly population. Almost every session of Congress reviews the Social Security Act, especially noting how social insurance benefits relate to current prices. Details of social security and provisions of the Medicare Act have been described previously, in Chapter 26.

The Community Health Services and Facilities Act of 1961 authorized new programs for out-of-hospital community services for the chronically ill and the aged. It increased federal grants for nursing-home construction, health research facilities, and experimental hospital and medical care facilities.

The housing acts provide funds for low- and moderate-cost houses, both rural and urban, for the elderly. The Drug Amendments of 1962 and the work of the Food and Drug Administration are designed to protect elderly people against false claims for medicines. Older persons are the heaviest users of drugs, but they have no money to waste on ineffective drugs and medicines. The Institute of Child Health and Human Development includes programs of research on health problems of the aging.

Because numerous departments within the federal government had responsibilities and programs related to the nation's older population, the Administration on Aging was established in 1965 to coordinate and strengthen government action. The Older Americans Act of 1965 and the amendment to it in 1967 were designed to encourage individual states to instigate programs meeting the needs of their residents. Federal funds supply 60 per cent of the monies for approved state programs. The Foster Grandparent Program proved highly successful. In this, people over 60 with low incomes were hired at the minimum wage to bring personal attention and affection to deprived and handicapped children. Services encouraged under the Older Americans Act are designed to establish senior centers, improve employment opportunities, increase incomes, provide homemaker and supportive services, improve nutrition, and help meet problems of transportation and the use of leisure time. Although federal funds are used for the planning of programs, success depends on the initiative and work done by state and local people.

Community Services for the Elderly

The highest and most worthy aims of the federal legislators depend on the individual citizen to carry them out. The licensed practical nurse can be a valuable aid in seeing that needy elderly people receive the help legislators plan for them.

Too often, personal and medical problems of old people are dismissed with

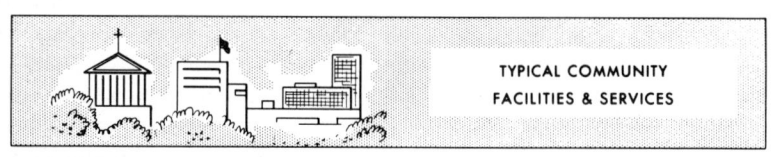

TYPICAL COMMUNITY FACILITIES & SERVICES

EDUCATIONAL
Adult education centers and courses
Nutrition courses
Retirement preparation seminars
Counseling services

EMPLOYMENT
Employment services
Sheltered workshops and work centers
Vocational training
Craft product sales program

RELIGIOUS
Religious services
Special group activities

RECREATIONAL & SOCIAL
Recreation facilities
Organizations of older people
Sponsored clubs
Multipurpose activity centers
Camping
Activity programs in housing
 developments and institutions

HEALTH & WELFARE
Outpatient services
Central information and referral services
Adult health and mental hygiene clinics
Home services
Rehabilitation activities and centers
Hospitals and nursing homes
Homes for the aged
Facilities for veterans

Figure 35. *The challenge to society is to create a climate for meaningful maturity. To home services may be added visiting nurses, homemaker services, home care, and meals-on-wheels. (1961 White House Conference on Aging,* Chart Book, *Chart 65, p. 78, Federal Council on Aging.)*

a shrug and the comment, "He is too old." Old people can be helped to solve their problems and to be relieved of physical suffering and helplessness.

Nurses are in a unique position to detect the problems of the elderly. Evidence indicates that they are more ready to tell their troubles to the nurse than to the more distant, more "specialized" physician or social worker.[2] A nurse should be aware of the existing services in her community for elderly people. She should become sensitive to the unspoken needs of elderly patients in order to be able to refer them where they can secure help.

Outpatient services are increasing in every community. The elderly person particularly benefits from receiving the necessary medical attention, then returning to his own home.

The visiting nurse services permit thousands of elderly people to remain in their own home rather than be institutionalized. The patient is often happier, and less funds are required — private and public.

Organized home care allows the elderly person to remain in his home, yet have the services of hospital care. The expense is less, and the elderly person does not have to make the tremendous adjustment to hospital life. But the household of the elderly person must be prepared to cooperate with the health service team. For example, is there enough space for the sick-room? Family relations may be strained; it is particularly hard to watch the slow decline of a loved one. The family members do not have the objectivity of the professional person, and they become more emotionally involved. The family members need encouragement and assurance that help will come when emergencies arise.

Homemaker services, where available, permit an elderly couple to remain together in their home. They also enable a single person to continue living in his apartment or home. Someone to buy groceries, cook a wholesome meal, and clean the house — this may be all the assistance that many elderly people require. Housekeeper programs provide cleaning services only. Often frail elderly people have been forced into institutional living because no homemaker service was available.

The meals-on-wheels program is vitally needed in many communities. An elderly person may not be really sick, but he does not have the energy required to cook a balanced meal. If one hot meal a day is brought to him, he has nourishment, plus contact with the outside world. Nurses frequently see a malnourished elderly person admitted to a hospital or nursing home.

Foster homes are available in some areas for elderly people. These arrangements seem to be more satisfactory when the family and the aged one have in common a religious faith or nationality. Among the aged in America, there are more than three million people who migrated from Europe to the United States. A Lithuanian elderly person might be welcomed more readily in a home of Lithuanian ancestry than one of Italian ancestry. Special boarding

[2] Barbara Henley, "Helping the Elderly Find Community Services," *Am. J. Nursing* (April 1963), p. 89.

arrangements are often made by some departments of public welfare and family service agencies.

Family agencies frequently have special plans for assisting elderly people. The nurse who is familiar with the family agencies in her community and who gets acquainted with the elderly person can often direct him to the right source of help. A Catholic patient can be helped by the Catholic charities; a Jewish patient should be directed to the Jewish social services. The American Cancer Society has many kinds of aid for patients with a malignancy.

Social workers can help elderly people with emotional problems if case loads permit. The public health nurse might give referral to persons with deep-seated anxieties covered by defenses, patients who need more protection or supervision, persons with strained household or family relationships, those who need changes in living arrangements, and those for whom "time hangs heavy." Personal problems can be just as real and as distressing to the elderly person as to the younger person. The nurse and the social worker have many bases for cooperation.

However, nurses should be cautious that "protective" services do not cause more harm than good. Too much help may result in earlier admission to an institution, and less time living independently. It requires careful judgment to know when help is really needed.

Importance of the Community

No discussion of the community and its elderly people is complete without pinpointing the importance of the community to the elderly person. As his ability to get around decreases, the importance of his neighborhood increases. The elderly person's immediate neighborhood may be his whole world. Minor inconveniences become major problems. The community services and recreational facilities in his neighborhood may be the only ones available to him. His use of services elsewhere is influenced by the public transportation available and the traffic dangers involved. The extent of his independence may be related to the conveniences of his own community.

His neighbors are the people he sees most. Friendly neighbors help the person continue living as near-normal a life as possible. All studies support the fact that continuing good social relationships help one to adjust to retirement.

A Look to the Future

As more people become interested and involved in making life worth living for elderly people, progress will slowly come.

For example, children's books may be rewritten to picture elderly people as wise, kind, and helpful — not stingy, crabby, or vulturous. The symbols of old age — gray hair, bifocals, and rocking chairs — may be replaced by images of retirees who are continuing their education, community service, or hobby pursuits. A child who grows up loving an elderly great-grandparent will likely look upon all elderly people with increased affection and understanding.

We will not try to segregate elderly people or to lump them together in one homogeneous group. We will realize that a roomful of elderly people have one characteristic in common — their age. We will recognize that varied solutions must be offered for different problems, such as the choice from among several kinds of living arrangements.

The emphasis on growing old will help people to accept the process of aging with dignity.

To the Nurse

Perhaps no other kind of nursing service is more needed, or more rewarding personally, than that of caring for elderly people.

If you choose geriatric nursing, you will gradually learn how to get along with the geriatric patient. You ask an older person to take his medicine, not tell him to do so. You may notice that the quality of the time you spend with the elderly patient is more important than the quantity of time. Listen to him intently and give him your undivided attention. You soon realize that you cannot change his way of thinking or his personal habits. If you show him that you truly accept him as a worthy individual, he will look upon you as a friend. To please a friend, he is more likely to try the exercises the physical therapist recommends, to eat the nutritious, attractive meals served him, and to do as much as possible of his own personal grooming.

The nurse who understands the work of other members of the health team, the needs of her patient, and the relationship of the patient's family has the capacity to become the competent, "big-hearted" nurse. Are you equal to the challenge?

Questions for Discussion

1. Take a field trip to visit (1) a good nursing home and/or (2) a senior citizens' day center.
2. Observe the planning for elderly people in your church. Report to the class any unique programs that have proved successful.
3. What are the requirements to obtain a license for a nursing home in your state?

4. To help get acquainted with the facilities for elderly people in your community, let each member of the class select one agency or resource to visit in person and then report to the rest of the class. The list might include:

Senior citizens' club	Visiting nurse service
Counseling or service center	Home care service
Public housing for elderly	Outpatient services
Home for the aged	Homemaker service
County home	Meals-on-wheels
Family agencies	Foster home care

Additional Readings

BOOKS

Burgess, Ernest W., ed., *Aging in Western Society, A Survey of Social Gerontology*. Chicago: The University of Chicago Press, 1960.

Leeds, Morton. *The Aged, The Social Worker, and the Community*. Section II, "The Professional"; Section III, "The Community, Small and Large." Cleveland: Howard Allen, Inc., 1961.

Moss, Bertram B. *Caring for the Aged*. Chap. 9, "Will a Nursing Home be Necessary?" Chap. 10, "What to Look for in a Nursing Home." Garden City, N.Y.: Doubleday & Company, Inc., 1966.

Shock, Nathan W. *Trends in Gerontology*. 2nd ed. Stanford, Calif.: Stanford University Press, 1957.

HOUSING LISTS

Lists of housing and nursing homes with information but no ratings or accreditation:

National Directory on Housing for Older People. National Council on Aging, 49 West 45th Street, New York, N.Y. 10036.

U.S. Guide to Nursing Homes. Edition A: West Coast Region; Edition B: Midwest Region; Edition C: East Coast Region. Parade, P.O. Box No. 130, Kensington Station, Brooklyn, N.Y. 11218.

SOURCES OF PAMPHLETS

Administration on Aging. For list of their publications, write to: Director, Public Information Staff, Administration on Aging, 330 Independence Avenue, S.W., Washington, D.C. 20201.

National Council on Aging. Write to: Director, National Council on Aging, 49 West 45th Street, New York, N.Y. 10036.

Social Security Administration. Price list of publications available from Superintendent of Documents, Washington, D.C. 20402.

State Commissions on Aging have various publication for residents of their state.

Recommended Audiovisual Aids

FILM

Environmental Health Aspects of Nursing Homes (13 min., U.S. Public Helath Service, produced under supervision of Michigan Department of Health, Color, 1962)

This film would interest the practical nurse who wants to work in or to operate a nursing home. It shows the planning required for a good nursing-home facility: blueprint plans, proper location, sanitation measures, and facility setup such as waiting room, cooking area, patient rooms, geriatric safety equipment, and laundry facilities and practice.

Appendix

ALPERN-BOLL DEVELOPMENTAL

SKILL-AGE INVENTORY

The Developmental Skill-Age Inventory provides a measurement of a child's functioning in five areas of human growth: physical, self-help, social, academic, and communication.

SCORING INSTRUCTIONS

Scoring is accomplished by the rater assigning a plus (+) or minus (−) for each item of each scale. The number of plus's for each scale is the subject's score for that scale (raw score).

The raw score for each scale is transformed to a Developmental Age Score by means of the table following. The child's accomplishments are thus compared to normative data, that is, the specific age at which children usually have mastered a skill.

The following scoring rules must be considered in all ratings:

a. In order for an item to be rated plus (+), the child's performance should be relatively consistent and dependable, *not* the result of unusual urging, luck or special circumstances.
b. If a child passes an advanced item in a scale (e.g., "speaking" in the Communication Scale), it is assumed that activities typically necessary for his development that appear earlier in the scale (e.g., "babbling") have been performed and are scored plus. This is true even though the earlier activity is no longer performed. In general, the rater should always recheck very carefully scale failures that are followed by later passes.
c. Physical and other handicaps of a permanent nature are not adjusted for in the scale. If a child has an orthopedic handicap, his physical skills score will be affected by his real locomotion difficulties. On the other hand, temporary handicaps (e.g., a broken leg expected to heal) are ignored. Activities known to be in the child's repertoire when not handicapped (e.g., skipping) are scored plus.

[1] The form of the Developmental Skill-Age Inventory contained in this book is a special version produced especially for this volume with the permission of Gerald D. Alpern, Ph.D., Director of Research, Child Psychiatry Services, Indiana University Medical Center, Indianapolis, Indiana 46202, and Thomas J. Boll, Ph.D., Research Psychologist, Child Development & Mental Retardation Center, University of Washington, Seattle, Washington 98105. The adaptation represents an abridgment of the experimental form employed for the standardization of the full inventory, which was designed to evaluate children from birth to 12 years of age.

CONVERSION OF RAW SCORES TO DEVELOPMENTAL AGE SCORES

Raw Score	Physical Age	Self-Help Age	Social Age	Academic Age	Communication Age
	Years Mos.	Years Mos.	Years Mos.	Years Mos.	Years Mos.
1	− 1mo.	− 1mo.	− 1mo.	− 2 mo.	− 1mo
2	− 3	− 3	− 3	− 4	− 3
3	− 4	− 5	− 5	− 6	− 4
4	− 6	− 7	− 7	− 8	− 6
5	− 7	− 9	− 9	−11	− 8
6	− 9	−11	−11	1− 2	− 9
7	−10	1− 1	1− 1	1− 4	−11
8	−11	1− 3	1− 3	1− 6	1− 0
9	1− 0	1− 4	1− 5	1− 8	1− 2
10	1− 2	1− 7	1− 7	1−11	1− 3
11	1− 4	1− 9	1− 9	2− 2	1− 5
12	1− 6	1−11	1−11	2− 4	1− 6
13	1− 9	2− 1	2− 0	2− 6	1− 8
14	1−11	2− 3	2− 3	2− 8	1− 9
15	2− 0	2− 5	2− 6	2−11	1−11
16	2− 2	2− 7	2− 9	3− 2	2− 0
17	2− 4	2− 9	2−11	3− 4	2− 3
18	2− 6	2−11	3− 0	3− 6	2− 4
19	2− 9	3− 0	3− 4	3− 8	2− 6
20	2−11	3− 4	3− 8	3−11	2− 8
21	3− 0	3− 8	3−11	4− 2	2− 9
22	3− 3	3−11	4− 0	4− 4	2−11
23	3− 6	4− 0	4− 4	4− 6	3− 0
24	3− 9	4− 4	4− 8	4− 8	3− 3
25	3−11	4− 8	4−11	4−11	3− 5
26	4− 0	4−11	5− 1	5− 0	3− 7
27	4− 2	5− 1	5− 3	5− 2	3− 9
28	4− 3	5− 3	5− 5	5− 4	3−11
29	4− 4	5− 5	5− 7	5− 6	4− 0
30	4− 6	5− 7	5− 9	5− 8	4− 6
31	4− 8	5− 9	5−11	5−10	4−11
32	4− 9	5−11	6− 0	5−11	5− 0
33	4−10	6− 0	6− 2	6− 0	5− 3
34	4−11	6− 2	6− 4	6− 2	5− 6
35	5− 0	6− 4	6− 6	6− 4	5− 9
36	5− 2	6− 6	6− 8	6− 6	5−11
37	5− 4	6− 8	6− 9	6− 8	6− 0
38	5− 5	6− 9	6−11	6−10	6− 4
39	5− 6	6−11		6−11	6− 8
40	5− 7			7− 0	6−11
41	5− 9				
42	5−11				
43	6− 0				
44	6− 3				
45					

Alpern-Boll Developmental Skill-Age Inventory

The rating may be done by the person who knows the child; that is, a teacher may evaluate her pupil or the nurse evaluate her little patient. Or the information may be obtained by interview; such as the public health nurse interviews the child's mother.

It should be remembered that the inventory is not a test in the usual sense, so attempts should not be made to have the child perform all the activities required. However, if the rater does not have enough knowledge, then one of the following is appropriate:

1. Ask someone who may know.
2. Attempt to have the child perform.
3. Estimate on the basis of other information.

The inventory will require about twenty minutes to administer and score.

IQ EQUIVALENCY SCORE

The intelligence quotient (IQ) has been accepted as the best known way of depicting by a single value a child's intellectual abilities. For several and varied reasons, the IQ concept has been justifiably challenged by knowledgeable educators and psychologists. Nevertheless, when the child's mental abilities are within normal limits, the IQ is representative and useful.

FUNCTIONING INTELLIGENCE COMPUTATION

1. Compute the child's Chronological Age in years and months. Chronological Age = ___ yrs. ___ mos.
2. Convert Chronological Age into months. Chronological Age in mos. = _____ mos.
3. Convert Academic Age into months. Academic Age = _____ mos.
4. Divide Academic Age (AA) by Chronological Age (CA). CA or AA ÷ CA = AA
5. Multiply step 4 answer by 100 which gives the Functioning Intelligence Quotient.

_____ (answer from 4)
   x 100

Functioning Intelligence Quotient = _____

Physical Developmental Age Scale

0 MONTHS TO 11 MONTHS

1. When child lies on stomach, he holds up his head, unassisted, for one minute.

2. Lies on stomach and rolls over on back (and vice versa) unassisted.
3. Sits upright on firm surface and maintains balance for at least one minute without support.
4. Can get to one place from another by any fashion of creeping or crawling.
5. Uses thumb and one or two fingers to pick things up, as opposed to grasping with his whole hand.
6. Comes to standing position by holding on to some object (not a person), pulling self upright.
7. Can stand unsupported, and maintains his balance for one minute.
8. Has established control of saliva so that mouth or chin does not ordinarily require wiping except when eating.

1 YEAR 0 MONTHS TO 1 YEAR 11 MONTHS

9. Walks for a purpose. Takes steps not merely for motor activity, but to reach an object. (No credit for walking to "Mommy" only when coaxed.)
10. Gets to a standing position without holding onto a person or an object, and remains standing for at least one minute without falling. (Balance may be unsteady.)
11. Walks up stairs using a wall, bannister, or person's hand. (Not necessary to alternate feet on the steps.)
12. Walks well enough that he does not need to be constantly watched to prevent his hurting himself.
13. Unwraps an object such as candy or gum.
14. Enough hand control to use pencil or crayon to scribble, or hand tool such as a hammer to hammer.

2 YEARS 0 MONTHS TO 2 YEARS 11 MONTHS

15. Can run. That is, moves on his feet at a more rapid pace than walking, for more than ten steps.
16. Picks up objects from the floor without falling over. (Bends at the knees or waist.)
17. Pitches or flings objects for at least three feet in the intended direction.
18. Uses scissors to cut paper or cloth. (Not necessary to be accurate, but cuts rather than tears.)
19. Can copy a straight line using a pencil, crayon or paintbrush.
20. Can turn the handle and open most interior doors.

3 YEARS 0 MONTHS TO 3 YEARS 11 MONTHS

21. Climbs upstairs alternating feet. May still go downstairs putting two feet on each step.

Alpern-Boll Developmental Skill-Age Inventory

22. Can jump down from bottom stair, both feet together (or from any other object eight inches off the floor.)
23. Rides tricycle using pedals for at least ten feet, and turns wide corners.
24. In attempting to copy a circle, at least makes a circular motion.
25. Turns handle and opens most exterior doors.

4 YEARS 0 MONTHS TO 4 YEARS 11 MONTHS

26. Moves by successive jumping or leaping with both feet together, for at least ten feet.
27. Can hop on one foot, for at least five feet.
28. Usually walks upstairs and downstairs alternating feet.
29. Catches a playground ball (large rubber ball) thrown by an adult standing five feet away. Catching means success 50 percent of the time.
30. Can throw a large rubber ball to an adult five feet away; enough accuracy that the adult usually catches the ball.
31. Can ride a tricycle with considerable skill. Specifically, can weave around boxes and trees without hitting them.

5 YEARS 0 MONTHS TO 5 YEARS 11 MONTHS

32. Marches to music. Moves feet up and down, with rhythm, imitating marching for at least two minutes.
33. Hops on either foot, and covers a distance of ten feet without stopping.
34. Can jump rope at least twice on either one or both feet; *or* can jump over a series of obstacles (eight inches high) in his path without stopping.
35. Skips for at least ten feet.
36. Can use a pair of scissors to cut out a two-inch square drawn on paper without being more than a quarter of inch off the line.
37. Can use a key to open and lock a small padlock.
38. Can make a solid snowball and throw it for at least eight feet.
39. Can safely climb on monkey bars or other climbing apparatus to a height of six feet without help.
40. Can throw a ball overhand with sufficient accuracy that an adult ten feet away could, without moving his legs, catch it at least 50 percent of the time.

6 YEARS 0 MONTHS TO 6 YEARS 11 MONTHS

41. Actually rides bicycle without training wheels (not just maintains balance).
42. Uses scissors to cut out a printed circle the size of a silver dollar, without being off more than a quarter of an inch.

43. Plays hopscotch, following rules. That is, able to hop on one foot to designated spot on the floor, hop, turn around and repeat the jump.
44. Can hammer a standard two-inch nail all the way into soft wood (without bending more than 50 percent of the nails).

Self-Help Developmental Age Scale

0 MONTHS TO 11 MONTHS

1. Attempts to reach objects nearby but beyond reach.
2. Bites, gnaws or chews solid or semi-solid foods.
3. Grasps hold of person or object by clutching with fist, fingers, or thumb and finger. Holds momentarily or longer.
4. Drinks from bottle, holding it with hands and/or feet. If breast-fed, holds breast during feeding.
5. Helps with dressing by holding out arm for sleeve, and foot for shoe.
6. Drinks from cup or glass with some assistance.

1 YEAR 0 MONTHS TO 1 YEAR 11 MONTHS

7. Removes socks, stockings or shoes unassisted if unfastened, to help undress and not merely as play.
8. Goes about the house without requiring constant supervision; needs only occasional checking.
9. Uses cup or glass, unassisted, for drinking, by grasping handle or by using either or both hands on sides of glass; no serious spilling.
10. Uses spoon to feed self without assistance and with only minimal spilling.
11. Usually discriminates between substances which are edible and those which are not. May put unedible materials in his mouth, but usually does not chew and swallow them.
12. Uses objects as useful tools, such as climbing on a stool or chair to reach something; or using a basket or a bag for carrying objects.

2 YEARS 0 MONTHS TO 2 YEARS 11 MONTHS

13. Removes his own coat without assistance when it is unfastened.
14. Usually uses a fork for eating solid foods.
15. Ordinarily obtains a drink for himself in familiar surroundings without help. (Gets cup or glass, turns the tap water on or off without serious messing.)
16. Dries own hands acceptably without help. Hands may be washed for him.

Alpern-Boll Developmental Skill-Age Inventory

17. Understands and avoids common dangers. (Tries to avoid falling from high places; or shows awareness of the danger of things such as broken glass, busy streets, or strange animals.)
18. Can put on own coat without help. (Need not button.)

3 YEARS 0 MONTHS TO 3 YEARS 11 MONTHS

19. Unfastens own clothing, such as large buttons, snaps, shoe laces and zippers.
20. Puts on shoes but not necessarily on correct foot.
21. Completely feeds himself using fork, spoon, and glassware correctly.
22. Puts on own coat, and manages buttons or zipper without help.

4 YEARS 0 MONTHS TO 4 YEARS 11 MONTHS

23. Goes to toilet alone without help. Performs all necessary operations. (May need help with difficult clothing such as back buttons.)
24. No more than one toileting accident per month, including both bowel and bladder accidents.
25. Typically washes his own face and hands acceptably and dries them without help.
26. Dresses himself completely except for tying shoe laces or other complicated devices. Must manage regular shirt or blouse size buttons.

5 YEARS 0 MONTHS TO 5 YEARS 11 MONTHS

27. Goes to school or other familiar places outside of immediate neighborhood "on his own." May go with friends, but no one is in direct charge of him.
28. Dresses self completely including shoe tying.
29. Takes money and makes store purchases when directed to do so. Gets object requested, without losing money. (Does not need to understand correct change.)
30. Puts toys away in an acceptable fashion when directed to do so.
31. Plays safely with such semi-hazard toys as skates, sleds, or wagons when unsupervised and outside of his own yard.
32. Can fix a bowl of dry cereal for himself.

6 YEARS 0 MONTHS to 6 YEARS 11 MONTHS

33. Uses table knife under ordinary circumstances for spreading bread with butter or jam.
34. Takes bath unassisted except for preparing bath or washing and drying hair.

35. Performs bedtime operations without help: goes to room alone, undresses, attends toilet, turns out light, etc. according to family routine. May be "tucked in" but requires no actual assistance.
36. Puts on and properly fastens boots, rubbers and other footgear.
37. Hangs up clothes and puts them away when directed to do so. Does so rather regularly, with only minimal reminders.
38. Answers telephone with proper greeting; notifies the person to whom the caller wishes to speak, or gives correct information as to his availability.
39. Uses knife for cutting meat. May be assisted occasionally with difficult meat.

Social Developmental, Age Scale

0 TO 11 MONTHS

1. Demonstrates desire to be picked up or held by parent or other familiar person. Shows this by holding up his arms; or by crying, which ceases when he is picked up.
2. Indicates desire for attention. Shows this by reaching for people, cooing at them, or by ceasing to cry or fuss when a person "talks" to him.
3. Waves "bye-bye," or claps hands, pat-a-cake fashion, in imitation of someone else.
4. Babbles or uses inarticulate speech in an apparent attempt to communicate. (Not just crying when uncomfortable.)
5. Responds in some clearly different way to strangers than to familiar people, such as showing preference to mother over strangers.
6. Is capable of responding negatively to strangers, urging or unpleasant situations. May refuse undesired foods, rebel at resented routines, or reject unwelcome overtures.
7. Uses movements as substitutes for vocal communication, such as shakes head "no," or holds out arms when he wants to be picked up.

1 YEAR 0 MONTHS TO 1 YEAR 11 MONTHS

8. Performs useful errands on request, such as taking or bringing named objects to or from nearby places. Carries out commands such as "bring it here" or "take it to Mommy."
9. Comes when called. Understands request, and cooperates at least 25 percent of time.
10. Plays independently alongside of others of approximately same age without creating antagonism (parallel play). Activity is individual rather than cooperative, but he "gets along" with other children.
11. Reveals some sense of ownership about people or property. Shows

understanding of "my" (but not necessarily "yours") in regard to parent, pet or toy.
12. Seems actively interested in exploring new places, such as a friend's home.
13. Jealous of attention shown to other children, especially sisters or brothers.

2 YEARS 0 MONTHS TO 2 YEARS 11 MONTHS

14. Occupies himself contentedly for a period of 15 minutes or more with simple activities such as TV, coloring, marking with pencil, building, or looking at pictures. May do this by himself or with others, but requires no constant adult supervision.
15. Indicates need for toileting through words or gestures (not mere fidgeting).
16. Associative play, i.e., interest in playing with same objects as other children though not capable of real cooperative (take turns) play.
17. Capable of playing with an easily breakable toy without destroying it the first time. Tries to use the toy as it was designed.
18. Demonstrates knowledge of his own sex or the sex of others by naming others as boy or girl, or man or woman; or chooses sex appropriate toys or clothing.

3 YEARS 0 MONTHS TO 3 YEARS 11 MONTHS

19. Participates in coordinated group activity, such as kindergarten circle games, with adult direction.
20. Understands taking turns; can wait for someone else to go first 75 percent of the time.
21. Likes to "help" in small ways about the house or yard, such as running errands, picking up things, helping to set or clear table, feeding pets, dusting.
22. Uses pencils or crayons to produce recognizable drawings of a person. (Need not be complete nor precise.)

4 YEARS 0 MONTHS TO 4 YEARS 11 MONTHS

23. Plays in his own neighborhood unsupervised (or in rural areas, the equivalent of one-half a city block). Does not include crossing the street on his own.
24. Engages in group activities with other children such as tag, hide-and-seek, jump-rope, hopscotch, marbles, or other locally popular games without needing constant adult supervision.
25. Has "special" friends, even though temporary.
26. Sometimes expresses sympathy and concern when a playmate, sibling or animal is injured or punished.

5 YEARS 0 MONTHS TO 5 YEARS 11 MONTHS

27. Responds sometimes to music by singing, marching, or dancing *with others*.
28. Able to help another child of similar age in a project such as building with toy bricks or logs, or making a castle or roads in the sand, for at least one-half hour of sustained interest.
29. Plays games such as follow-the-leader which require imitating the actions of the leader. May be the leader or follower.
30. Performs actually useful tasks for parent or teacher. May run errands, pick up or put away items.
31. Knows "mine" and "yours" and observes prerogatives regarding them. Asks for something instead of taking it.
32. Observes care in use of things. Generally refrains from damaging or misusing objects or materials.

6 YEARS 0 MONTHS TO 6 YEARS 11 MONTHS

33. Engages in extended (for 15 minutes or more) imaginative play. Plays roles of nurse, parent or other figures. Does so singly or in groups. Mimics. Dresses up.
34. Plays simple table games such as checkers, Old Maid, Candy Land or Lotto with a friend of approximately the same age. Observes the rules, takes his turn, and recognizes a "winner."
35. Able to fit into a routine similar to a first-grade classroom in which specific periods are set aside for activity and non-activity. (Need not always conform but his behavior is not generally disruptive.)
36. Has asked questions regarding his own body; e.g. heartbeat, where food goes, or the differences between his own and the other sex.
37. Uses the terms "thank you," "please" and "you're welcome" appropriately.
38. Realizes the money people earn is related to their job; that is, a doctor or lawyer earns more than a shoe shiner or a janitor.
39. Understands the concept of voting; that things will be done according to the way that the majority "votes."

Academic Developmental Age Scale

0 TO 11 MONTHS

1. Picks up things by himself that are within reach.
2. Reacts, by being more or less active, to changes such as being picked up or a person entering the room.

Alpern-Boll Developmental Skill-Age Inventory

3. Shows signs that he actually recognizes people or things.
4. Shows he likes or dislikes particular people, objects, or surroundings (other than food).
5. Shows active interest in an object or person (other than food objects) for at least one minute.

1 YEAR 0 MONTHS TO 1 YEAR 11 MONTHS

6. Looks in correct place for toys which roll out of sight (or similar object).
7. Uses pencil, crayon or marking utensil to scribble or scratch (as fore-runner of writing or drawing).
8. When asked, points to at least one body part (arm, eye) on himself or on a doll.
9. Entertains himself by turning pages in a book, or looking at or pointing to pictures in the book.
10. While playing, sometimes groups items by color, form or size.

2 YEARS 0 MONTHS TO 2 YEARS 11 MONTHS

11. Copies a vertical line in imitation of one drawn by an adult.
12. Takes things apart as a matter of curiosity rather than willful destruction. Such as: cuts with scissors, unwraps things, tears or cuts paper in an exploratory way.
13. If asked, will give you "one more" of something or take "one more" spoonful of food.
14. Can name, or points to when named, at least 20 objects or pictures of objects.
15. Recognizes himself in a photograph.

3 YEARS 0 MONTHS TO 3 YEARS 11 MONTHS

16. Uses the words "big" or "little" consistently and correctly.
17. Understands the concept of three; that is, will hand you three pieces of candy.
18. Copies a circle.
19. When asked, points correctly to at least two colors.
20. Draws a human with a head and at least one other part (e.g., two eyes, two arms, mouth).

4 YEARS 0 MONTHS TO 4 YEARS 11 MONTHS

21. Offers genuine word rhyme to simple words such as "tree," "cap," "head."

22. Can mold with clay or clay-like material, crude but recognizable shapes (except for a snake).
23. Counts to six meaningfully. That is, could usually count correctly six objects in front of him.
24. Recognizes time of day or night, and relates time to any one of the ordinary experiences such as getting up, meals, or bedtime.
25. Draws recognizable forms such as person, house, tree, animal or landscape.
26. Can draw a cross (one vertical and one horizontal line) after an adult demonstrates.

5 YEARS 0 MONTHS TO 5 YEARS 11 MONTHS

27. Will copy or draw a square with right angle corners and equal sides.
28. Prints or writes his first name or at least three other words *without copying*.
29. Copies or spontaneously draws a triangle. The sides of the triangle need not be equilateral but should be generally symmetrical.
30. Knows and will tell you correctly in what month his birthday falls.
31. Names or recognizes by name a penny as distinguished from a nickel and dime. (Need not know numerical values.)
32. Can name or point to at least eight colors.
33. Draws picture of recognizable man with head, trunk, arms and legs. (May be stick figure form.)

6 YEARS 0 MONTHS TO 6 YEARS 11 MONTHS

34. Can name the days of the week.
35. Can write the numbers from 1 to 25. (A few irregularities permissible.) permissible.)
36. Counts objects meaningfully up to 13.
37. Recognizes directions of "right" and "left."
38. Does simple number additions to 10 with apparent understanding. May use fingers.
39. Writes or prints legibly a dozen or more simple words with correct spelling. Does so without copying. May include proper names.
40. Recognizes at least 15 printed words. Understands their meaning.

Communication Developmental Age Scale

0 TO 11 MONTHS

1. Makes vocal noises other than crying or fussing. Spontaneously gurgles or coos with apparent pleasure.

Alpern-Boll Developmental Skill-Age Inventory

2. Uses his voice for self-satisfaction. Plays with inflexion or makes certain sounds other than crying or whimpering.
3. Babbles or makes inarticulate sounds as though he imitates words or pretends to talk.
4. Turns and looks toward a speaker or other source of sound rather consistently.
5. Hesitates or refrains from performing activity upon being told "no-no."
6. Occasionally repeats words such as "da-da" or "ma-ma." (Need not know the meaning.)
7. Uses movements as substitutes for vocal communication, such as shakes head "no," or holds out arms when he wants to be picked up.

1 YEAR 0 MONTHS TO 1 YEAR 11 MONTHS

8. Uses gestures in response to verbal speech, such as waving hand "bye-bye" to indicate departure, shaking head up and down for "yes," or shaking head side to side for "no."
9. Uses simple speech equivalents (real words, word-like sounds, or grunts) to indicate his needs and wants, or to make social contact (other than crying or whining).
10. Uses words for at least five familiar objects or actions (not including persons).
11. Recognizes the names of a dozen or more common objects when he hears them.
12. Carries out commands of show, come, go or get. (Such as "go to Ma-Ma" or "get the spoon.")
13. Uses at least 15 words to express himself.
14. Enjoys nursery rhymes, repeats certain parts, and tries to join in verbally.
15. Spontaneously or on request, will name (not merely repeat) at least 20 objects as he leafs through picture book.

2 YEARS 0 MONTHS TO 2 YEARS 11 MONTHS

16. Communicates the idea of "another" or "more" by asking for another cookie or indicating by gesture that he wants more.
17. Uses 50 or more recognizable words, not merely understands their meaning. Uses them in conversational speech.
18. Puts two or more words together to form simple sentences, such as "Me go" or "You give." Always using the same two words would indicate they are one word to him.
19. Correctly uses such pronouns as "I," "me," "you," "he," and "she." May occasionally substitute "I" for "me," but never substitutes "me" for "you."

20. Occasionally will give his first and last name on request.
21. Can say at least two nursery rhymes or songs such as "Happy Birthday" or "Jingle Bells." Knows at least one verse.
22. Tells you by word or gestures that he "reads" picture action. If he tells you that the boy is running, he understands the action depicted in the pictures.

3 YEARS 0 MONTHS TO 3 YEARS 11 MONTHS

23. Will *usually* offer his full name when asked by adults.
24. Talks in short sentences, of at least three words, to offer information or answer questions.
25. Tells you whether he is a boy or girl, consistently and correctly, when asked.
26. Has sung a song of at least 30 words in front of another person.
27. Generally uses plurals correctly.
28. Asks questions using "what," "where," or "who."

4 YEARS 0 MONTHS TO 4 YEARS 11 MONTHS

29. Tells a familiar story as he looks at a picture book, such as "The Three Bears," or "Little Red Riding Hood." Story corresponds to pictures as he goes through the book. May leave out portions not represented by pictures.
30. Ninety-five percent of his speech intelligible to strangers. Most adults easily understand what he says.
31. Sometimes speaks in sentences with as many as eight words.

5 YEARS 0 MONTHS TO 5 YEARS 11 MONTHS

32. Can converse on the telephone. Listens for comments, answers them, and waits until the other person stops talking before speaking.
33. Can communicate (by gesture, pointing, speech) to a salesperson what he wants to buy and completes the transaction.
34. Can tell you (by gesture or using fingers) how old he is now, how old he was last year and how old he will be next year.
35. Recognizes at least five written words (such as stop, go, run, push) and demonstrates understanding of their meaning by actions.
36. Will sometimes ask the meaning of an unfamiliar word, and then includes the word in his vocabulary.

Alpern-Boll Developmental Skill-Age Inventory

6 YEARS 0 MONTHS TO 6 YEARS 11 MONTHS

37. Reads aloud a simple story so that listener can follow the story.
38. Can dial a number or request a number on the telephone when he wants to speak to someone.
39. Can recite (without pictures as aids) at some length a familiar story such as "Little Red Riding Hood" or "The Three Bears."
40. Can correctly recite the entire "Pledge of Allegiance," or any 25-word prayer or poem he has memorized (other than songs).

ADDRESSES FOR AUDIOVISUAL AIDS

(Note: many of the films listed in this book are available from your state board of health.)

Columbia Broadcasting System, Inc.
51 West 52nd Street
New York, N.Y. 10019

Churchill Films
662 North Robertson Blvd.
Los Angeles, California 90069

Coronet Films
65 East South Water Street
Chicago, Illinois 60601

General Mills
Consumer Relations Division
9200 Wayzee Blvd.
Minneapolis, Minnesota 55440

Guidance Associates
Harcourt, Brace & Jovanovich
Pleasantville, New York 10570

International Film Bureau
332 South Michigan Avenue
Chicago, Illinois 60604

McGraw-Hill Book Company, Inc.
Text-Film Division
330 West 42nd Street
New York, N.Y. 10036

Metropolitan Life Insurance Company
Health and Welfare Division
One Madison Avenue
New York, N.Y. 10010

New York State Dept. of Commerce
Film Library
West Mall Plaza
845 Central Avenue
Albany, New York 12206

Addresses for Audiovisual Aids

J. C. Penney Company, Inc.
Educational & Consumer Relations
1301 Avenue of Americas
New York, N.Y. 10019

Chas. Pfizer & Company, Inc.
235 East 42nd Street
New York, N.Y. 10017

Filmstrip of the Month Club
Audiovisual Division
Popular Science Publishing Company, Inc.
335 Lexington Avenue
New York, N.Y. 10017

Prentice-Hall, Inc.
Englewood Cliffs, New Jersey 07631

QED productions
Division of Cathedral Films, Inc.
available from
Singer Education & Training
1345 Diversey Parkway
Chicago, Illinois 60614

Stanley-Bowmar Company, Inc.
4 Broadway
Valhalla, New York 10595

3M Company, 3M Center
Visual Products Division
St. Paul, Minnesota 55101

U.S. Public Health Service
National Medical Audiovisual Facility
Atlanta, Georgia 30333

GENERAL REFERENCES

Aldrich, C. Anderson, and Mary M. Aldrich. *Babies Are Human Beings*, Rev. ed. New York: The Macmillan Company, 1962.

Bettelheim, Bruno. *Dialogues with Mothers*. New York: Macmillan-Free Press, 1962.

de Schweinitz, Karl. *Growing Up*. 4th ed. New York: The Macmillan Company, 1968.

Erikson, Erik. *Childhood and Society*. Rev. ed. New York: W. W. Norton and Company, Inc., 1964.

Ginott, Haim G. *Between Parent and Child*. New York: The Macmillan Company, 1965.

Jersild, Arthur T. *The Psychology of Adolescence*. 2nd ed. New York: The Macmillan Company, 1963.

Mead, Margaret, and Ken Heyman. *Family*. New York: The Macmillan Company, 1965.

Noyes, Arthur P., William P. Camp, and Mildred van Sickel. *Psychiatric Nursing*. 6th ed. New York: The Macmillan Company, 1964.

Rapier, Dorothy Kelley, and others. *Practical Nursing*. 4th ed. St. Louis: The C. V. Mosby Company, 1970.

Rasmussen, Sandra. *Foundations of Practical and Vocational Nursing*. New York: The Macmillan Company, 1970.

Robinson, Corrine. *Basic Nutrition and Diet Therapy*. 2nd ed. New York: The Macmillan Company, 1970.

Rubin, Theodore Isaac. *Jordi*. New York: The Macmillan Company, 1960.

Rubin, Theodore Isaac. *Lisa and David*. New York: The Macmillan Company, 1961.

Ruslink, Doris. *Family Health and Home Nursing*. New York: The Macmillan Company, 1963.

Scott, Lou. *Programmed Instruction and Review for Practical and Vocational Nurses*. 2 vols. New York: The Macmillan Company, 1968.

Spock, Benjamin, and Marion O. Lerrigo. *Caring for Your Disabled Child*. New York: The Macmillan Company, 1965.

INDEX

Academic age, 317
Accident prevention, aged, 284–85
   baby, 59–60
   preschool child, 90–94
Accident-prone children, 94
Acne, 160
Activity, adults, 192–95
   aged, 242–47
   children's creative, 120–21
   new baby, 54
   overweight child, 140
   schoolchild, 136–37
   sick child, 119–23
   underweight child, 141
Adjustment, to aging, 264–65
   to marriage, 20–23
   to middle age, 184–86
   to work, 176–77
Administration on Aging, 211, 305
Adolescent(s), 152–73
   definition, 152
   delinquents, 165–67
   diversions, 168–69
   grooming, 159–60
   health habits, 158–64
   illness, 167
   motherhood, 164–65
   nutrition, 160–64
   physical development, 44, 46, 155–57
   posture, 160
   social acceptance, 154–55
   understanding physical changes, 157–58
Adult, extra, 237
   mature (middle age), 184–96
      alone again, 187
      food needs, 191–92
      health consultation, 190
      health routines, 190–91
      male climacteric, 189
      menopause, 188–89
      physical changes, 187–88
      rediscovery, 184–87
      use of leisure time, 192–95
   single, 180–81
   young, 174–83
      activities, 174
      choice of career, 175–76
      choice of life partner, 177–78
      engagement, 178–79
      illness, 181–82

      maturity, 179–80
      from school to work, 176–77
Adult education, for aged, 246–47
Aged, activity, 242–48, 280–81
   challenge to nursing, 6, 309
   community resources, 301–10
   community responsibility for, 297–301
   definition, 232–33
   employment, 242–44
   finances, 287–96
   independence, 240
   love, 239–40
   mental and personality changes, 264–70
   number today, 229–30
   personal hygiene, 273–86
   physical changes, 251–63
   proportion of population, 225, 229
   reasons for increase, 230–32
   relative term, 233
   religious faith, 241
   in rural life, 236
   social and emotional needs, 236–50
Aging, definition, 232
Aid to Families with Dependent Children (AFDC), 13, 213
Alpern, Dr. Gerald, 46–47, 217, 315
Anemia, adolescent girls, 161
   aged, 255, 267, 276
Annuity, 294
Anxiety, aged, 268
   new parents, 30
   pediatric patient, 118
   postpartum, 30
   schoolchild, 145–46
Anxiety fears, 107, 110, 118
Arteriosclerosis, causes, 254–55
   definition, 254
   effect on aged, 254, 255, 257
Arthritis, in aged, 253
Associated Hospital Service of New York, 219
Atherosclerosis, definition, 254

Baby, 53–64
   developmental highlights, 54–55
   newborn, 4, 30, 53
   sitting up, 39, 54
   standing alone, 39, 55

333

Baby care, clothes, 57–58
  daily schedule, 56
  feeding schedule, 55–56
  food, 55–56
  laundering baby clothes, 58–59
  play and playthings, 60–62
  play space, 60
  safety, 59–60
  toys, 61
Basal metabolism, adolescent, 161
  aged, 275–76
  middle-aged, 191–92
  young adult, 181
Bathing, geriatric patient, 282
Bed rest, dangers, 280
Bedsores, aged, 275, 280
Behavior, preschool child, 82–84
  schoolchild, 142–43
  two-year-old, 66
Biological age, 44
Birth, illegitimate, 8, 153
Birth rate, 7–8, 231
Bismarck, 233
Bladder control, 64–65. *See also* Toilet control
Blind Assistance Program, 214
Blind patient, diversion, 193
Blood, circulation of, 132, 254–55
Blood pressure, aged, 254–55
  schoolchild, 132
Blue Cross, 219
Body cells, 252
Body proportions, adolescence, 44, 156–57
  changes, 38, 44
  newborn, 38, 44
Boll, Thomas, 46–47, 315
Bone development, 44, 156
  effect of bed rest, 280
  facial, 159
  ossification, 44, 253–54
  wrist bone, 44
Books, adolescent, 169
  adult patient, 246
  schoolchild, 149
Booster inoculations, 89
Borinstein Home for the Jewish Aged, Indianapolis, Indiana, 303
Bortz, Dr. Edward L., 237, 251
Brain, cells of, 259
  functioning in aged, 252, 267–68, 270
Breakfast, adolescent, 162
  schoolchild, 139
Broken families, 24–26
  death, 25
  desertion, 25
  divorce, 24–25
Brothers and sisters, 4, 31–32, 43
Budget, retired couple, 287, 292

Calcium, for adolescent, 161
  for aged, 276
  for middle-aged, 191
  utilization, aged, 253, 256
Calories, adolescent, 161
  aged, 275–76
  middle-aged, 191–92
  schoolchild, 140–41
Career choice, 175–76
Cataracts, 260
Cerebellum, aging, 259
Cerebral accident, 268
Cerebral arteriosclerosis, 267
Child, emotionally disturbed, 216–17
  battered, 67–68, 209
  fear of hospitals, 4, 107–15
  five-year-old, 88–97
  food, 98–106
  four-year-old, 81–87
  recreation for sick, 117–26
  three-year-old, 73–79
  two-year-old, 64–72
Child Development, Office of, 211, 262
Child guidance clinic, 216–17
Child labor laws, 209
Child Study Center at Yale University, 113
Child welfare services, 213
Childbirth, increased safety, 231
Children's Bureau, 211
Chronic diseases, beginning, 190
Chronological age, 317
Churchill, Sir Winston, 270
Circulatory system, aging, 254–55
  schoolchild, 136
Cleanliness, adolescent, 159–60
  aged, 282–83, 284
  four-year-old, 81
  three-year-old, 73
Climacteric, male, 39, 259
Clothes, adolescent, 155
  aged, 283
  baby, 57–58
  laundering baby clothes, 58–59
  preschool child, 77–78
Cole, Luella, 46
Communications, family members, 16
  middle-aged couple, 186
  two-year-old, 109
Community, definition, 197
  family contributions, 205
  health, 198–99
  influences family, 199
  rural, 199–201
  stable, 202–203
  suburban, 201–202
  urban, 6, 7, 153, 197, 199–201, 203
Community Health Services and Facilities Act of 1961, 305

Index

Community responsibility for aged, 208, 244, 297–311
Community resources, 208–22
  for aged, 301–10
  for aid to families with dependent children, 213
  blind assistance, 214
  child guidance clinic, 216–17
  child welfare, 213
  Family Service Association, 217
  foster care, 213, 214, 307
  home-care programs, 219–20, 307
  homemaker services, 220–21, 307
  local agencies, 218
  meals-on-wheels, 221, 307
  medical assistance, 214
  national voluntary health agencies, 218
  old-age assistance, 214
  prospective parents, 29
  public health nursing, 215
  rehabilitation centers, 218–19
  services for crippled children, 214
  visiting nurses, 215–16
Community service, of aged, 244
Companions, 85, 88, 94–95
Companionship, aged, 237–38
Constipation, in aged, 257, 280, 281–82
Cooperation, adolescent patient, 168
  geriatric patient, 273
  mother of sick child, 114
  pediatric patient, 115
  schoolchild patient, 133, 146
Cooperative play, 41, 69, 78, 94
Counseling, guidance, 175–76
  premarital, 177
  services for aged, 304–305, 308
Craftwork. *See* Diversions
Crippled Children's Services, 214
Cultural, definition, 196
  differences in marriage, 24
Curiosity, four-year-old, 86
  preschool child, 92
  schoolchild, 133, 146
  two-year-old, 64, 70

Day center for retired people, 304–305
Death, attitude of aged, 241
  in family, 25
Delinquent teenagers, 165–67
  neurotic, 165–67
  sociopathic, 165–67
  subcultural, 165–66
Dental care, aged, 278
  schoolchild, 141
Dentures, 262, 278
Dependence, aged, 264, 268–69, 273. *See also* Independence

Depression, aged, 266
Desertion, 25, 203
Development, 37–49
  adolescent, 155–57
  age for certain tasks, 39
  characteristic traits of different stages, 40–41
  definition, 38
  environment, 43
  girls compared to boys, 40
  heredity influences, 41–42
    environment, 42
  maturation and learning, 37–38
  muscle system, 46
  skeletal system 44
  teeth, 45
Developmental highlights for baby, 54–55
Developmental skill-age inventory, 46–47, 315–29
Developmental trends, 40
Diabetes, in aged, 258, 282
  diversions for patient, 194
Diapers, care of, 58–59
Diet. *See* Food; Nutrition
Digestive system, aging, 256–57
Discipline, home, 16
  pediatric ward, 83–84
  preschool child, 82–84
  and punishment, 83
  schoolchild, 142–43
Diversions, adolescent, 168–69
  adult patient, 193–95
  aged, 245–46
  and physical condition, 193–94
  preschool child, 117–26
  schoolchild, 146–49
Divorce, 20, 23–25
Donahue, Dr. Wilma, 300
Drugs, teenagers use of, 158–59
Duvall, Evelyn Millis, 15, 19

Ears. *See* Hearing
Eating, between meals, adolescent, 162
  aged, 277
  overweight schoolchild, 141
  preschool child, 103–104
  See also Food; Nutrition; Overweight; Underweight
Economic Opportunity Act of 1964, 212
Edentia, 275
Eisenhower, President Dwight, 238, 290
Elimination, aged, 257, 281–82
  learning control, 64–65
  See also Toilet control
Emotional control, aged 268
Emotional development, six through nine, 142–43

ten through twelve, 143-44
Employment, aged, 242-44
　young adult, 175-77
Endocrine glands, aging, 258-59
Endowment, 294
Engagement, 178-79
Enophthalmos, 260
Environment, growth and development, 42-44
Estrogen, 188-89
Examination physical, aged, 273-74
　periodical, in middle age, 197
　preschool child, 89-90
Exercise, adolescent, 160, 163
　adult, 191
　aged, 280-81
　schoolchild, 136-37
　See also Activity
Eyes, aging, 260-61
　life expectancy, 251
　"second sight," 260
　tests, five-year-old, 89
　　schoolchild, 142

Family, extended, 208, 297
　nuclear, 208, 297
　social unit, 10-11
Family life, 10-18
　adolescent influenced by, 8, 202-204
　affect of baby, 31-32
　affect on patient, 10-12
　breakdown, 12-13, 25
　changes, affecting aged, 236-37, 298-99
　　today, 6-8
　characteristics of success, 15-16
　community influences, 199
　dependence on community, 8, 204-205
　evaluating success, 14-15
　importance, 12
　religious influence, 16
　schoolchildren characteristics of, 129-30
　security, 12
　successful, 10-18
　unsuccessful, 12-13
Family Service Agency, Southwestern Illinois, 204
Family Service Association, 217
Family Service Association of Indianapolis, 203-204
Father, importance, to baby, 31
　to schoolchildren, 130
　to three-year-old, 78
Fatigue, adolescent, 160
　adult, 187, 191
　aged, 266, 278
　five-year-old, 85

schoolchild, 136
three-year-old, 74
two-year-old, 66
Fats, in diet of aged, 278
Fears of children, after hospitalization, 108-10
　anxiety, 107-108, 110
　conquering, 111-12
　of hospital, 108-109
　normal, 107-108
Federal government, and aged, 305-306
Feeding schedule, baby, 55-56
Fingernails, of aged, 261-62, 282
Five-year-old, 88-97
　accident-prone, 94
　companions, 94
　emotional development, 88
　health examination, 89-90
　muscle development, 46
　physical development, 88
　play, 94-95
　ready for school, 89
　safe environment, 92-94
　safety education, 90-92
　toys, 94-95
Fontanel, 53
Food, adolescent, 161-64
　aged, 274-278
　baby, 55-56
　schoolchild, 139-41
　toddler and preschool child, 98-105
　　appetite, 99
　　chronic vomiters, 101
　　eating between meals, 103-104
　　hospital meals, 104-105
　　meaning of food to child, 98
　　new to child, 102-103
　　pattern of normal eating, 99
　　preparation and serving, 101-102
　　setting the stage, 101
　　unsuitable for child, 103
Foot care, aged patient, 283
Foster care of children, 213-14
Foster Grandparent Program, 306
Foster homes for aged, 307-308
Four-year-old, 81-87
　behavior, 83-84
　companions, 85
　discipline, 82-83
　fears, 81
　independence, 82
　make-believe, 85
　personal habits, 81
　play, 85-86
　separation from parents, 81
　temper tantrums, 82
　toys, 85-86

Index

Franklin, Benjamin, 270
Frightened child, 110–11
Function, of hospitals, 3

Gallbladder, aging of, 256
Games, five-year-old, 94
   schoolchild, 148
   senior citizens' day center, 304–305
   sick child, 122
Gangs, adolescent, 154–55, 165
   schoolchild, 143–44
Gastric juice, 256
Genitals, aging, 259
Geriatric patient, nursing, 273, 309
Geriatrician, definition, 233
Geriatrics, 233
Gerontology, 233
Gesell, Arnold, 54
Ghetto, definition, 198
Glands, aging of endocrine, 225
   apocrine sweat, 159
   influence on growth, 42
   sebaceous, 159–60, 261
Glasses, bifocals, 188
   schoolchild, 142
Gonads, 259
Grooming, adolescent, 159–60
   aged, 284
Group life, adolescent, 154–55
   aged, 237–38
   schoolchild, 143–44
Growth and development, 37–51. *See also* Development
Growth record chart, boy, 134
   girl, 135
Guilt, 244

Hair, aging, 261
   care of aged, 282
   newborn, 53
Handicapped Children's Home/Service in New York City, 118
Happiness, aged, 267, 287
Head Start Program, 212
Health examination, aged, 273–74
   children, 89–90
   middle-age, 190
   preschool, 89–90
Health facility, 301
Health habits, adolescent, 158–64
Health needs, schoolchild, 137–42
   young adult, 181
Health services, child, 89
   community, 208–22
   federal, 210–12
   maternal, 28–29
   need for aged, 287–96
   state, 213–14
Hearing, aged, 251, 260–61
   middle-age, 188
   newborn, 53
   schoolchild, 142
Heart, aging, 254–55
   childhood, 131
Height, adolescent, 155–56
   aged, 254
   growth record charts, 134, 135
   newborn, 53
Helfner, Ray E., 68
Heredity, 41–42
Hobbies, adolescent, 168–69
   aged, 245–46
   retired people, day center, 304–305
   schoolchild, 144–45
Holmes, Oliver Wendell, 270
Homebound child, 117–18, 148–49
Home-care program, 219–20
   for aged, 307
Homemaker services, 220–21
   for aged, 307, 308
Homeostasis, 252
Hospitalization, adolescent, 152, 168
   aged, 234
   preparation of child, 112–13
   preschool child, 64, 73, 88, 108–18
   schoolchild, 133
Hostility, 94, 109
Housing, aged, 295, 298–301
   family with schoolchildren, 131
   improvement, 202
   urban and rural, 202
Hyperactive patient, diversion for, 194
Hypertension, definition, 254

Illness, adolescent, 167
   cost for aged, 290–93
   disruption of home life, 131
   preschool child, 107–16
   schoolchild, 4, 145–46
   young adult, 181–82
Imagination, five-year-old, 88, 95
   four-year-old, 84–85
   schoolchild, 149
Immunity, in aged, 253
Immunization, 89
Incontinent patient, 268, 280, 282
Independence, adolescent, 162
   aged, 234, 240, 248, 298–99
   five-year-old, 88
   four-year-old, 82
   two-year-old, 66
Inflation, 294–95

Insomnia, aged, 279
Intelligence, influence on development, 41–42
Investments, for aged, 294–95
Iron, deficiency, of adolescent, 161, 163
   of aged, 276
   sources, 161

Jealousy, in marriage, 22
   of new baby, 32
Juvenile delinquency, 7, 13, 153, 165–67

Kempe, C. Henry, 67–68
Kidneys, aged, 257
Kyphosis, 251

Larynx, aging, 255
Learning, ability in aged, 259–60
   cause of development, 37–38
   speed in aged, 260
Leisure time, aged, 242, 245–47
   middle-age, 192–93
Life expectancy, 225–28
   eyes, 251
   nonwhite population, 225
   skin, 251
Liver, aging, 256
Love, aged couple, 239–40
Lungs, aging, 256
   childhood, 136

Malnutrition, adolescent, 161
   aged, 257, 267, 274–76
Malocclusion, 141, 262
Marriage, cause of failure, 23–24
   choice of partner, 177–78
   preparation, 19–20, 178
Marriage adjustments, 20–24
   middle-age, 184–86
Maturation, definition, 37
Maturity, emotional, 179
Meals-on-wheels, 221
   for aged, 307
Medicaid, 209, 210, 211
Medical assistance program, 214
Medical care, costs for aged, 291
Medicare, 209, 290–92
Menopause, 188–89
Menstruation, 39, 44, 158
Mental abnormalities, aged, 265–66
Mental health, definition, 179
   maintenance in aged, 235
Mental illness, 42

Michelangelo, 270
Middle age, 184–96
Mortality rate, infant, 231
   maternal, 231
   schoolchild, 137
Mother, of hospitalized child, 114
   middle-aged, 185
   of newborn, 30, 55
   teenage, 164–65
"Mothering" of new baby, 12, 54
Mouth care, aged, 278
Mouth changes with age, 256
Muscular coordination, adolescent, 15
   schoolchild, 137
   three-year-old, 73
   two-year-old, 64, 70
Muscular system, adolescent, 46
   aging, 254
   development, 46
   five-year-old, 46
   schoolchild, 133, 136
   three-year-old, 73

Nails, aging, 261–62
   care, 282–83
Nerve cells, 252
Nervous system, aging, 252, 258–59
   newborn, 53
Newborn baby, description, 53
Newlywed, 19–27
   adjustments, 20–23
   broken families, 24–25
   death, 25
   desertion, 25
   divorce, 23–24
   married love, 19
   preparation for marriage, 19–20
   romantic love, 19
Nose, development, 157
   newborn, 53
Nuclear family, 8, 208, 297
Nursing care, adolescent patient, 168
   aged, 273, 309
   mature adult, 191–92
   new mother, 30, 55
   preschool child, 114–15
   schoolchild, 145–46
   teenage mother, 164–65
Nursing homes, 301–304
Nutrition, adolescent, 161–64
   aged, 274–76. *See also* Food

Obese, definition, 140
Occupational therapy, in nursing homes, 303

Index

Old-age assistance program, 214, 292
Older Americans Act of 1965, 305–306
Oral hygiene, aged, 278
Oral temperatures, aged, 253
Organs, definition, 252
Ossification, cartilages in aged, 254
    definition, 44
Osteoporosis, in adult, 189
    in aged, 253
Outpatient services for aged, 307
Overprotection, aged, 240, 308
Overweight, adolescent, 161–63
    aged, 251, 276
    definition, 140
    schoolchild, 139–41

Pancreas, aging, 258
Pediatrics, new trends, 113–14
Peer relationships, adolescents, 154–55
    aged, 237–38
    schoolchild, 142–44
Periodontal disease, in aged, 262
Pharynx, aging, 255
Physical changes, adolescence, 44, 46, 155–58
    aged, 251–63
    See also Development
Physical examination, *See* Health examination
Physical therapy, in nursing homes, 303
Play, dramatic, 121–22
    imitative, 121–22
    importance to child, 69–70, 117
    stages, 41
Play space, baby, 60
Playmates, 85, 94
Playtime at the hospital, 118
Pope John XXIII, 235
Posture, adolescent, 160
    aged, 251, 254
Preadolescent, 143–44
Pregnancy, adjustment for couple, 30
Privacy, adolescent, 168
    patient in nursing home, 301
    schoolchild, 131, 145
Progressive patient care, 301
Psychosomatic illness, children, 216
Puberty, 152, 156, 159
Public Health Nursing, Bureau of, 215
Public welfare, state department, 213–14
Punishment, preschool child, 83

Rebellion, 61, 72, 165, 273
Recognition, for aged, 238–39

Recreation, aged, 304–305
    family, 130
    sick child, 117–26
    See also Diversions; Hobbies; Play
Rediscovery, 5–6, 184–87
Referrals, to child guidance clinic, 217
    of elderly people, 308
Regression, from bed rest, 280
    with illness, 117–19
    toward senility, 268–69
Rehabilitation, adolescent, 167
    aged, 280–81
    families with complex problems, 203–204
    middle-age, 193–95
    nursing home patient, 280–81
    schoolchild, 146
    young adult, 182
Rehabilitation centers, 218–19
Reproductive system, aging, 154
Respiratory system, aging, 255–56
Rest, adolescent, 160
    aged, 278–79, 280
    bed, 280
    five-year-old, 88
    four-year-old, 81
    schoolchild, 133, 136, 138
Retarded children, 42
Retirement, 242–43, 264
    incomes, 287–89, 293
    man, 245, 304–305
    villages, 300
Rigidity, aged, 265
Robertson, James, 107

Safety, aged, 284–85
    baby, 59–60
    preschool child, 90–94
Sandburg, Carl, 270
Savings, aged, 289, 294
Schedule, daily, baby, 56
Schizophrenia, 42
Schoolchild, 133–51
Sedatives, for aged, 261, 267, 269
Senility, definition, 232
    symptoms, 268–69
Senior Citizen's Charter, 248
Senn, Dr. Milton, 113–14
Separation from parents, 108
    four-year-old, 81
    schoolchild, 133
    three-year-old, 73
    two-year-old, 64
Sex education, adolescent, 157–58
    preschool child, 78
    schoolchild, 144

Index

Sexual activity, in aged, 259
Sharing, 69
Six- to twelve-year-old, 133–51
   dental care, 141
   diversions, 146–49
   food habits, 139
   health needs, 137–42
   hobbies and play, 144–45
   illness and the hospital, 145–46
   muscle development, 133, 136
   organic development, 136
   overweight, 139–41
   perfecting skills, 137
   physical growth, 133–36
   social and emotional development, 142–44
   underweight, 141
Skeletal system, aging, 253–54
   development, 44
Skin, of aged, 251, 261
Sleep, aged, 278–79
   baby, 57
   child in hospital, 75–76
   preschool child, 74, 81
   schoolchild, 138
Smell, aged, 251
   newborn, 53
Snacks, adolescent, 162
   aged, 227
   preschool child, 103–104
Social and Rehabilitation Services, 211
Social Security Administration, 209, 210, 211
Social Security Amendments, 1965, 291–92
Social Security payments, 289–90
Speech, five-year-old, 88
   four-year-old, 78
   three-year-old, 78
   two-year-old, 68–69
Storyhour in hospital, 124–25

Teeth, aging, 262
   care, during childhood, 141
      during old age, 274, 278
Temperature, aged, 253
Three-year-old, 73–80
   clothes, 77
   learning to dress, 76
   muscular development, 73
   nighttime at the hospital, 75
   other learnings, 78
   personal habits, 73
   play and toys, 78–79
   poor sleep, 74
   sex interest, 78

   sleep habits, 74
Thyroid, aging, 258
Tissues, definition, 252
   epithelial, 252
   rate of replacement, 252
Titian, 270
Toenails, aging, 261–62
   care of aged, 283
Toilet control, 64–65, 73
   age for learning, 39
Toys, for baby, 60–62
   five-year-old, 94–95
   four-year-old, 85–86
   sick child, 120–22
   three-year-old, 78–89
   two-year-old, 69–71
Tranquilizers, 269
Two-year-old, 64–73
   battered child, 67–68
   learning to talk, 68–69
   negative stage, 66
   play and toys, 69
   sharing, 69–71
   temper tantrums, 65
   toilet control, 64–65

Underweight, adolescent, 162
   schoolchild, 141
Urban community, 199–201, 203–204
Urbanization, definition, 200
Urinary system, aging, 257
U.S. Department of Health, Education and Welfare, 210, 211

Vascular system, aging, 254–55
Vision, aged, 250, 260
Visiting nurse, 215
Vomiters, chronic, 101

Weight, adolescent, 161–62
   aged, 251, 275–76
   newborn, 53
   overweight, aged, 251, 275–76
   schoolchild, 139–41
Wesley, John, 270
White, Robert G., 241, 267
White House Conference on Aging, 1961, 244, 305
   1971, 211
Withdrawal, aged, 242

Young children in hospitals, 113